PERIPHERAL ARTERIAL DISEASE

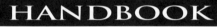

HANDBOOK

PERIPHERAL ARTERIAL DISEASE

HANDBOOK

WILLIAM R. HIATT
ALAN T. HIRSCH
JUDITH REGENSTEINER

CRC Press
Boca Raton   London   New York   Washington, D.C.

Library of Congress Cataloging-in-Publication Data

Peripheral arterial disease handbook / [edited by] William R. Hiatt, Judith G.
Regensteiner, Alan T. Hirsch.
    p. ; cm.
  Includes bibliographical references and index.
  ISBN 0-8493-8413-3
  1. Peripheral vascular diseases. 2. Arteries--Diseases. 3. Arterial occlusions.
I. Hiatt, William R. II. Regensteiner, Judith G. III. Hirsch, Alan T. (Alan Tick)
[DNLM: 1. Peripheral Vascular Diseases. WG 500 P4422 2001]
RC694 .P475 2001
616.1′31—dc21
                                         2001025110
                                              CIP

Visit the CRC Press Web site at www.crcpress.com

© 2001 by CRC Press LLC

No claim to original U.S. Government works
International Standard Book Number 0-8493-8413-3
Library of Congress Card Number 2001025110
Printed in the United States of America   2 3 4 5 6 7 8 9 0
Printed on acid-free paper

Dedication

We hope that this book will be used to improve the health of persons who suffer from the consequences of peripheral arterial disease and other vascular disorders.

It is dedicated with love to:

Susan W. Hiatt
Kelsey M. Hiatt
William H. and Luana R. Hiatt

Kenneth Schneider
Alyssa P. Schneider
Max O. and Dorothy L. Regensteiner

Laurie E. Curtis
Rebecca K. Hirsch
Jonathan I. Hirsch
Robert A. and Margot T. Hirsch

Acknowledgments

The editors would like to acknowledge the excellent editorial assistance of David Jepsen and Sylvia Wood in preparing this book for publication.

Introduction

Peripheral arterial diseases (PAD) affect a substantial percentage of the adult population in the United States. Specifically, peripheral arterial occlusive disease has an age-adjusted prevalence of 12% and increases to more than 20% in the geriatric population. Although less common, critical leg ischemia (CLI) may affect as many as 500,000 to 1,000,000 individuals each year. As a group, these patients have a high risk of cardiovascular morbidity and mortality. The risk of fatal and nonfatal ischemic events in patients with claudication is similar to that for patients with known coronary disease. In patients with CLI, the risk of mortality can be as high as 25% per year. Therefore, as a group, these patients deserve intensive cardiovascular risk modification and aggressive use of anti-platelet therapies. In addition to their high event rates, patients with PAD have significant impairments in quality of life and performance of the activities of daily living. Patients with CLI also have pain at rest in their limbs and may have non-healing ulcers and gangrene with the threat of limb loss. Thus, additional management strategies are required to improve ambulatory capacity and prevent limb loss in this disabled population.

Diseases of the abdominal aorta are also common and often asymptomatic. For most of these patients, management is directed toward early detection and appropriate surgical intervention to prolong survival by preventing aneurysm rupture. Other diseases of the aorta can lead to atheroemboli with the blue toe syndrome and ischemic digits in the lower extremity.

Cerebrovascular diseases are a major cause of stroke in the United States. Patients experiencing these disorders are often asymptomatic. Again, screening and early detection are needed to plan appropriate interventions to prevent ischemic stroke. In symptomatic patients, carefully considered use of both medical and surgical approaches to management is critical.

Visceral arterial diseases are less common, but have both distinct presentation and management strategies. Related to these disorders is the high prevalence of renal vascular disease in patients with other forms of atherosclerosis. Because these diseases also are often under-recognized, physicians may need to consider surgical or interventional radiology procedures among their treatment options.

In addition to the major diseases described above, this *Peripheral Arterial Disease Handbook* reviews peripheral manifestations of vasculitis, vasospastic disorders in Raynaud phenomenon, and unusual vascular disease syndromes. Throughout these discussions, our primary focus is to establish critical aspects of epidemiology and pathophysiology and then present appropriate diagnostic and management strategies. Thus, this handbook is targeted to the practical needs of medical students, house officers, and fellows considering or participating in vascular disease training programs. We hope that this discussion will be both practical and useful in the daily management of patients with PAD.

The final goal of this handbook is to discuss the importance of integrated vascular care. No longer can the management of a patient with vascular disease be conducted in isolation. For example, an appropriate angioplasty approach to a diseased arterial segment may treat the manifestations in that regional circulation but ignore the systemic risk factors that contributed to the development of the disease. Therefore, the integration of vascular medicine, vascular surgery, interventional radiology, nursing, and technology is critical to the optimal management of these patients. Thus, the last chapter of this book presents important strategies regarding integrated vascular care.

In summary, with its practical focus on epidemiology and pathophysiology as well as critical issues of prevention, detection, and strategies for care, it is hoped that the *Peripheral Arterial Disease*

Handbook will be a useful addition to the armamentarium for the diagnosis and management of patients with common PAD.

William R. Hiatt, M.D.
Judith G. Regensteiner, Ph.D.
Alan T. Hirsch, M.D.

Contributors

Warren P. Bundens, M.D., Ph.D
University of California San Diego
La Jolla, CA

Lori L. Cindrick, M.D.
Glenside, PA

Jay D. Coffman, M.D.
Professor of Medicine
Section of Vascular Medicine
Boston University Medical Center
Boston, MA

Anthony J. Comerota, M.D.
Chief, Section of Vascular Surgery
Department of Surgery
Temple University Hospital
Philadelphia, PA

John P. Cooke, M.D., Ph.D.
Division of Cardiovascular Medicine
Stanford University School of Medicine
Stanford, CA

Mark A. Creager, M.D.
Cardiovascular Division
Brigham and Women's Hospital
Boston, MA

Michael H. Criqui, M.D., M.P.H.
University of California, San Diego
La Jolla, CA

Beatrice A. Golomb, M.D., Ph.D.
University of California San Diego
School of Medicine
La Jolla, CA

Alden H. Harken, M.D.
Professor and Chairman
Department of Surgery
University of Colorado Health Sciences Center
Denver, CO

Kenneth Harris, M.D.
Division of Vascular Surgery
London Health Sciences Centre
London, Ontario, Canada

Kathryn L. Hassell, M.D.
Associate Professor
Hematology Research Administration
University of Colorado Health Sciences Center
Denver, CO

William R. Hiatt, M.D.
Novartis Professor for Cardiovascular Research
Divisions of Geriatrics and Cardiology
Vascular Medicine Section
University of Colorado Health Sciences Center
President, Colorado Prevention Center
Denver, CO

Alan T. Hirsch, M.D.
Director
Vascular Medicine Program
Cardiovascular Division
University of Minnesota Hospital
Minneapolis, MN

David W. Hunter, M.D.
Professor of Radiology
Fairview–University Medical Center
University of Minnesota
Minneapolis, MN

Michael R. Jaff, D.O.
The Heart and Vascular Institute
  of New Jersey
Morristown, NJ

William C. Krupski, M.D.
Professor of Surgery
Chief, Section of Vascular Surgery
University of Colorado Health Sciences Center
Denver, CO

Gregory Landry, M.D.
Division of Vascular Surgery
Oregon Health Sciences University
Portland, OR

Emile R. Mohler III, M.D.
Director, Vascular Medicine
Cardiovascular Section
Presbyterian Medical Center
Philadelphia, PA

J. Ernesto Molina, M.D.
Professor of Surgery
Department of Surgery
University of Minnesota Medical School
Minneapolis, MN

Gregory L. Moneta
Division of Vascular Surgery
Oregon Health Sciences University
Portland, OR

Helen Moore, B.Sc.
Department of Surgery
Lutheran General Hospital
Park Ridge, IL

Marsha Neumyer, B.S., R.V.T.
Hershey Medical Center
Vascular Studies Section
College of Medicine
University of Pennsylvania
Hershey, PA

Mark R. Nehler, M.D.
Assistant Professor of Surgery
University of Colorado Health Sciences Center
Denver, CO

Jeffrey W. Olin, D.O.
Director
The Heart and Vascular Institute
  of New Jersey
Morristown, NJ

John M. Porter, M.D.
Division of Vascular Surgery
Oregon Health Sciences University
Portland, OR

Judith G. Regensteiner, Ph.D.
Associate Professor of Medicine
Division of Internal Medicine
Vascular Medicine Section
University of Colorado Health Sciences CenterDenver, CO

Thom W. Rooke, M.D.
Mayo Clinic Rochester
Rochester, MN

Lloyd M. Taylor, Jr., M.D.
Division of Vascular Surgery
Oregon Health Sciences University
Portland, OR

Diane Treat-Jacobson, R.N., Ph.D.
Cardiovascular Division
University of Minnesota Hospital
Minneapolis, MN

Paul A. Tunick, M.D., F.A.C.C., F.A.C.P.
Professor of Clinical Medicine
NYU School of Medicine
Non-Invasive Cardiology Laboratory
NYU Medical Center
New York, NY

M. Eileen Walsh, R.N., M.S.N., C.V.N.
Vascular Clinic Nurse Specialist
Toledo, OH

John V. White, M.D.
Chairman, Department of Surgery
Lutheran General Hospital
Park Ridge, IL

Contents

Section I
Pathophysiology of Arterial Disease

Chapter 1
Mechanisms of Atherosclerosis in Peripheral
Arterial Diseases 3
John P. Cooke

Chapter 2
Arterial Hemostasis and Thrombosis..21
Kathryn L. Hassell

Chapter 3
Endothelial Function in Atherosclerosis 31
Mark A. Creager

Section II
Peripheral Arterial Diseases

Chapter 4
Peripheral Arterial Disease 57
*Beatrice A. Golomb, Michael H. Criqui,
and Warner P. Bundens*

Chapter 5
Clinical and Vascular Laboratory Evaluation
of Peripheral Arterial Disease..81
Michael R. Jaff and William R. Hiatt

Chapter 6
Claudication: The Primary Symptom of Peripheral
Arterial Disease 95
Judith G. Regensteiner and Alan T. Hirsch

Chapter 7
Critical Limb Ischemia 119
Helen L. Moore and John V. White

Chapter 8
Acute Arterial Ischemia 147
Kenneth A. Harris

Chapter 9
Extracranial Carotid Artery Disease 169
Anthony J. Comerota and Lori L. Cindrick

Section III
Abdominal Arterial Diseases

Chapter 10
Visceral Arterial Disease 191
*Lloyd M. Taylor, Jr., Gregory L. Moneta, Gregory Landry,
and John M. Porter*

Chapter 11
Etiology, Prevalence, and Natural History
of Atherosclerotic Renal Artery Stenosis 219
Michael R. Jaff

Section IV
Diseases of the Aorta

Chapter 12
Abdominal Aortic Aneurysms..241
William C. Krupski

Chapter 13
Aortic Dissection...283
Mark R. Nehler and Alden Harken

Chapter 14
Aortic Disease: Atheroembolism
and Thromboembolism...299
Paul A. Tunick

Section V
Vasculitis and Vasospasm

Chapter 15
Thromboangiitis Obliterans (Buerger Disease)........................323
Jeffrey W. Olin

Chapter 16
Vasculitis..339
Emile R. Mohler III

Chapter 17
Raynaud Phenomenon..363
Jay D. Coffman

Section VI
Less Common Vascular Diseases and Syndromes

Chapter 18
Unusual Vascular Diseases of the Extremities.........................387
Jeffrey W. Olin

Chapter 19
Compression Syndromes of the Thoracic Outlet 413
J. Ernesto Molina

Chapter 20
Upper Extremity Arterial Disease...437
Thom W. Rooke

Section VII
Integrated Vascular Care

Chapter 21
The Vascular Health Care Team: Teamwork Devoted
to the Optimal Care of Peripheral Arterial Disease...............457
Alan T. Hirsch, Anthony J. Comerota, David Hunter,
M. Eileen Walsh, Diane Treat-Jacobson,
and Marsha Neumyer

Appendix 1
Selected Professional and Educational Resources
for Vascular Professionals 481

Index..487

Section I

**Pathophysiology
of Arterial Disease**

1 Mechanisms of Atherosclerosis in Peripheral Arterial Diseases

John P. Cooke

CONTENTS

1.1 Introduction...3
1.2 Pathogenesis of Atherosclerosis 4
    1.2.1 Atherogenesis...4
        1.2.1.1 Role of Endothelial Dysfunction 5
        1.2.1.2 Angiogenesis and Plaque Growth....................7
    1.2.2 Antiatherogenic Mechanisms..8
    1.2.3 Plaque Vulnerability and Rupture.....................................11
        1.2.3.1 Macrophages and Inflammation.....................12
        1.2.3.2 Role of Infection 13
        1.2.3.3 Imaging Vulnerable Plaque 13
    1.2.4 Precipitating Vascular Events 15
1.3 Conclusion 15
References...16

1.1 INTRODUCTION

Atherosclerosis is the major cause of death and disability in the United States, accounting annually for approximately 750,000 deaths, largely due to myocardial infarction (MI) and stroke (respectively, the first

0-8493-8413-3/01/$0.00+$1.50
© 2001 by CRC Press LLC

and third major causes of mortality). Other vascular events, such as rupture of vascular aneurysms, catastrophic atheroembolization, and mesenteric and renal ischemia also contribute to the morbidity of this disease.

Individuals predisposed to atherosclerosis can often be identified as having one or more risk factors. The accepted risk factors, determined from large epidemiologic studies, are age, diabetes mellitus, tobacco use, hypercholesterolemia, hypertension, and family history. Myocardial infarctions are much less common in countries where dietary intake of cholesterol and serum cholesterol levels are low than in countries where individuals consume a Western diet and have higher cholesterol levels. The recent Westernization of the diet in Asia, together with the popularity of tobacco, has been associated with a dramatic increase in atherosclerotic vascular disease. In some Asian/Pacific countries (e.g., the Philippines) coronary events are now the greatest cause of mortality. In addition to the traditional risk factors, a number of putative risk factors have been proposed. These include obesity, estrogen deficiency, and elevated blood levels of homocysteine, fibrinogen, C-reactive peptide, lipoprotein(a), and asymmetric dimethylarginine, as well as the constellation of metabolic abnormalities associated with insulin resistance. The mechanisms by which these risk factors initiate and promote atherogenesis are being elucidated, and will likely lead to new therapeutic strategies.

As discussed in detail below, many of the risk factors appear to exert their effect on the vessel wall by inducing endothelial injury. This may be a common pathway by which these factors initiate and accelerate atherogenesis.

1.2   PATHOGENESIS OF ATHEROSCLEROSIS

1.2.1   ATHEROGENESIS

Atherosclerosis has been called a "response to injury of the endothelium."[1] Recent data from our laboratory and others indicate that there may be a common pathway by which the known risk factors affect endothelial function. Experimental models of hypertension, hypercholesterolemia, diabetes mellitus, or tobacco exposure are characterized by common endothelial abnormalities. There may be increased generation of superoxide anion and reduced bioactivity or synthesis of endothelium-derived nitric oxide (NO).[2–5] These alterations in endothelial biology trigger a series of events that precipitate and promote atherogenesis.

1.2.1.1   Role of Endothelial Dysfunction

The endothelium of vessels exposed to hypercholesterolemia, hyperglycemia, hyperhomocysteinemia, hypertension, or tobacco begin to generate increased amounts of oxygen-derived free radicals within days, or even hours, of exposure to these stimuli. Oxidative stress perturbs the cell membrane and increases endothelial permeability. Moreover, within the endothelial cell, oxidant-sensitive transcriptional proteins are activated, most notably nuclear factor–κB (NF-κB). Activated NF-κB translocates to the nucleus, where it induces the expression of adhesion molecules (e.g., vascular cell adhesion molecule [VCAM-1]) and chemokines (e.g., monocyte chemoattractant peptide [MCP-1]) that permit monocyte adhesion and infiltration.[6,7] The expression of these adhesion molecules and chemokines explains the observation that within several days of a high-cholesterol diet, monocytes adhere to the endothelium, particularly at intercellular junctions.[1]

    The monocytes then migrate into the subendothelium. They are attracted in part by low-density lipoprotein (LDL) cholesterol that has become trapped, and subsequently oxidized, in the subendothelial matrix. The oxidation of LDL particles in the subintimal space promotes foam cell formation.[1] Oxidized LDL cholesterol is recognized as foreign, thus stimulating an immune response. Indeed, in individuals with vascular disease, antibodies directed against oxidized LDL cholesterol can be found in the serum and in plaque.[8] Oxidized LDL cholesterol is taken up via the scavenger receptor. Unlike the receptor for native LDL, the scavenger receptor is not downregulated by intracellular cholesterol. Accordingly, oxidized LDL is abundantly consumed by the macrophages via the scavenger receptors, with the result that the macrophages become grossly swollen with lipid, giving them a characteristic "foamy" appearance by microscopy. Accumulating foam cells distend the overlying endothelium to form the fatty streak. These macrophages release mitogens and chemoattractants that recruit additional macrophages as well as vascular smooth muscle cells into the lesion. In addition, they generate reactive oxygen species that increase local oxidative stress.

Foam cells may rupture through the endothelial surface.[1] In these areas of endothelial ulceration, platelets adhere to the vessel wall, releasing epidermal growth factor, platelet-derived growth factor, and other mitogens and cytokines that promote smooth muscle migration and proliferation. Vascular smooth muscle cells migrating into the lesion undergo a change in phenotype from contractile to secretory cells. These secretory vascular smooth muscle cells elaborate extra-cellular matrix (e.g., elastin), which transforms the lesion into a fibrous plaque. Extracellular matrix may contribute significantly to growth of the lesion. Indeed, a genetic variant of the stromelysin promoter that causes reduced degradation of extracellular matrix is associated with accelerated progression of atherosclerosis.[9] In addition to elaborating extracellular matrix, the smooth muscle cells may also become engorged with lipid to form foam cells.

The lesion grows with the recruitment of more cells, the elabora-tion of extracellular matrix, and the accumulation of lipid until it is transformed from a fibrous to a complex plaque. The complex plaque is typically characterized by a fibrous cap that overlies a necrotic core. ("Necrotic" may be a misnomer, because apoptosis undoubtedly con-tributes significantly to cell death and is likely involved in the forma-tion of the cell-free, lipid-rich area in the interior of a complex plaque.) The necrotic core is composed of cell debris and cholesterol, and contains a high concentration of the thrombogenic tissue factor secreted by macrophages. In later-stage lesions, calcification may occur. Calcifying vascular cells (CVC) in the vessel wall can transform into osteoblastlike cells and secrete such bone proteins as osteopon-tin.[10] Histologic examination of these areas reveals similarities to bone tissue. Oxidized lipoprotein stimulates the CVC to elaborate bone protein. By contrast, oxidized lipoprotein reduces bone formation by osteoblasts.[10] This intriguing finding may account for the clinical observation that, in some patients with atherosclerosis, the radiogram discloses a calcified aorta and an osteopenic spine.

In addition to inducing endothelial dysfunction due to oxidative stress, the known risk factors also have other effects that may contribute to atherogenesis. Homocysteine, for example, works through a variety of putative mechanisms.[11] Homocysteine is an amino acid that can react with LDL cholesterol to form oxidized LDL cholesterol, which is often found in foam cells and early atherosclerotic lesions. Through the formation of reactive oxygen species, homocysteine can promote endothelial dysfunction, proliferation of vascular smooth muscle cells, lipid peroxidation, and, as discussed above, oxidation of LDL cholesterol. It is also a well-recognized risk factor for thrombophlebitis and thus promotes both venous and arterial thrombosis.

Aging is also associated with increased oxidative stress. Senescent endothelial cells generate more superoxide anion, have less NO bioactivity, and express higher levels of endothelial adhesion molecules. Atherosclerosis can be thought of as a form of focal senescence, in that the rate of endothelial turnover and telomere shortening is accelerated at bends, branches, and bifurcations of the vessel. Local delivery of genes to reverse the endothelial aging process (e.g., telomerase transfection) might be a novel strategy for treating atherosclerosis.[12]

1.2.1.2   Angiogenesis and Plaque Growth

Recent evidence strongly suggests that neovascularization of plaque is required for its continued growth. In genetically hypercholesterolemic mice, the growth of vascular lesions was retarded by administration of angiogenesis inhibitors.[13] This finding is consistent with previous observations in humans of intense neovascularization of large complex plaques.[14] These small capillaries are derived from the vasa vasorum in the adventitia. It is a characteristic feature of atherosclerotic vessels to manifest an increase in adventitial vascularity.

Plaque vessels may serve as conduits for inflammatory cells, as well as providing oxygen and nutrition to cells in the plaque. These capillaries express endothelial adhesion molecules that may recruit inflammatory cells into lesions.[15] Furthermore, neovascularization may predispose to plaque hemorrhage or rupture. Many of the processes involved in angiogenesis are similar to those that are preconditional for plaque rupture, most notably metalloproteinase activation and matrix degradation.[16] Indeed, there is an increased prevalence of neovascularization in lesions with plaque rupture, mural hemorrhage, or unstable angina.[17] These data raise some concerns about therapeutic angiogenesis as a treatment strategy for atherosclerotic diseases.

1.2.2 ANTIATHEROGENIC MECHANISMS

A number of endogenous mechanisms oppose atherogenesis. High-density lipoprotein (HDL) cholesterol particles may participate in reverse cholesterol transport (i.e., from the vessel to the liver) and also contain enzymes that metabolize platelet-activating factor (i.e., paraoxonase and platelet-activating factor acetylhydrolase).[18] Tissue plasminogen activator is produced by endothelial cells,[19] and, by inducing fibrinolysis, may reduce the local accretion of thrombus. Intracellular superoxide dismutase detoxifies superoxide anion. Endothelium-derived NO and prostacyclin (PGI_2) inhibit several atherogenic processes.[20] In addition to their action as vasodilators, they inhibit the adherence of platelets and leukocytes to the endothelium. Furthermore, both NO and PGI_2 inhibit the proliferation of vascular smooth muscle cells and macrophages and suppress the generation of oxygen-derived free radicals. The latter action suppresses activation of oxidant-responsive genes (e.g., MCP-1 and VCAM-1) that mediate monocyte binding and infiltration into the vessel wall.

Hypercholesterolemia reduces the bioactivity of endothelium-derived NO.[20] In parallel, the endothelium begins to generate superoxide anion.[2] This increased endothelial generation of superoxide anion induced by hypercholesterolemia in rabbit models (Figures 1.1

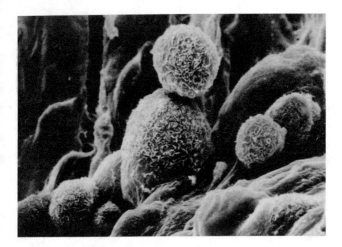

FIGURE 1.1 Scanning electron microphotograph of the luminal surface of the left main coronary artery from a New Zealand White rabbit fed a high-cholesterol diet for 2 weeks. Note the monocytes adhering to the endothelium. Monocyte adherence to the endothelium is the first step in atherogenesis. (From the American College of Cardiology, *J. Am. Coll. Cardiol.*, 23, 452, 1994. With permission.)

and 1.2) can be reversed by placing the animal on a low-cholesterol diet.[21] The reduction in superoxide anion generation is associated with an improvement in endothelium-dependent vasodilator function. In addition to inducing the generation of superoxide anion, hypercholesterolemia causes a decline in tissue glutathione levels, thereby increasing susceptibility to oxidative damage.[22]

Multiple mechanisms may account for the abnormalities in the L-arginine–NO pathway induced by hypercholesterolemia. These include: reduced availability of L-arginine, abnormalities of endothelial receptor–G protein coupling, decreased levels of cofactors such as tetrahydrobiopterin, reduced NO synthase expression and activity, and increased degradation of NO by superoxide anion or

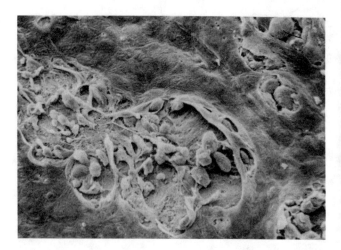

FIGURE 1.2. Scanning electron microphotograph of the luminal surface of the left main coronary artery from a New Zealand White rabbit fed a high-cholesterol diet for 12 weeks. Macrophages have ruptured through the endothelial lining leaving an ulceration that becomes a nidus for thrombus formation.

oxidized lipoproteins or a circulating inhibitor of NO synthase.[23] Accumulating evidence indicates that endogenous methylarginines inhibit the activity of NO synthase. One of these, asymmetric dimethylarginine (ADMA), is a competitive inhibitor of NO synthase and is elevated in patients with atherosclerosis or its risk factors.[24] The elevation in ADMA probably explains the observation that administration of L-arginine to individuals with atherosclerosis (or risk factors for atherosclerosis) restores endothelial vasodilator function and can even reduce symptoms of coronary or peripheral arterial disease (PAD).[25–27] Chronically, L-arginine supplementation enhances vascular NO production, reduces superoxide anion generation, suppresses monocyte adherence, and inhibits (or even reverses) intimal lesion formation in hypercholesterolemic rabbits.[23,28] By contrast, pharmacologic inhibition of NO synthase or genetic deletion of the enzyme accelerates atherogenesis in animal models.

1.2.3 PLAQUE VULNERABILITY AND RUPTURE

Plaque rupture is accepted as the major cause of acute coronary syndromes,[29] aortic atheroembolism, and symptomatic carotid artery disease. Plaque rupture and thrombosis are often asymptomatic but contribute to the rapid growth of lesions as the thrombus undergoes fibrosis. Histopathologic studies reveal that, at the site of a coronary thrombosis, plaque rupture is noted in two thirds of cases.[29] The remaining cases appear to be caused by thrombosis occurring at the site of endothelial denudation. Areas of endothelial denudation are typically associated with collections of macrophages subjacent to the injured endothelium. In these areas, macrophages appear to be emerging through micro-ulcerations in the endothelial surface.

A number of characteristics differentiate stable plaque from plaque that is likely to rupture, i.e., vulnerable plaque. A common feature of vulnerable plaque is thinning of the overlying fibrous cap, which is largely composed of vascular smooth cells and extracellular matrix. In vulnerable or ruptured plaques, the fibrous cap appears to be eroded at the shoulder of the lesion (where the fibrous cap meets the intima of the normal segment of the vessel wall). This, the area that is impacted by the greatest hemodynamic stress, is where rupture typically occurs.[29,30]

Another commonality is a large necrotic core filled with lipid and cell debris. The lipid core has a semifluid consistency at body temperature that likely plays a role in plaque stability: the more fluid the core, the greater mechanical stress the fibrous plaque must bear.[30] Another characteristic feature of the ruptured plaque is intraplaque and intraluminal thrombosis.[31] Angioscopic studies have revealed that patients with unstable angina characteristically have complex ulcerated lesions with associated thrombosis. In contrast, those with stable angina typically have obstructive lesions with an unperturbed endothelial surface.[32] Finally, another common feature of ruptured plaque is an intense infiltration of the plaque with macrophages.[29] A wealth of data now indicate that macrophages within the plaque play a key role in plaque vulnerability.

1.2.3.1 Macrophages and Inflammation

Accumulating evidence indicates that macrophages are responsible for characteristic features of the vulnerable plaque, including the endothelial disruption, thin fibrous cap, large acellular core, and thrombogenicity of the plaque contents. In the normal vessel, the synthesis and degradation of extracellular matrix is glacially slow, with collagen turnover being measured in years. However, in the diseased vessel, extracellular matrix degradation is increased and can lead to structural weakening of the fibrous cap. An intense infiltration of macrophages is invariably observed at the site of plaque rupture, where the fibrous cap appears to be undermined. In addition to cathepsins, these macrophages synthesize abundant amounts of metalloproteinases (MMP-1, MMP-3, and MMP-9). These MMPs degrade extracellular matrix, weakening the fibrous cap.[29]

In addition to an increased degradation of extracellular matrix, inflammatory cells may reduce the synthesis of collagen by vascular smooth muscle cells. T-cells in the region of the fibrous cap elaborate interferon (INF)-γ, a potent inhibitor of collagen synthesis. Furthermore, INF-γ is known to induce apoptosis of vascular smooth muscle cells.[33] Vascular smooth muscle cells may also be under attack by the free radicals hydrochlorous acid and peroxynitrate anion, produced by the macrophages, both of which may induce apoptosis.[34] The increased apoptosis may account for the observation that fibrous caps that have ruptured have half as many smooth muscle cells as intact fibrous caps.[35] Macrophages contribute to the thrombotic nature of the vulnerable plaque. The macrophages in the lesion are a rich source of tissue factor, which can be found in the acellular core as well as in the vascular smooth muscle of the fibrous cap.[36] Macrophage content and expression of tissue factor correlate with rupture of the human atherosclerotic plaque. Macrophage and tissue factor content is greater in coronary atherectomy specimens from patients with unstable angina than in those who have stable angina.

1.2.3.2   Role of Infection

Mounting circumstantial evidence implicates infection in the progression of atherosclerosis.[37] There is seroepidemiological and immunohistochemical evidence that such infectious agents as cytomegalovirus, herpes viruses, and *Chlamydia pneumoniae* are associated with atherosclerotic vascular disease and vascular events. Such infections may trigger plaque rupture by increasing hemodynamic stress (e.g., tachycardia and increased cardiac output that may accompany a febrile illness) or may directly affect the vascular biology of the plaque. Infection localizing to the plaque may activate endothelial cells to express adhesion molecules, may stimulate vascular cells to undergo proliferation, or induce resident inflammatory cells to elaborate cytokines that promote further local inflammation. The local inflammation that precipitates plaque rupture may be part of a systemic process. In coronary artery disease, markers of inflammation have been associated with the development of atherosclerosis and plaque rupture. Elevation of C-reactive protein is a marker of systemic inflammation. In the Physician's Health Study, an elevated C-reactive protein was a risk factor for the development of symptomatic PAD and also a risk for peripheral revascularization.[38] Elevations in fibrinogen are a putative risk factor for vascular events. Hyperfibrinogenemia may also be a marker for systemic inflammation, as well as a contributor to increased blood viscosity and hypercoagulability.

1.2.3.3   Imaging Vulnerable Plaque

It is apparent from the above discussion that an imaging modality to detect vulnerable plaque would be useful for the identification (and appropriate management) of those patients at greatest risk for a catastrophic vascular event. Unfortunately, there currently are no adequate imaging modalities to detect vulnerable plaque. Angiography can detect stenoses, but this information is not useful in predicting vulnerability to rupture.[39,40] Indeed, 50% to 75% of plaque ruptures leading to coronary thrombosis occur at sites where the plaque caused less than 50% narrowing of the lumen.[39] Furthermore, intravascular ultrasound studies reveal that the volume of the intimal lesion may often be underestimated by angiography.[41] Intravascular ultrasound is superior to angiography in assessing plaque burden, and can provide some information regarding characteristics of the lesion; however, two-dimensional visual images cannot yet provide tissue characterization that can reproducibly differentiate stable from unstable atheroma. Whereas angioscopy and intravascular ultrasound can identify the presence of thrombosis and some of the lipid-rich plaques, these techniques are invasive and not practical in evaluating the prognosis in most individuals with minimal or no symptoms. Noninvasive tests are needed to determine the risk of acute coronary syndromes, but current noninvasive tests are neither sensitive nor specific. In one study of patients with coronary artery disease, subjects were prospectively evaluated with angiography, exercise testing, and ambulatory monitoring. However, none of these tests, singly or combined, was effective in predicting acute events.[42] This is probably because stenosis severity, which is assessed by these technologies, is unrelated to acute events.[43]

Ultrafast computed tomography is noninvasive and useful in measuring calcium content in the vessel wall, but there are no clinical studies indicating a positive correlation between calcium content and clinical events. Indeed, in patients with stroke, the risk of recurrent vascular events is negatively correlated with aortic calcium content.[44] Magnetic resonance angiography may replace angiography to detect stenoses, but is currently ineffective at detecting vulnerable plaques. However, a recent study of carotid artery lesions before endarterectomy using surface coils indicates that magnetic resonance imaging, with future refinements, may be capable of effectively discriminating lipid core, fibrous caps, calcification, and normal media and adventitia.[45]

1.2.4 PRECIPITATING VASCULAR EVENTS

There is a circadian pattern of acute MI and sudden death, with most heart attacks occurring in the morning during arousal from sleep or shortly thereafter.[46] A similar circadian pattern is observed in certain physiological parameters, with increases in heart rate, blood pressure, and platelet aggregability also occurring in the morning hours.[46] The circadian variation in hemodynamic stress and blood coagulability probably accounts for the increase in vascular events in the morning hours, and is likely driven by increased sympathetic nerve flow during arousal from sleep. In addition to this circadian variation, there is a weekly variation, with increased events occurring on Monday in workers but not retired persons.

The sympathetic nervous system is also activated by fear, anger, and strenuous exertion, possibly accounting for the increased risk of MI with emotional or physical stress. A study by Muller and colleagues[46] revealed that the risk of MI was elevated about twofold after an outburst of anger, heavy exertion, or sexual activity. Several other external events have been reported as possible triggers, including earthquakes, blizzards, heat waves, and missile strikes. All of these triggers likely exert their effects via the sympathetic nervous system, which may explain the observation that β-adrenergic antagonists confer longevity in patients with atherosclerotic coronary artery disease.

1.3 CONCLUSION

We have learned a great deal about the pathogenesis of atherosclerosis in the last 25 years. During that time, it was discovered that atherosclerosis is a highly complex and dynamic phenomenon that involves an array of cell types and processes. Atherosclerosis begins as an endothelial injury, or, perhaps more accurately, as an alteration in endothelial function. The derangement in endothelial functions leads to the expression of adhesion molecules and chemokines that begin the inflammatory process. The terminal event in atherosclerosis, plaque rupture, is also caused by an inflammatory process. Between the beginning and the end, a complex vascular pathobiology is set in motion by a number of risk factors, although it is highly modifiable by rectification of those risk factors. New insights into the cellular and molecular mechanisms of atherogenesis will result in new therapeutic strategies that will relegate this disease to the 20th century.

REFERENCES

1. Ross, R., Cellular and molecular studies of atherosclerosis, *Atherosclerosis,* 131, S3, 1997.
2. Ohara, Y., Peterson, T.E., and Harrison, D.G., Hypercholesterolemia increases endothelial superoxide anion production, *J. Clin. Invest.,* 91, 2546, 1993.
3. Rajagopalan, S., Kurz, S., Munzel, T., et al., Angiotensin II-mediated hypertension in the rat increases vascular superoxide production via membrane NADH/NADPH oxidase activation: contribution to alterations of vasomotor tone, *J. Clin. Invest.,* 97, 1916, 1996.
4. Tesfamariam, B. and Cohen, R.A., Free radicals mediate endothelial cell dysfunction caused by elevated glucose, *Am. J. Physiol.,* 263, H321, 1992.
5. Tsao, P. S., Buitrago, R., Chang, H., et al., Effects of diabetes on monocyte–endothelial interactions and endothelial superoxide production in fructose-induced insulin-resistant and hypertensive rats, *Circulation,* 92, A266, 1995.
6. Tsao, P.S., Buitrago, R., Chan, J.R., et al., Fluid flow inhibits endothelial adhesiveness: nitric oxide and transcriptional regulation of VCAM-1, *Circulation,* 94, 1682, 1996.
7. Tsao, P.S., Wang, B., Buitrago, R., et al., Nitric oxide regulates monocyte chemotactic protein-1, *Circulation,* 96, 934,1997.
8. Steinberg, D., Low-density lipoprotein oxidation and its pathobiological significance, *J. Biol. Chem.,* 272, 20963, 1997.
9. Ye, S., Eriksson, P., Hamsten, A., et al., Progression of coronary atherosclerosis is associated with a common genetic variant of the human stromelysin-1 promoter, which results in reduced gene expression. *J. Biol. Chem.,* 271, 13055, 1996.

10. Parhami, F., Morrow, A.D., Balucan, J., et al., Lipid oxidation products have opposite effects on calcifying vascular cell and bone cell differentiation: a possible explanation for the paradox of arterial calcification in osteoporotic patients, *Arterioscler. Thromb. Vasc. Biol.,* 17, 680, 1997.

11. Welch, G.N. and Loscalzo, J., Homocysteine and atherothrombosis, *N. Engl. J. Med.,* 338, 1042, 1998.

12. Yang, J., Chang, E., Cherry, A.M., et al., Human endothelial cell life extension by telomerase expression, *J. Biol. Chem.*, 274, 26141,1999.

13. Moulton, K.S., Heller, E., Konerding, M.A., et al., Angiogenesis inhibitors endostatin or TNP-470 reduce intimal neovascularization and plaque growth in apolipoprotein E–deficient mice, *Circulation,* 99, 1726, 1999.

14. Barger, A.C., Beeuwkes, R., Lainey, L., et al., Hypothesis: vasa vasorum and neovascularization of human coronary arteries, *N. Engl. J. Med.*, 310, 175, 1984.

15. O'Brien, K.D., McDonald, T.O., Chait, A., et al., Neovascular expression of E-selectin, ICAM-1, and VCAM-1 in human atherosclerosis and their relation to intimal leukocyte content, *Circulation,* 93, 672, 1996.

16. Gross, J.L., Moscatelli, D., and Rifkin, D.B., Increased capillary endothelial cell protease activity in response to angiogenic stimuli *in vitro,* *Proc. Natl. Acad. Sci. USA.*, 80, 2623, 1983.

17. Tenaglia, A.N., Peters, K.G., Sketch, M.H., Jr., et al., Neovascularization in atherectomy specimens from patients with unstable angina. *Am. Heart. J.,* 135, 10, 1998.

18. Zimmerman, G.A., McIntyre, T. M., and Prescott, S.M., Adhesion and signaling in vascular cell-cell interactions, *J. Clin. Invest.,* 100, S3, 1997.

19. Vaughan, D.E., The renin-angiotensin system and fibrinolysis, *Am. J. Cardiol.,* 79, 12,1997.

20. Cooke, J.P. and Dzau, V. J., Nitric oxide synthase: role in the genesis of vascular disease, *Annu. Rev. Med.,* 48, 489, 1997b.

21. Ohara, Y., Peterson, T.E., Sayegh, H.S., Subramanian, R.R., et al., Dietary correction of hypercholesterolemia in the rabbit normalizes endothelial superoxide anion production, *Circulation,* 92, 898, 1995.

22. Ma, X.L., Lopez, B.L., Liu, G.L., et al., Hypercholesterolemia impairs a detoxification mechanism against peroxynitrite and renders the vascular tissue more susceptible to oxidative injury, *Circ. Res.,* 80, 894, 1997.

23. Cooke, J.P. and Dzau, V.J., Derangements of the nitric oxide synthase pathway, L-arginine, and cardiovascular diseases. *Circulation*, 96, 379, 1997a.

24. Boger, R.H., Bode-Boger, S.M., Szuba, A., et al., Asymmetric dimethylarginine (ADMA): a novel risk factor for endothelial dysfunction: its role in hypercholesterolemia, *Circulation*, 98, 1842, 1998.

25. Boger, R.H., Bode-Boger, S.M., Thiele, W., et al., Biochemical evidence for impaired nitric oxide synthesis in patients with peripheral arterial occlusive disease, *Circulation*, 95, 2068, 1997.

26. Bode-Boger, S.M., Boger, R.H., Alfke, H., et al., L-arginine induces nitric oxide-dependent vasodilation in patients with critical limb ischemia: a randomized, controlled study, *Circulation*, 9, 85,1996.

27. Lerman, A., Burnett, J.C.J., Higano, S.T., et al., Long-term L-arginine supplementation improves small-vessel coronary endothelial function in humans, *Circulation*, 97, 2123,1998.

28. Candipan, R.C., Wang, B.Y., Buitrago, R., et al., Regression or progression: dependency on vascular nitric oxide, *Arterioscler. Thromb. Vasc. Biol.*, 16, 44, 1996.

29. Fuster, V. and Lewis, A., Conner Memorial Lecture: Mechanisms leading to myocardial infarction: insights from studies of vascular biology [published erratum appears in *Circulation* 1995 Jan. 1; 91 (1); 256], *Circulation*, 90, 2126–2146, 1994.

30. Loree, H.M., Tobias, B.J., Gibson, L.J.,et al., Mechanical properties of model atherosclerotic lesion lipid pools, *Arterioscler. Thromb.*, 14, 230, 1994.

31. Stary, H.C., Chandler, A.B., Dinsmore, R.E., et al., A definition of advanced types of atherosclerotic lesions and a histological classification of atherosclerosis, a report from the Committee on Vascular Lesions of the Council on Arteriosclerosis, American Heart Association, *Arterioscler. Thromb. Vasc. Biol.*, 15, 1512, 1995.

32. Sherman, C.T., Litvack, F., Grundfest, W., et al., Coronary angioscopy in patients with unstable angina pectoris, *N. Engl. J. Med.*, 315, 913, 1986.

33. Geng,Y.J., Wu, Q., Muszynski, M., et al., Apoptosis of vascular smooth muscle cells induced by *in vitro* stimulation with interferon-gamma, tumor necrosis factor-alpha, and interleukin-1 beta, *Arterioscler. Thromb. Vasc. Biol.*, 16, 19, 1996.

34. Heinecke, J.W., Mechanisms of oxidative damage of low-density lipo-protein in human atherosclerosis, *Curr. Opin. Lipidol.*, 8, 268, 1997.

35. Falk, E., Why do plaques rupture?, *Circulation*, 86, III-30, 1992.

36. Marmur, J.D., Thiruvikraman, S.V., Fyfe, B.S., et al., Identification of active tissue factor in human coronary atheroma, *Circulation*, 94, 1226, 1996.

37. Libby, P., Egan, D., and Skarlatos, S., Roles of infectious agents in atherosclerosis and restenosis: an assessment of the evidence and need for future research, *Circulation*, 9, 4095, 1997.

38. Ridker, P.M., Cushman, M., Stampfe, M.J., et al., Plasma concentra-tion of C-reactive protein and risk of developing peripheral vascular disease, *Circulation*, 97, 425,1998.

39. Ambrose, J.A., Winters, S.L., Arora, R.R.,et al., Coronary angio-graphic morphology in myocardial infarction: a link between the pathogenesis of unstable angina and myocardial infarction, *J. Am. Coll. Cardiol.*, 6, 1233, 1985.

40. Little, W.C., Constantinescu, M., Applegate, R.J., et al., Can coronary angiography predict the site of a subsequent myocardial infarction in patients with mild-to-moderate coronary artery disease?, *Circulation*, 78, 1157, 1988.

41. Pinto, F.J., Chenzbraun, A., Botas, J., et al., Feasibility of serial intracoronary ultrasound imaging for assessment of progression of intimal proliferation in cardiac transplant recipients, *Circulation*, 90, 2348, 1994.

42. Mulcahy, D., Husain, S., Zalos, G., et al., Ischemia during ambulatory monitoring as a prognostic indicator in patients with stable coronary artery disease, *JAMA*, 277, 318, 1997.

43. Mann, J.M. and Davies, M.J., Vulnerable plaque: relation of charac-teristics to degree of stenosis in human coronary arteries, *Circulation*, 94, 928, 1996.

44. Cohen, A., Tzourio, C., Bertrand, B., et al., Aortic plaque morphology and vascular events: a follow-up study in patients with ischemic stroke, FAPS Investigators (French Study of Aortic Plaques in Stroke), *Circulation*, 96, 3838, 1997.

45. Toussaint, J.F., Lamuraglia, G.M., Southern, J.F., et al., Magnetic resonance images lipid, fibrous, calcified, hemorrhagic, and throm-botic components of human atherosclerosis *in vivo*, *Circulation*, 94, 932, 1996.

46. Muller, J.E., Tofler, G.H., and Stone, P.H., Circadian variation and triggers of onset of acute cardiovascular disease, *Circulation,* 79, 733, 1989.

2 Arterial Hemostasis and Thrombosis

Kathryn L. Hassell

CONTENTS

2.1 Arterial Hemostasis and Thrombosis 21
    2.1.1 Platelet-Dependent Thrombosis...21
    2.1.2 Fibrin-Rich Thrombosis..23
    2.1.3 Endogenous Anticoagulants..25
    2.1.4 Fibrinolysis..25
2.2 Hemostatic Risk Factors and Peripheral Vascular Disease 26
    2.2.1 Fibrinogen 27
    2.2.2 Plasminogen Activator Inhibitor-1................................27
    2.2.3 Factor VII 27
    2.2.4 Von Willebrand Factor 28
2.3 Conclusions...28
References...28

2.1 ARTERIAL HEMOSTASIS AND THROMBOSIS

The mechanisms of thrombosis in the arterial system center on two phases: (1) formation of a platelet-rich thrombus (platelet-dependent thrombosis), followed by (2) thrombin activation leading to development of a fibrin deposition (fibrin-rich thrombus).[1,2] Balancing forces include endogenous anticoagulant and fibrinolytic systems.

2.1.1 PLATELET-DEPENDENT THROMBOSIS

Under normal conditions, the arterial vessel wall is lined with intact endothelium, to which platelets do not adhere. Figure 2.1 depicts the

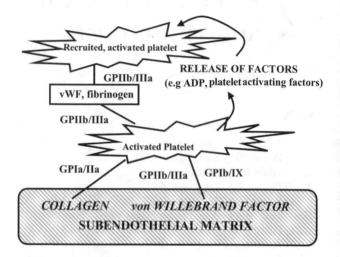

FIGURE 2.1 Sequence of events involved in generation of platelet-dependent thrombosis. ADP = adenosine dinucleotide phosphate; GP = glycoprotein; plt = platelet; vWF = von Willebrand factor.

events that occur to generate platelet-dependent thrombosis. If there is disruption of the endothelial surface, with exposure of the subendothelial matrix, medial, or adventitial layers, then platelet adhesion occurs spontaneously. This adhesion is mediated by integrin receptors on the platelet surface, including glycoprotein (GP) Ia/IIa, which binds to collagen. Collagen may be the most important component of the subendothelial matrix for initiation of platelet adhesion.[3] GP Ib/IX, another platelet receptor, binds to von Willebrand factor (vWF) embedded or attached to the subendothelial matrix, preferentially recognizing this immobilized vWF over that in the plasma.[1,4] Adhesion to subendothelial matrix, especially via vWF, appears to be significantly augmented at higher shear stresses.[5] These receptor-ligand interactions result not only in platelet adhesion, but also in platelet activation. Subsequent intracellular processes within the platelet are thought, in turn, to activate the integrin

GP IIb/IIIa on the platelet surface. GP IIb/IIIa binds a variety of adhesive proteins, including vWF, fibrinogen, fibronectin, and vitronectin, and recognizes the amino acid sequence arginine-glycine-aspartate, further augmenting adhesion.[6]

Adhesion of platelets induces platelet activation, which results in shape change; release of platelet aggregation agents from platelet storage granules, including adenosine diphosphate, fibrinogen, collagen, fibronectin, thrombospondin, epinephrine, platelet-activating factor, serotonin, and vWF; and stimulation of the production and release of thromboxane A_2.[1,2] Platelet aggregation rapidly follows, resulting in a platelet-rich thrombus adherent to the area of injury or exposure of subendothelium. There is controversy about the role that thrombin plays in the development of the platelet-rich thrombus. Thrombin, via a specific thrombin receptor, is a potent platelet agonist, inducing aggregation and recruitment of platelets.[7] Some authors argue that because platelet adhesion, aggregation, and accumulation occur within milliseconds, there is insufficient time for thrombin generation and subsequent fibrin formation to play a role in the process.[1,8] Alternatively, platelet deposition in thrombus formation has been attenuated in experimental models by treatment with direct antithrombin agents.[2,9] In this initiation of arterial thrombosis, it may be that small quantities of thrombin play a role as platelet agonist, but not as an inducer of fibrin clot. Platelet-dependent thrombosis may more readily occur and promote pathologic thrombosis when arterial stenosis results in elevated shear stress or when an atherosclerotic plaque ruptures and releases adhesive GPs (e.g., vitronectin and fibronectin).

2.1.2 Fibrin-Rich Thrombosis

It is clear from histopathologic and experimental observation that the formation of a fibrin-rich thrombus is an important second phase in arterial thrombosis. Basic events are depicted in Figure 2.2. Activation and efficient propagation of blood coagulation occurs on a phospholipid surface. When activated, the platelet phospholipid membrane is altered and phosphotidylserine is flipped to the outside of the membrane, creating a procoagulant surface.[10] Damage to the endothelium may result

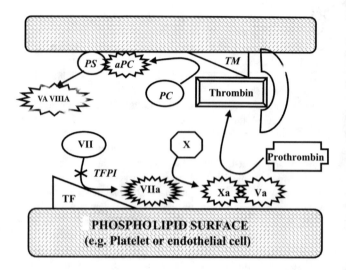

FIGURE 2.2 Basic events involved in formation of fibrin-rich thrombus. Abbreviations represent various factors.

in exposure of circulating blood to smooth muscle cells in the media, which elaborate tissue factor (TF) when stimulated by agonists such as platelet-derived growth factor,[11] and to the adventitia, where TF is present in normal vessels.[12] On these procoagulant surfaces, TF/factor VIIa complexes form, initiating coagulation by the extrinsic pathway. Factor Xa is generated, which, when complexed with factor Va, converts prothrombin (factor II) to thrombin (factor IIa). Thrombin has a multitude of effects, including the conversion of fibrinogen into fibrin, which is cross-linked by factor XIII to form a stable fibrin clot. Thrombin also activates factors V (including the factor V released from activated platelet granules) and VIII in a positive feedback loop. In arterial thrombosis, the generation of thrombin is thought to occur predominantly on the phospholipid surface of the accumulated platelets and is highly dependent on the presence of platelet deposition.[13,14] Increased elaboration of tissue factor by the smooth muscle cells and monocytes/macrophages involved in the development of the atherosclerotic plaque, especially when stimulated by inflammatory mediators, likely enhances the risk for development of arterial thrombosis.[2]

2.1.3 ENDOGENOUS ANTICOAGULANTS

Regulation of thrombin-associated coagulation is mediated by antithrombin, protein C, protein S, and tissue factor pathway inhibitor (TFPI). Antithrombin binds and inactivates the activated clotting factors, especially factors Xa and IIa (thrombin), in the presence of heparinlike glycosaminoglycans associated with vascular endothelium.[15] Protein C is activated by a complex of thrombin bound to thrombomodulin on the surface of endothelial cells. Activated protein C then binds to protein S on a phospholipid surface; this complex inactivates factors Va and VIIIa.[16] TFPI is produced by endothelium and directly binds to and inhibits factor Xa. TFPI/factor Xa complexes then bind to TF/factor VIIa complexes, forming a quatenary structure that renders all these factors inactive.[17] Resistance to protein C, conferred most commonly by a mutation in factor V called factor V Leiden, is a common genetic polymorphism that results in reduced endogenous anticoagulant activity.[18] Although these factors may limit the secondary phase of fibrin-rich thrombosis, there is little consistent evidence that deficiencies of or resistance to these anticoagulant factors increase the risk of arterial thrombotic disease.[1] This is supported by the observation that antiplatelet treatment strategies are consistently more effective than antithrombin treatment strategies, at least in some models of arterial thrombosis.[2]

2.1.4 FIBRINOLYSIS

Fibrinolysis is initiated when plasminogen binds to the fibrin present in a thrombus. Endothelial cells near the site of vessel injury secrete tissue plasminogen activator (tPA) at an increased rate, stimulated in part by fibrin itself, by thrombin bound in the thrombus, and by vessel occlusion.[19] Then tPA binds to fibrin and converts the plasminogen bound to fibrin into plasmin. Plasmin cleaves both the un-cross-linked and cross-linked fibrin to which it is bound, generating fibrin split products. Digestion of fibrin opens additional binding sites for plasminogen. Fibrinolysis is further stimulated as digestion of fibrin opens additional binding sites for plasminogen, and plasmin cleaves tPA into a 2-chain molecule, which has a greater affinity for fibrinogen, resulting in amplification of the fibrinolytic process.[19] Endothelial cells have surface receptors for tPA, urokinase-like plasminogen activator (uPA), and plasminogen, and can thus facilitate conversion of plasminogen to plasmin.[20]

Major physiologic inhibitors of fibrinolysis include α_2-antiplasmin and plasminogen activator inhibitor-1 (PAI-1). α_2-Antiplasmin binds and inhibits plasminogen, and PAI-1 binds and inhibits both tPA and uPA. α_2-Antiplasmin is made in the liver; PAI-1 is made in endothelial cells, adipose tissue, liver, and platelets, and is released from platelets during platelet aggregation.[21] PAI-1 is also present in the subendothelial matrix, limiting fibrinolysis at the site of vessel injury.[22]

The overall net effect of the fibrinolytic system in response to vessel injury is to limit thrombolysis at the site of injury (subendothelial matrix) but facilitate thrombolysis to limit the extent of thrombosis at the surface of the clot (on fibrin) and on the surface of intact endothelial cells more distant from the site of injury. The inadequate release of fibrinolytic activators or excessive release of inhibitors—as has been characterized in patients with obesity, insulin resistance, tobacco use, and abnormal lipid profiles—may shift the balance and allow perpetuation and propagation of thrombosis.[19]

2.2   HEMOSTATIC RISK FACTORS AND PERIPHERAL VASCULAR DISEASE

Much of the available information about hemostatic risk factors in arterial vascular disease centers on coronary artery disease, or does not distinguish between subjects with isolated peripheral vascular disease and those who have coronary or cerebral vascular disease as well as peripheral vascular disease. A number of studies have investigated the more commonly recognized hemostatic risk factors.

2.2.1 FIBRINOGEN

Multiple studies have demonstrated statistically significant higher levels of fibrinogen in patients with coronary artery disease.[23] Although most investigations have not distinguished patients with isolated peripheral arterial disease (PAD), several studies have found a positive correlation between fibrinogen levels and severity of PAD, as measured by ankle–brachial pressure index, imaging, symptoms, and treadmill testing in both diabetic and nondiabetic subjects.[24–27] A strong independent correlation of fibrinogen with severity of PAD was demonstrated in a study that controlled for the presence of coronary or cerebral vascular disease.[28] Several studies have also demonstrated increased D-dimer levels in patients with arterial vascular disease, suggesting activation of the fibrinolytic system, presumptively in response to increased fibrin generation in these patients.[24,27] It is not clear whether the elevation in fibrinogen is part of the pathophysiologic process in arterial disease or simply a marker of underlying inflammation that is thought to contribute significantly to artherosclerotic disease.

2.2.2 PLASMINOGEN ACTIVATOR INHIBITOR-1

Impaired fibrinolysis might be expected to exacerbate PAD, limiting the ability to clear fibrin deposition and control thrombus extension. Elevated levels of PAI-1 have been associated with arterial vascular disease, although it has not been established as a variable independent of insulin resistance or obesity.[29] In patients with peripheral vascular disease without known coronary artery disease, PAI-1 levels did not correlate with severity of disease, independent of body mass index and age.[28]

2.2.3 FACTOR VII

As a significant factor in the secondary phase of arterial thrombosis, factor VII and VIIa levels have been investigated in patients with arterial disease. Although a correlation between factor VII levels and significant coronary artery disease can be demonstrated, weak or no correlation has been documented between factor VII levels and peripheral vascular disease.[26,28]

2.2.4 VON WILLEBRAND FACTOR

Both as a potential marker of inflammation and of endothelial injury, and as a mediator of platelet aggregation, elevated levels of vWF might be expected in patients with arterial disease. However, studies have failed to demonstrate a relation between elevated vWF and atherothrombotic events or severity of arterial disease.[1]

2.3 CONCLUSIONS

Arterial hemostasis and thrombosis are initiated and principally mediated by platelet adhesion, activation, and aggregation. A secondary phase of thrombin and fibrin generation produces fibrin deposition into the thrombus, facilitated by the activated platelet phospholipid surface. Control of the propagation and extension of thrombosis is mediated to some extent by endogenous anticoagulants and by the fibrinolytic system. Many aspects of procoagulant, anticoagulant, and fibrinolytic mechanisms are altered in peripheral vascular disease. These derangements include heightened shear stresses due to stenotic vessels, leading to enhanced platelet adhesion and activation; increased tissue factor elaboration along damaged vessels, resulting in increased thrombin generation; and imbalances in the fibrinolytic system that limit the capacity to control thrombosis. Therapeutic intervention is directed at inhibiting platelet function and coagulation, and enhancing fibrinolysis to compensate for these derangements.

REFERENCES

1. Stormorken, H., Hemostatic risk factors in arterial thrombosis and atherosclerosis: the thrombin-fibrin and platelet vWF axis, *Thromb. Res.*, 88, 1, 1997.
2. Eisenberg, P.R., Platelet-dependent and procoagulant mechanisms in arterial thrombosis, *Int. J. Cardiol.*, 68(Suppl 1), S3, 1999.
3. Kirchhofer, D., Role of collagen-adherent platelets in mediating fibrin formation in flowing whole blood, *Blood*, 86, 3815, 1995.

4. Turitto, V.T., Factor VIII/von Willebrand factor in subendothelium mediates platelet adhesion, *Blood*, 65, 823, 1985.

5. Ruggeri, Z.M., The role of von Willebrand factor and fibrinogen in the initiation of platelet adhesion to thrombogenic surfaces, *Thromb. Haemost.*, 74, 460, 1995.

6. Hawiger, J., Adhesive interactions of platelets and their blockade, *Ann. N. Y. Acad. Sci.*, 614, 270, 1991.

7. Eidt, J.F., Thrombin is an important mediator of platelet aggregation in stenosed canine coronary arteries with endothelial injury, *J. Clin. Invest.*, 84, 18, 1989.

8. Luscher, E.F., The formation of the haemostatic plug—a special case of platelet aggregation, *Thromb. Haemost.*, 70, 234, 1993.

9. Harker, L.A., Thrombin hypothesis of thrombus generation and vascular lesion formation, *Am. J. Cardiol.*, 75, 12B, 1995.

10. Zwaal, R.F.A., Pathophysiologic implications of membrane phospholipid asymmetry in blood cells, *Blood*, 89, 1121, 1997.

11. Schecter, A.D., Tissue factor expression in human arterial smooth muscle cells. TF is present in three cellular pools after growth factor stimulation, *J. Clin. Invest.*, 100, 2276, 1997.

12. Barstad, R.M., Procoagulant human monocytes mediate tissue factor/factor VIIa-dependent platelet-thrombus formation when exposed to flowing nonanticoagulated human blood, *Arterioscler. Thromb. Vasc. Biol.*, 15, 11, 1995.

13. Ghigliotti, G., Prolonged activation of prothrombin on the vascular wall after arterial injury, *Arterioscler. Thromb. Vasc. Biol.*, 18, 250, 1998.

14. Eisenberg, P.R., Importance of platelets in arterial clot-associated procoagulant activity, *Circulation*, 92, 803, 1995.

15. Marcum, J.A., Anticoagulantly active heparin-like molecules from vascular tissue, *Biochemistry*, 32, 1730, 1984.

16. Esmon, C.T., The protein C anticoagulant pathway, *Arterioscler. Thromb.*, 12, 135, 1992.

17. Broze, G.J., Jr., The lipoprotein-associated coagulation inhibitor that inhibits factor VII-tissue factor complex also inhibits factor Xa: insight into its possible mechanism of action, *Blood*, 71, 335, 1988.

18. Martinelly, I., Heightened thrombin generation in individuals with resistance to activated protein C, *Thromb. Haemost.*, 75, 703, 1996.

19. Francis, C.W., *Hemostasis and Thrombosis*, J.B. Lippincott, Philadelphia, 1994, 1085.

20. Plow, E., *Thrombosis and Hemorrhage*, Williams & Wilkins, Baltimore, 1998, Chap. 18.

21. Kruithof, E.K., Studies on the release of a plasminogen activator inhibitor by human platelets, *Thromb. Haemost.*, 55, 201, 1986.

22. Mimuro, J., Extracellular matrix of cultured bovine aortic endothelial cells contains functionally active type I plasminogen activator inhibitor, *Blood*, 70, 721, 1987.

23. Ernst, E., Fibrinogen as a cardiovascular risk factor: a meta-analysis and review of the literature, *Ann. Intern. Med.*, 118, 956, 1993.

24. Lassila, R., Severity of peripheral artherosclerosis is associated with fibrinogen and degradation of cross-linked fibrin, *Arterioscler. Thromb.*, 13, 1738, 1993.

25. Tkac, I., Fibrinogen and albuminuria are related to the presence and severity of peripheral arterial disease in women with type 2 diabetes mellitus, *Angiology*, 48, 715, 1997.

26. Cortellaro, M., The PLAT study: a multidisciplinary study of hemostatic function and conventional risk factors in vascular disease patients, *Arteriosclerosis*, 90, 109, 1991.

27. Lee, A.J., The role of haematological factors in diabetic peripheral arterial disease: the Edinburgh artery study, *Br. J. Haematol.*, 105, 648, 1999.

28. Philipp, C.S., Association of hemostatic factors with peripheral vascular disease, *Am. Heart J.*, 134, 978, 1997.

29. Juhan-Vague, I., PAI-1, obesity, insulin resistance, and risk of cardiovascular events, *Thromb. Haemost.*, 78, 656, 1997.

3 Endothelial Function in Atherosclerosis

Mark A. Creager

CONTENTS

3.1 Introduction..31
3.2 The Inflamed Endothelium.......................................32
3.3 Endothelium-Derived Nitric Oxide 33
3.4 Mechanisms of Endothelial Dysfunction 37
3.5 Treatment of Endothelial Dysfunction.....................41
    3.5.1 Clinical Implications of Treating
        Endothelial Dysfunction 43
3.6 Conclusions..44
References..44

3.1 INTRODUCTION

The endothelium is a single layer of cells that comprises the inner lining of blood vessels and serves as an interface between the circulating blood and subjacent vascular smooth muscle. In the healthy state, the endothelium synthesizes biologically active substances that modulate vasomotor tone and regulate coagulation. The endothelium is ideally situated as a protective barrier, preventing the blood vessel from undergoing pathologic changes in response to injury. Atherosclerosis is the most common form of vascular disease, causing morphologic disruption of the blood vessel wall that includes lipid deposition, vascular smooth muscle proliferation, and fibrosis. Atherosclerosis begins when the endothelium's protective properties are overcome by injurious factors such as high cholesterol, tobacco smoke, diabetes mellitus, and high blood pressure.

3.2 THE INFLAMED ENDOTHELIUM

One of the first steps in atherogenesis is the expression of leukocyte adhesion molecules, such as intercellular adhesion molecule–1 (ICAM-1) and vascular cell adhesion molecule–1 (VCAM-1), on the endothelial surface.[1] These molecules, along with chemokines such as monocyte chemoattractant protein–1 (MCP-1), facilitate the capture and migration of leukocytes from circulating blood into the vascular wall.[1] Thus begins the process of monocyte transformation into lipid-rich macrophages and the cascade of events that leads to vascular smooth proliferation, alterations in collagen synthesis and degradation, thickening of the intima, and obliteration of the vascular lumen.

Common to most, if not all, known risk factors for atherosclerosis is increased oxidative stress. Hypercholesterolemia, hyperglycemia, and angiotensin II, for example, activate one or more cellular enzyme systems, such as lipoxygenase, cyclooxygenase, reduced nicotinamide adenine dinucleotide phosphate (NADPH) oxidase, and xanthine oxidase, that produce oxygen-derived free radicals.[2,3] When oxidative stress overcomes endogenous antioxidants, such as superoxide dismutase, glutathione peroxidase, ascorbate, and α-tocopherol, the vascular milieu is altered. The resulting oxidative stress activates redox-sensitive signaling pathways and transcription factors, such as nuclear factor–κB (NF-κB) and activator protein-1 (AP-1), that result in expression of a number of cytokines and cellular adhesion molecules intrinsic to the atherogenic process (Figure 3.1).[4,5] An important constituent of the endothelium, nitric oxide (NO), may mitigate the effects of oxidative stress and inhibit vascular inflammatory gene expression by reducing superoxide generation, preventing oxidation of low-density lipoprotein (LDL), and stabilizing NF-κB.[5–7]

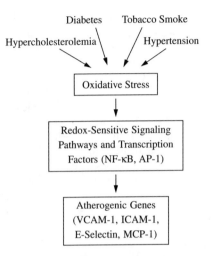

FIGURE 3.1 Oxidative stress activates redox-sensitive signaling pathways that result in expression of cytokines and cellular adhesion molecules that participate in atherogenesis. AP-1 = activator protein-1; ICAM-1 = intercellular adhesion molecule–1; MCP-1 = monocyte chemoattractant protein–1; NF-κB = nuclear factor–κB; VCAM-1= vascular cell adhesion molecule–1. (Adapted from Kunsch, C., and Medford, R. M., *Circ. Res.*, 1999. With permission.)[5]

3.3   ENDOTHELIUM-DERIVED NITRIC OXIDE

In 1980, Furchgott and Zawadzki first reported that endothelium synthesizes and releases a substance that relaxes blood vessels, for which they coined the term endothelium-derived relaxing factor (EDRF).[8] They found that preconstricted rings of rabbit thoracic aorta with intact endothelium relaxed when exposed to increasing concentrations of acetylcholine; however, the rings constricted when the endothelium had been denuded. Subsequent studies by these and other investigators determined that EDRF was also NO.[9,10] The Nobel Prize in medicine in 1998 was awarded to Rolbert Furchgott, Louis Ignarro, and Ferid Murad, for their respective research involving the discovery of EDRF and the elucidation of NO-signaling mechanisms. Endothelium-derived NO is synthesized from the precursor, L-arginine, by the constitutive enzyme NO synthase (eNOS) via a series of electron transfers that result in formation of NO and L-citrulline (Figure 3.2).[11] The reaction takes place in the presence of several cofactors, including calcium, tetrahydrobiopterin, NADPH, and flavin adenine dinucleotide. A variety of biochemical and pharmacologic stimuli such as serotonin, thrombin, bradykinin, and acetylcholine stimulate receptors on the endothelial surface that mediate transport of calcium into the cell, thus initiating this enzymatic process. Shear stress also activates specific receptors to promote the intracellular transport of calcium and subsequent production of NO.[19]

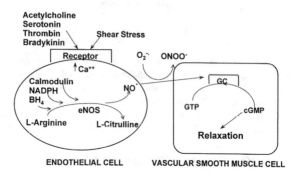

FIGURE 3.2 Synthetic pathway for endothelium-derived nitric oxide (NO). A variety of biochemical and pharmacologic stimuli, as well as shear stress, facilitate calcium (Ca^{++}) influx into the endothelium, in the presence of several cofactors, including calmodulin, reduced nicotinamide adenine dinucleotide phosphate (NADPH), and tetrahydrobiopterin (BH_4). L-arginine is metabolized via the constitutive enzyme NO synthase (e-NOS) to NO. NO activates guanylyl cyclase (GC), the enzyme responsible for the production of cyclic guanosine monophosphate (cGMP) from guanosine 5' triphosphate (GTP). (For other abbreviations, see Figure 3.1.)

Nitric oxide moves rapidly to the underlying vascular smooth muscle, where it activates guanylyl cyclase (which increases cyclic guanosine monophosphate [cGMP]), and, through subsequent signaling mechanisms, causes vascular relaxation. By acting on comparable receptors of platelets, NO can reduce platelet adhesiveness and platelet aggregation.[13,14]

The importance of NO in regulating vasomotor tone in humans was initially reported by Ludmer and colleagues, who found that intracoronary administration of acetylcholine caused epicardial coronary vasodilation in smooth-appearing coronary arteries but coronary vasoconstriction in atherosclerotic coronary arteries (Figure 3.3).[15] Thus, extending the *in vitro* experiments of Furchgott and Zawadzki,

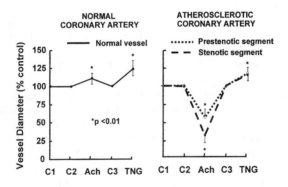

FIGURE 3.3 Responses of human coronary arteries to acetylcholine (Ach). *Left panel:* Intracoronary infusion of Ach causes dilation of normal epicardial coronary arteries compared with control conditions (C1, C2, C3). Nitroglycerin (TNG) also causes coronary artery dilation. *Right panel:* In the prestenotic and stenotic segments of atherosclerotic coronary arteries, Ach causes coronary vasoconstriction, whereas TNG causes vasodilation, indicating loss of endothelium-dependent vasodilation. (From Ludmer, P.L., Selwyn, A., Shook, T.L., et al., *N. Engl. J. Med.*, 1986. With permission.[15])

acetylcholine appeared to release a relaxing factor from the endothelium in healthy states, but acted directly on muscarinic receptors of vascular smooth muscle to induce vasoconstriction in atherosclerosis. The importance of this observation can be extrapolated to the pathophysiology of myocardial ischemia, because endogenous substances such as serotonin, thrombin, and norepinephrine (via 2-receptors) are likely to cause vasodilation in healthy vessels but vasoconstriction in atherosclerotic arteries. Thus, endothelial abnormalities may disrupt the critical relation between coronary blood flow and myocardial oxygen demand, resulting in myocardial ischemia. Indeed, coronary vasoconstriction has been shown to occur in coronary artery disease patients exposed to exercise or mental stress.[16,17] Taken together, these observations suggest that the bioavailability of endothelium-derived NO is reduced in atherosclerotic vessels, preventing the normal modulation of vasomotor tone.

As noted previously, NO has other important physiologic properties that protect the blood vessel from injury. Specifically, by inhibiting vascular inflammatory gene expression, NO may protect the vessel from atherogenic processes.[6,7,18,19] Conversely, if the bioavailability of NO were decreased, transcription factor activation might proceed unchecked, resulting in the expression of inflammatory cytokines and cellular adhesion molecules that initiate atherosclerosis. Indeed, in experimental models and in humans with atherosclerotic risk factors, endothelium-dependent vasodilation is impaired, implicating reduced bioavailability of NO. There is impaired endothelium-dependent relaxation of arteries from hypercholesterolemic animals, even in the absence of atherosclerosis and in forearm resistance vessels of patients with hypercholesterolemia who do not have clinical manifestations of atherosclerosis (Figure 3.4).[20–23] Similar findings have been made with other risk factors for atherosclerosis, including type 1 and type 2 diabetes mellitus, cigarette smoking, and hypertension.[24–27] Hyperhomocysteinemia, an independent risk factor for atherosclerosis, also is associated with impaired endothelial function.[28,29] Even aging, a nonmodifiable risk factor for atherosclerosis, is associated with abnormal endothelium-dependent vasodilation that increases with each decade of life (Figure 3.5).[30,31]

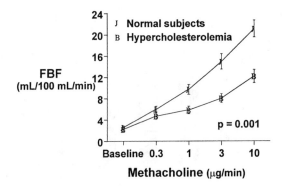

FIGURE 3.4 Forearm blood flow (FBF) response to the endothelium-dependent vasodilator methacholine in normal subjects and patients with hypercholesterolemia. Endothelium-dependent vasodilation is less in the patients with hypercholesterolemia. (From Ting, H.H., Timimi, F.K., Haley, E.A., et al., *Circulation*, 1997. With permission.[23])

3.4 MECHANISMS OF ENDOTHELIAL DYSFUNCTION

Multiple mechanisms may contribute to endothelial dysfunction and reduce the bioavailability of NO by decreasing its synthesis or increasing its degradation (Table 3.1). Decreased synthesis of NO could occur because of abnormal endothelial cell receptor function and signal transduction, reduced levels of L-arginine or competition for eNOS by an arginine analog, decreased cofactors such as tetrahydrobiopterin, and impaired expression or activity of eNOS.

Administration of L-arginine improves endothelium-dependent vasodilation in hypercholesterolemic rabbits and in patients with hypercholesterolemia.[32–35] Although these findings initially raised the possibility that there was insufficient L-arginine to drive the enzymatic reaction resulting in the production of NO, it was subsequently learned that plasma concentrations of L-arginine in these individuals approximate

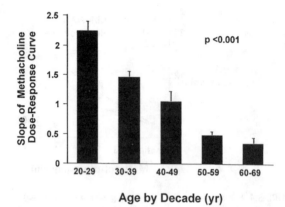

FIGURE 3.5 Effect of age on endothelium-dependent vasodilation. Bars represent the slope of the dose-response curve to methacholine chloride. The slope decreases with each decade of age, indicating an age-related impairment of endothelium-dependent vasodilation. (From Gerhard, M., Roddy, M.-A., Creager, S.J., et al., *Hypertension*, 1996. With permission.[31])

TABLE 3.1
Mechanisms of Endothelial Dysfunction

"Decreased" intracellular L-arginine

Endogenous eNOS inhibitor (ADMA)

Abnormal endothelial receptor signaling

Deficiency of tetrahydrobiopterin

Reduced expression or activity of eNOS

Inactivation of NO by superoxide anion

ADMA = asymmetric dimethylarginine; eNOS = constitutive
  enzyme, NO synthase; NO = nitric oxide.

60 to 100 μmol/L and that the Michaelis constant (K_m) for eNOS is 2.9 μM, indicating sufficient levels of this amino acid.[36] Recent studies have supported the notion of an endogenous arginine analog, asymmetric dimethylarginine (ADMA), that competitively inhibits NO synthesis and reduces its formation.[37,38] This finding is of potential importance, as administration of N^G-monomethyl-L-arginine (L-NMMA), an eNOS inhibitor, promotes the development of atherosclerosis in cholesterol-fed rabbits,[39,40] whereas administration of L-arginine attenuates atherosclerosis in this model.[39] Abnormal endothelium-dependent vasodilation in hypercholesterolemia has also been associated with abnormalities in endothelium receptor–signaling pathways[41,42] and has been corrected by the administration of the cofactor tetrahydrobiopterin.[43] Liao and colleagues have reported that oxidized LDL reduces the expression of eNOS.[44]

Increased degradation of NO could occur in the presence of excess superoxide anions, which oxidize NO to peroxynitrite.[45–47] Inactivation of NO by reactive oxygen species, specifically superoxide anion, has been demonstrated with virtually all risk factors for atherosclerosis. Superoxide anion formation is increased in animal models of hypercholesterolemia,[3] and lipoxygenases may promote LDL oxidation.[48,49] Hyperglycemia may increase oxidative stress in diabetic patients via glucose auto-oxidation, arachidonic acid metabolism, and superoxide formation from eNOS.[4] Angiotensin II, a pathogenetic feature of some forms of hypertension, activates reduced nicotine adenine dinucleotide (NADH) and NADPH oxidases to produce superoxide anion.[51,52] Tobacco smoke contains oxidizing substances, and homocysteine increases oxidative stress by lipid peroxidation and suppression of glutathione peroxidase.[53–55]

The importance of superoxide anion as a cause of endothelial dysfunction can be inferred from studies that have examined the effect of antioxidants on endothelium-dependent vasorelaxation. Administration of superoxide dismutase improves endothelium-dependent relaxation in the hypercholesterolemic rabbit,[56] and α-tocopherol and probucol improve endothelium-dependent vasodilation in hyperchlesterolemic rabbits.[57,58] Similarly, in diabetic animals, endothelium-dependent relaxation improves with superoxide dismutase.[59]

Studies in humans have used a variety of antioxidants such as ascorbic acid (vitamin C), α-tocopherol (vitamin E), and probucol to study the contribution of oxidative stress to endothelial dysfunction. Ascorbic acid is a water-soluble antioxidant that scavenges superoxide anion, spares glutathione from oxidation, and prevents the oxidation of LDLs. *In vitro*, ascorbic acid concentrations of 1 to 10 mM have been shown to scavenge superoxide anion.[60] In humans, intra-arterial administration of vitamin C, sufficient to achieve these concentrations, has been shown to improve endothelium-dependent vasodilation in forearm resistance vessels of patients with hypercholesterolemia, type 1 diabetes mellitus, type 2 diabetes mellitus, hypertension, and in cigarette smokers.[23,61–64] Also, ascorbic acid, when administered orally at a dose of 2 g, improves endothelium-dependent vasodilation of the brachial arteries of normal subjects with methionine-induced hyperhomocysteinemia.[65] Oral vitamin C also improves endothelium-dependent vasodilation of the brachial artery in patients with coronary artery disease and a variety of atherosclerotic risk factors.[66] Studies using vitamin E as the antioxidant, either alone or in combination with vitamin C, have yielded conflicting results. The combination of vitamin C, 1,000 mg and vitamin E, 800 U has been shown to prevent the impairment of endothelium-dependent vasodilation that follows ingestion of a high-fat meal.[67] Chronic administration of vitamin E improved endothelium-dependent vasodilation in hypercholesterolemic smokers.[68] Yet, several studies have not detected beneficial effects on endothelium-dependent vasodilation resulting from the chronic administration of these antioxidant vitamins.[69–71] The combination of lipid-lowering and antioxidant therapy with lovastatin and probucol improved endothelium-dependent vasodilation in atherosclerotic coronary arteries more than lipid-lowering therapy alone with lovastatin and cholestyramine.[72] In this study, the susceptibility of LDLcholesterol to oxidation was significantly reduced in the lipid-lowering antioxidant group compared with the lipid-lowering group alone, thus further supporting the contention that increased oxidative stress impairs endothelial function in patients with hypercholesterolemia.

3.5 TREATMENT OF ENDOTHELIAL DYSFUNCTION

It stands to reason that therapies designed to modify risk factors of atherosclerosis might result in clinical benefits, in part by increasing the bioavailability of NO. Restoration of NO could potentially attenuate the atherogenic process and improve the vasodilator responsiveness of atherosclerotic vessels to reduce myocardial ischemia. Therapeutic interventions that have been shown to improve endothelial function include lipid-lowering therapy, estrogen-replacement therapy, and angiotensin-converting enzyme (ACE) inhibitors. Antioxidant treatment was discussed above.

Treatment of hypercholesterolemic patients with 3-hydroxy-3-methylglutaryl coenzyme A (HMG-CoA) reductase inhibitors ("statins") or cholestyramine for 6 to 12 months has been shown to improve coronary endothelial function.[73–75] Endothelium-dependent vasodilation of forearm resistance vessels improves as early as 1 to 3 months after initiation of statin therapy.[76,77] Moreover, forearm endothelium-dependent vasodilation has been shown to improve immediately after LDL apheresis in patients with severe hypercholesterolemia.[78] Beneficial effects on endothelial function can be attributed to the lipid-lowering effects of these drugs; however, it is noteworthy that HMG-CoA reductase inhibitors have been shown in experimental models to improve the activity of eNOS, irrespective of their effects on lipids.[79] Improvement in coronary vasomotor reactivity resulting from restoration of endothelium-dependent vasodilation may partly account for reduction of myocardial ischemia, assessed by ambulatory ischemia monitoring, in patients treated with lovastatin compared with placebo.[80]

Estrogen administration improves endothelium-dependent vasodilation in oophorectomized rabbits and *Cynomolgus* monkeys.[81,82] In humans, acute administration of Premarin®* or estradiol

---

* Registered trademark of Wyeth-Ayerst, Radnor, PA.

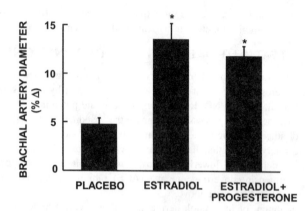

FIGURE 3.6 Effect of estradiol and progesterone on endothelium-dependent vasodilation in postmenopausal women. In a randomized crossover placebo-controlled trial, both transdermal estradiol and the combination of transdermal estradiol and intravaginal natural progesterone improve flow-mediated endothelium-dependent vasodilation of the brachial artery compared with placebo (*asterisks*). These observations indicate that estrogen has favorable effects on endothelial function in postmenopausal women. (From Gerhard, M., Walsh, B.W., Tawakol, A., et al., *Circulation*, 1998. With permission.[87])

improves coronary and forearm endothelium-dependent vasodilation.[83-85] Such improvement cannot be explained by reductions in cholesterol because it is unlikely to occur immediately after a single dose of estrogen. Chronic administration of estrogen for a period of approximately 2 months also improves flow-mediated endothelium-dependent vasodilation of the brachial artery.[86] The addition of natural progesterone does not attenuate this favorable response (Figure 3.6).[87]

ACE inhibitors might favorably affect the bioavailability of NO by one of two mechanisms. By blocking the degradation of brady-kinin, these drugs may increase its concentration, which, in turn, stimulates the production of NO. Alternatively, angiotensin-converting inhibitors, by blocking angiotensin II, could prevent superoxide formation and inactivation of NO.[2] Quinapril has been shown to improve coronary and brachial artery endothelium-dependent vasodilation in patients with coronary artery disease.[88,89] In patients with hypertension, ACE inhibition has been shown to improve endothelium-dependent vasodilation of forearm resistance vessels in some studies but not in others.[90–92]

3.5.1 CLINICAL IMPLICATIONS OF TREATING ENDOTHELIAL DYSFUNCTION

It remains to be established whether strategies designed to improve endothelial function will benefit clinical outcome by reducing adverse cardiovascular events. Lipid-lowering therapy has been proven to reduce fatal and nonfatal myocardial infarction in patients with coronary artery disease.[93–95] Plaque stabilization probably accounts for much of this benefit. The ability of estrogen-replacement therapy to reduce adverse cardiovascular events, as suggested by epidemiologic surveys and case-control studies, has yet to be confirmed in a prospective trial. The Heart and Estrogen/Progestin Replacement Study (HERS) failed to find any benefit of estrogen and medroxyprogesterone treatment on cardiovascular events in postmenopausal women.[96] ACE inhibitor therapy has been shown to reduce coronary events in patients with heart failure.[97–99] In the Heart Outcomes Prevention Evaluation (HOPE) study, ramipril significantly reduced the incidence of adverse cardiovascular events in patients with atherosclerosis.[100] The Cambridge Heart Antioxidant Study found that vitamin E reduced nonfatal myocardial infarction but not total mortality.[101] In the GISSI-3 (Gruppo Italiano per lo Studio della Streptochinasi nell'Infarto Miocardio–3) substudy, vitamin E did not prevent cardiovascular events.[102] In the HOPE study, vitamin E, 400 IU, produced no benefit.[100]

3.6 CONCLUSIONS

The endothelium regulates healthy blood vessel homeostasis. However, when overcome by injurious stimuli, the endothelium participates in an inflammatory process that results in atherosclerosis. NO is a fundamental endothelium-derived substance that protects the blood vessel from injury and contributes to normal vasomotor tone. Its bioavailability is reduced in patients with risk factors for atherosclerosis. Mechanistic insight into the causes of endothelial dysfunction has suggested a variety of effective therapeutic strategies including lipid-lowering drugs, antioxidants, estrogen-replacement therapy, and ACE inhibition to improve endothelial function by preserving NO. The final proof that improvement in endothelial function prevents atherosclerosis and reduces adverse cardiovascular events awaits large prospective clinical trials.

REFERENCES

1. Ross, R., Cellular and molecular studies of atherogenesis, *Atherosclerosis*, 131 (Suppl), S3, 1997.
2. Rajagopalan, S., Kurz, S., Munzel, T., et al., Angiotensin II-mediated hypertension in the rat increases vascular superoxide production via membrane NADH/NADPH oxidase activations: contribution to alterations of vasomotor tone, *J. Clin. Invest.*, 97, 1916, 1996.
3. Ohara, Y., Peterson, T.E., and Harrison, D.G., Hypercholesterolemia increases endothelial superoxide anion production. *J. Clin. Invest.*, 91, 2546, 1993.
4. Berliner, J.A., Navab, M., Fogelman, A.M., et al., Atherosclerosis: basic mechanisms—oxidation, inflammation, and genetics, *Circulation*, 91, 2488, 1995.
5. Kunsch, C. and Medford, R.M., Oxidative stress as a regulator of gene expression in the vasculature, *Circ. Res.*, 85, 753, 1999.
6. De Caterina, R., Libby, P., Peng, H.B., et al., Nitric oxide decreases cytokine-induced endothelial activation: nitric oxide selectively reduces endothelial expression of adhesion molecules and proinflammatory cytokines, *J. Clin. Invest.*, 96, 60, 1995.

7. Peng, H.B., Libby, P., and Liao, J K., Induction and stabilization of IκB-α by nitric oxide mediates inhibition of NF-κB, *J. Biol. Chem.*, 270, 14214, 1995.

8. Furchgott, R.F. and Zawadzki, J.V., The obligatory role of endothelial cells in the relaxation of arterial smooth muscle by acetylcholine, *Nature,* 288, 373, 1980.

9. Palmer, R.M.J., Ferridge, A.G., and Moncada, S., Nitric oxide release accounts for the biological activity of endothelium-derived relaxing factors, *Nature*, 327, 524, 1987.

10. Ignarro, L.J., Byrns, R.E., Buga, G.M., et al., Endothelium-derived relaxing factor from pulmonary artery and vein possesses pharmacologic and chemical properties identical to those of nitric oxide radical, *Circ. Res.*, 61, 866, 1987.

11. Vane, J.R., Anggard, E.E., and Botting, R.M., Regulatory function of the vascular endothelium, *N. Engl. J. Med.,* 323, 27, 1990.

12. Cooke, J.P., Rossitch, E., Jr., Andon, N.A., et al., Flow activates an endothelial potassium channel to release an endogenous nitrovasodilator, *J. Clin. Invest.*, 88, 1663, 1991.

13. Radomski, M.W., Palmer, R.M., and Moncada, S., An L-arginine/nitric oxide pathway present in human platelets regulates aggregation, *Proc. Natl. Acad. Sci. USA*, 87, 5193, 1990.

14. Stamler, J.S., Mendelsohn, M.D., Amarante, P., et al., N-acetylcysteine potentiates platelet inhibition by endothelium-derived relaxing factor, *Circ. Res.*, 65, 789, 1989.

15. Ludmer, P.L., Selwyn, A.P., Shook, T.L., et al., Paradoxical vasoconstriction induced by acetylcholine in atherosclerotic coronary arteries. *N. Engl. J. Med.*, 315, 1046, 1986.

16. Gordon, J.B., Ganz, P., Nabel, et al., Atherosclerosis and endothelial function influence the coronary vasomotor response to exercise, *J. Clin. Invest.*, 83, 1946, 1989.

17. Yeung, A.C., Vekshtein, V.I., Krantz, D.S. et al., The effect of atherosclerosis on the vasomotor response of coronary arteries to mental stress, *N. Engl. J. Med.*, 325, 1551, 1991.

18. Zeiher, A.M., Fisslthaler, B., Schray-Utz, B. et al., Nitric oxide modulates expression of monocyte chemo-attractant protein-a in cultured human endothelial cells, *Circ. Res.*, 76, 980, 1995.

19. Spiecker, M., Peng H.B., and Liao, J.K., Inhibition of endotheial vascular cell adhesion molecule-1 expression by nitric oxide involves the induction and nuclear translocation of IKBα, *J. Biol. Chem.*, 272, 30969, 1997.

20. Harrison, D.G., Armstrong, M.L., Freidman, P.C., et al., Restoration of endothelium-dependent relaxation by dietary treatment of atherosclerosis, *J. Clin. Invest.*, 80, 1808, 1987.

21. Cohen, R.A., Zitnay, K.M., Haudenschild, C.C., et al., Loss of selective endothelial cell vasoactive function in pig coronary arteries caused by hypercholesterolemia, *Circ. Res.*, 63, 903, 1988.

22. Creager, M.A., Cooke, J.P., Mendelsohn, M.E., et al., Impaired vasodilation of forearm resistance vessels in hypercholesterolemic humans, *J. Clin. Invest.*, 86, 228, 1990.

23. Ting, H.H., Timimi, F.K., Haley, E.A., et al., Vitamin C improves endothelium-dependent vasodilation in forearm resistance vessels of humans with hypercholesterolemia, *Circulation*, 95, 2617, 1997.

24. Johnstone, M.T., Creager, S.J., Scales, K.M., et al., Impaired endothelium-dependent vasodilation in patients with insulin-dependent diabetes mellitus, *Circulation*, 88, 2510, 1993.

25. Williams, S.B., Cusco, J.A., Roddy, M.-A., et al., Impaired nitric oxide-mediated vasodilation in patients with non-insulin-dependent diabetes mellitus, *J. Am. Coll. Cardiol.*, 27, 567, 1996.

26. Celermajer, D.S., Sorensen, K.E., Georgakopoulos, D., et al., Cigarette smoking is associated with dose-related and potentially reversible impairment of endothelium-dependent dilation in healthy young adults, *Circulation*, 88, 2149, 1993.

27. Panza, J.A., Quyyumi, A.A., Brush, J.E., Jr., et al., Abnormal endothelium-dependent vascular relaxation in patients with essential hypertension, *N. Engl. J. Med.*, 320, 22, 1990.

28. Lentz, S.R., Sobey, C.G., Piegors, D.J., et al., Vascular dysfunction in monkeys with diet-induced hyperhomocyst(e)inemia, *J. Clin. Invest.*, 98, 24, 1996.

29. Tawakol, A., Omland, T., Gerhard, M., et al., Hyperhomocyst(e)inemia is associated with impaired endothelium-dependent vasodilation in humans, *Circulation*, 95, 1119, 1997.

30. Celermajer, D.S., Sorensen, K.E., Spiegelhalter, D.J., et al., Aging is associated with endothelial dysfunction in healthy men years before the age-related decline in women, *J. Am. Coll. Cardiol.*, 24, 471, 1994.

31. Gerhard, M., Roddy, M.-A., Creager, S.J., et al., Aging progressively improves endothelium-dependent vasodilation in forearm resistance vessels in humans, *Hypertension*, 27, 849, 1996.

32. Girerd, X.J., Hirsch, A.T., Cooke, J.P., et al., L-arginine augments endothelium-dependent vasodilation in cholesterol-fed rabbits, *Circ. Res.*, 67, 1301, 1990.

33. Creager, M.A., Gallagher, S.J., Girerd, X.J., et al., L-arginine improves endothelium-dependent vasodilation in hypercholesterolemic humans, *J. Clin. Invest.*, 90, 1248, 1992.

34. Clarkson, P., Adams, M.R., Powe, A.J., et al., Oral L-arginine improves endothelium-dependent dilation in hypercholesterolemic young adults, *J. Clin. Invest.*, 97, 1989, 1996.

35. Cooke, J.P., Andon, N.A., Girerd, X.J., et al., Arginine restores cholinergic relaxation of hypercholesterolemic rabbit thoracic aorta, *Circulation*, 83, 1057, 1991.

36. Pollock, J.S., Forstermann, U., Mitchell, J.A., et al., Purification and characterization of particulate endothelium-derived relaxing factor synthase from cultured and native bovine aortic endothelial cells, *Proc. Natl. Acad. Sci. USA.*, 88, 10480, 1991.

37. Böger, R.H., Bode-Böger, S.M., Thiele, W., et al., Biochemical evidence for impaired nitric oxide synthesis in patients with peripheral arterial occlusive disease, *Circulation*, 95, 2068, 1997.

38. Miyazaki, H., Matsuoka, H., Cooke, J.P., et al., Endogenous nitric oxide synthase inhibitor: a novel marker of atherosclerosis, *Circulation*, 99, 1141, 1999.

39. Cooke, J.P., Singer, A.H., Tsao, P., et al., Anti-atherogenic effects of L-arginine in the hypercholesterolemic rabbit, *J. Clin. Invest.*, 90, 1168, 1992.

40. Naruse, K., Shimizu, K., Muramatsu, M., et al., Long-term inhibition of NO synthesis promotes atherosclerosis in the hypercholesterolemic rabbit thoracic aorta, *Arterioscler. Thromb.*, 14, 746, 1994.

41. Flavahan, N.A., Lysophosphatidylcholine modifies G protein-dependent signaling in porcine endothelial cells, *Am. J. Physiol.*, 264, H722, 1993.

42. Casino, P.R., Kilcoyne, C.M., Cannon, R.O. III, et al., Impaired endothelium-dependent vascular relaxation in patients with hypercholesterolemia extends beyond the muscarinic receptor, *Am. J. Cardiol.*, 75, 40, 1995.

43. Stroes, E., Kastelein, J., Cosentino, F., et al., Tetrahydrobiopterin restores endothelial function in hypercholesterolemia, *J. Clin. Invest.*, 99, 41, 1997.

44. Liao, J.K., Shin, W.S., Lee, W.Y., et al., Oxidized low-density lipoprotein decreases the expression of endothelial nitric oxide synthase, *J. Biol. Chem.*, 270, 319, 1995.

45. Mügge, A., Elwell, J.K., Peterson, T.E., et al., Release of intact endothelium-derived relaxing factor depends on endothelial superoxide dismutase activity, *Am. J. Physiol.*, 260, C219, 1991.

46. Rubanyi, G.M., and Vanhoutte, P.M., Oxygen-derived free radicals, endothelium, and responsiveness of vascular smooth muscle, *Am. J. Physiol.*, 250, H815, 1986.

47. Gryglewski, R.J., Palmer, R.M.G., and Moncada, S., Superoxide anion is involved in the breakdown of endothelium-derived vascular relaxation factor, *Nature*, 320, 454, 1986.

48. Yla-Herttuala, S., Rosenfeld, M.D., Parthasarathy, S., et al., Gene expression in macrophage-rich human atherosclerotic lesions: 15-lipoxygenase and acetyl LDL receptor mRNA colocalize with oxidation-specific lipid-protein adducts, *J. Clin. Invest.*, 87, 1146, 1991.

49. Wolle, J., Welch, K.A., Devall, L.J., et al., Transient overexpression of human 15-lipoxygenase in aortic endothelial cells enhances tumor necrosis factor-induced vascular cell adhesion molecule-1 gene expression, *Biochem. Biophys. Res. Commun.*, 220, 310, 1996.

50. Tesfamariam, B., and Cohen, R.A., Free radicals mediate endothelial cell dysfunction caused by elevated glucose, *Am. J. Physiol.*, 236, H321, 1992.

51. Griendling, K.K., Ushio-Fukai, M., Lassegue, B., et al., Angiotensin II signaling in vascular smooth muscle: new concepts, *Hypertension*, 29, 366, 1997.

52. Weir, M.R., and Dzau, V.J., The renin-angiotensin-aldosterone system: a specific target for hypertension management, *Am. J. Hypertens.*, 12, 205S, 1999.

53. Murohara, T., Kugiyama, K., Ohgushi, M., et al., Cigarette smoke extract contacts isolated porcine coronary arteries by superoxide anion-mediated degradation of EDRF, *Am. J. Physiol.*, 266, H874, 1994.

54. Reilly, M., Delanty, N., Lawson, J.A., et al., Modulation of oxidant stress *in vivo* in chronic cigarette smokers, *Circulation*, 94, 19, 1996.

55. Welch, G.N., and Loscalzo, J., Homocysteine and atherothrombosis [see comments], *N. Engl. J. Med.*, 338, 1042, 1998.

56. Mügge, A., Elwell, J. H., Peterson, T. E., et al., Chronic treatment with polyethylene-glycolated superoxide dismutase partially restores endothelium-dependent vascular relaxation in cholesterol-fed rabbits, *Circ. Res.*, 69, 1293, 1991.

57. Keaney, J.F., Jr., Xu, A., Cunningham, D., et al., Dietary probucol preserves endothelial function in cholesterol-fed rabbits by limiting vascular oxidative stress and superoxide generation, *J. Clin. Invest.*, 95, 2520, 1995.

58. Keaney, J.F., Jr., Gaziano, M., Xu, A., et al., Dietary antioxidants preserve endothelium-dependent vessel relaxation in cholesterol-fed rabbits, *Proc. Natl. Acad. Sci. USA.*, 90, 11880, 1993.

59. Langestroer, P., and Pieper, G.M., Regulation of spontaneous EDRF release in diabetic rat aorta by oxygen free radicals, *Am. J. Physiol.*, 263, H257, 1992.

60. Jackson, T.S., Xu, A., Vita, J.A., et al., Ascorbate prevents the interaction of superoxide and nitric oxide only at very high physiological concentrations, *Circ. Res.*, 83, 916, 1998.

61. Taddei, S., Virdis, A., Ghiadoni, L., et al., Vitamin C improves endothelium-dependent vasodilation by restoring nitric oxide activity in essential hypertension, *Circulation*, 97, 2222, 1998.

62. Ting, H.H., Timimi, F.K., Boles, K.S., et al., Vitamin C improves endothelium-dependent vasodilation in patients with non-insulin-dependent diabetes mellitus, *J. Clin. Invest.*, 97, 22, 1996.

63. Timimi, F.K., Ting, H.H., Haley, E.A., et al., Vitamin C improves endothelium-dependent vasodilation in patients with insulin-dependent diabetes mellitus, *J. Am. Coll. Cardiol.*, 31, 552, 1998.

64. Heitzer, T., Just, H., and Münzel, T., Antioxidant vitamin C improves endothelial dysfunction in chronic smokers, *Circulation*, 94, 6, 1996.

65. Kanani, P.M., Sinkey, C.A., Browning, R.L., et al., Role of oxidant stress in endothelial dysfunction produced by experimental hyperhomocyst(e)inemia in humans, *Circulation*, 100, 1161, 1999.

66. Levine, G.N., Frei, B., Koulouris, S.N., et al., Ascorbic acid reverses endothelial vasomotor dysfunction in patients with coronary artery disease, *Circulation*, 93, 1107, 1996.

67. Plotnick, G.D., Corretti, M.C., and Vogel, R.A., Effect of antioxidant vitamins on the transient impairment of endothelium-dependent brachial artery vasoactivity following a single high-fat meal, *JAMA*, 278, 1682, 1997.

68. Heitzer, T., Yla Herttuala, S., Wild, E., et al., Effect of vitamin E on endothelial vasodilator function in patients with hypercholesterolemia, chronic smoking, or both, *J. Am. Coll. Cardiol.*, 33, 499, 1999.

69. Green, D., O'Driscoll, G., Blanksby, B., et al., Lack of effect of vitamin E administration on basal nitric oxide function in male smokers and non-smokers, *Clin. Sci.*, 89, 343, 1995.

70. Duffy, S.J., Vita, J.A., and Keaney, J.F., Antioxidants and endothelial function, *Heart Failure*, 13, 135, 1999.

71. Gilligan, D.M., Sack, M.N., Guetta, V., et al., Effect of antioxidant vitamins on low-density lipoprotein oxidation and impaired endothelium-dependent vasodilation in patients with hypercholesterolemia, *J. Am. Coll. Cardiol.*, 24, 1611, 1994.

72. Anderson, T.J., Meredith, I.T., Yeung, A.C., et al., The effect of cholesterol-lowering and antioxidant therapy on endothelium-dependent coronary vasomotion, *N. Engl. J. Med.*, 332, 488, 1995.

73. Leung, W.H., Lau, C.P., and Wong, C.K., Beneficial effect of cholesterol-lowering therapy on coronary endothelium-dependent relaxation in hypercholesterolaemic patients, *Lancet*, 341, 1496, 1993.

74. Egashira, K., Hirooka, Y., Kai, H., et al., Reduction in serum cholesterol with pravastatin improves endothelium-dependent coronary vasomotion in patients with hypercholesterolemia, *Circulation*, 89, 2519, 1994.

75. Treasure, C.B., Klein, J.L., Weintraub, W.S., et al., Beneficial effects of cholesterol-lowering therapy on the coronary endothelium in patients with coronary artery disease, *N. Engl. J. Med.*, 332, 481, 1995.

76. Stroes, E.S., Koomans, H.A., de Bruin, T.W., et al., Vascular function in the forearm of hypercholesterolaemic patients off and on lipid-lowering medication, *Lancet*, 346, 467, 1995.

77. O'Driscoll, G., Green, D., and Taylor, R.R., Simvastatin, an HMG-coenzyme A reductase inhibitor, improves endothelial function within 1 month, *Circulation*, 95, 1126, 1997.

78. Tamai, O., Matsuoka, H., Itabe, H., et al., Single LDL apheresis improves endothelium-dependent vasodilatation in hypercholesterolemic humans, *Circulation*, 95, 76, 1997.

79. Laufs, U., La Fata, V., Plutzky, J., et al., Upregulation of endothelial nitric oxide synthase by HMG CoA reductase inhibitors, *Circulation*, 97, 1129, 1998.

80. Andrews, T.C., Raby, K., Barry, J., et al., Effect of cholesterol reduction on myocardial ischemia in patients with coronary disease, *Circulation*, 95, 324, 1997.

81. Gisclard, V., Miller, V.M., and Vanhoutte, P.M., Effect of 17 beta-estradiol on endothelium-dependent responses in the rabbit, *J. Pharmacol. Exp. Ther.*, 244, 19, 1988.

82. Williams, J.K., Honoré, E.K., Washburn, S.A., et al., Effects of hormone replacement therapy on reactivity of atherosclerotic coronary arteries in *Cynomolgus* monkeys, *J. Am. Coll. Cardiol.*, 24, 1757, 1994.

83. Gilligan, D.M., Badar, D.M., Panza, J.A., et al., Effects of estrogen replacement therapy on peripheral vasomotor function in postmenopausal women, *Am. J. Cardiol.*, 75, 264, 1995.

84. Collins, P., Rosano, G.M.C., Sarrel, P.M., et al., 17β-Estradiol attenuates acetylcholine-induced coronary arterial constriction in women but not men with coronary heart disease, *Circulation*, 92, 24, 1995.

85. Reis, S.E., Gloth, S.T., Blumenthal, R.S., et al., Ethinyl estradiol acutely attenuates abnormal coronary vasomotor responses to acetylcholine in postmenopausal women, *Circulation*, 89, 52, 1994.

86. Lieberman, E.H., Gerhard, M.D., Uehata, A., et al., Estrogen improves endothelium-dependent flow-mediated vasodilation in postmenopausal women, *Ann. Intern. Med.*, 121, 936, 1994.

87. Gerhard, M., Walsh, B.W., Tawakol, A., et al., Estradiol therapy combined with progesterone and endothelium-dependent vasodilation in postmenopausal women. *Circulation*, 98, 1158, 1998.

88. Mancini, G.B., Henry, G.C., Macaya, C., et al., Angiotensin-converting enzyme inhibition with quinapril improves endothelial vasomotor dysfunction in patients with coronary artery disease. The TREND (Trial on Reversing ENdothelial Dysfunction) Study, *Circulation*, 94, 258, 1996.

89. Anderson, T.J., Elstein, E., Haber, H., et al., Comparative study of ACE-inhibition, angiotensin II antagonism, and calcium channel blockade on flow-mediated vasodilation in patients with coronary disease (BANFF study), *J. Am. Coll. Cardiol.*, 35, 60, 2000.

90. Hirooka, Y., Imaizumi, T., Tagawa, T., et al., Effects of L-arginine on impaired acetylcholine induced and ischemic vasodilation of the forearm in patients with heart failure, *Circulation*, 90, 658, 1994.

91. Creager, M.A. and Roddy, M.-A., Effect of captopril and enalapril on endothelial function in hypertensive patients, *Hypertension*, 24, 499, 1994.

92. Kiowski, W., Linder, L., et al., Nuesch, R., Effects of cilazapril on vascular structure and function in essential hypertension, *Hypertension*, 27, 371, 1996.

93. Randomized trial of cholesterol lowering in 4444 patients with coronary heart disease: the Scandinavian Simvastatin Survival Study (4S), *Lancet*, 344, 1383, 1994.

94. Pfeffer, M.A., Sacks, F.M., Moye, L.A., et al., Cholesterol and recurrent events: a secondary prevention trial for normolipidemic patients: CARE Investigators, *Am. J. Cardiol.*, 76, 98C, 1995.

95. Prevention of cardiovascular events and death with pravastatin in patients with coronary heart disease and a broad range of initial cholesterol levels: the Long-Term Intervention with Pravastatin in Ischaemic Disease (LIPID) Study Group, *N. Engl. J. Med.*, 339, 1349, 1998.

96. Hulley, S., Grady, D., Bush, T., et al., Randomized trial of estrogen plus progestin for secondary prevention of coronary heart disease in postmenopausal women: Heart and Estrogen/progestin Replacement Study (HERS) Research Group, *JAMA*, 280, 605, 1998.

97. Pfeffer, M.A., Braunwald, E., Moye, L.A., et al., Effect of captopril on mortality and morbidity in patients with left ventricular dysfunction after myocardial infarction: results of the survival and ventricular enlargement trial_ The SAVE Investigators [see comments], *N. Engl. J. Med.*, 327, 669, 1992.

98. Yusuf, S., Pepine, C.J., Garces, C., et al., Effect of enalapril on myocardial infarction and unstable angina in patients with low ejection fractions [see comments], *Lancet*, 340, 1173, 1992.

99. Effect of ramipril on mortality and morbidity of survivors of acute myocardial infarction with clinical evidence of heart failure: the Acute Infarction Ramipril Efficacy (AIRE) Study Investigators, *Lancet*, 342, 821, 1993.

100. Yusuf, S., Sleight, P., Pogue, J., et al., Effects of an angiotensin-converting-enzyme inhibitor, ramipril, on cardiovascular events in high-risk patients: The Heart Outcomes Prevention Evaluation Study Investigators [published erratum appears in *N. Engl. J. Med.* 342, 748, 2000], *N. Engl. J. Med.*, 342, 145, 2000.

101. Stephens, N.G., Parson, A., Schofield, P.M., et al., Randomized controlled trial of vitamin E in patients with coronary artery disease: Cambridge Heart Antioxidant Study (CHAOS), *Lancet*, 3745, 781, 1996.

102. Gruppo Italiano per lo Studio della Sopravvivenza nell'Infarto miocardico, Dietary supplementation with n-3 polyunsaturated fatty acids and vitamin E after myocardial infarction: results of the GISSI-Prevenzione trial, *Lancet*, 354, 447, 1999.

Section II

Peripheral Arterial Diseases

4 Peripheral Arterial Disease

Beatrice A. Golomb, Michael H. Criqui, and Warner P. Bundens

CONTENTS

4.1 Introduction..57
4.2 Risk Factors for Peripheral Arterial Disease 61
4.3 Vascular Risk in Peripheral Arterial Disease Patients..............67
    4.3.1 Peripheral Arterial Disease Risk....................................68
    4.3.2 Coronary Artery Disease Risk..69
    4.3.3 Cerebrovascular Disease Risk...69
    4.3.4 Overall Cardiovascular Risk 70
    4.3.5 Overall Mortality Risk..70
4.4 Discussion..71
4.5. Conclusions...73
References..74

4.1 INTRODUCTION

At least 10 million people in the United States have peripheral artery disease, or PAD, which consists of partial or complete atherosclerotic obstruction of peripheral arteries, typically defined as those arteries supplying the lower extremities. Moreover, as many as 4 million Americans have symptomatic intermittent claudication (IC), which classically consists of pain in the lower extremities, typically induced by exercise and relieved by rest.[1,2] Although arteries to sites other than the legs, such as the brain, are also considered peripheral, the term

PAD in conventional usage refers expressly to reduced arterial blood flow to the legs. As is true of atherosclerotic disease to vessels supplying the heart, atherosclerotic disease in PAD may be asymptomatic (analogous to silent coronary ischemia), may produce symptoms with exercise (analogous to stable angina), or, in severe cases, may lead to symptoms at rest.

PAD has important morbidity and mortality implications, although the number of deaths directly ascribed to PAD is comparatively modest. Symptomatic disease affects quality of life and function by causing pain and restricting ambulation. Asymptomatic disease is also vitally important, as it may predict future risk of compromised ambulation, lower-extremity ulcers, and possible need for vascular surgery or amputation. Moreover, asymptomatic as well as symptomatic disease is a consistent and powerful independent predictor of coronary artery disease (CAD) and cerebrovascular disease (CBVD).

PAD incidence and prevalence are strongly age dependent, and PAD will continue to increase as a source of morbidity as the population continues to age. Currently, the prevalence of PAD is more than 20% in those older than 70 years of age. Data from subjects enrolled in the Framingham Study, one of the few studies to assess incidence by age and sex, reveal that onset of symptomatic disease (i.e., IC) increased 10-fold in men from ages 30 to 44 (six per 10,000) to ages 65 to 74 (61 per 10,000).[3] In women, incidence of PAD rose almost 20-fold from the younger (three per 10,000) to the older (54 per 10,000) age group.[3] Others have reported 5-year IC incidence rates of 7.5% in 55- to 74-year-old men and women.[4] These incidence data underestimate clinically relevant PAD, as they are confined to symptomatic disease; asymptomatic disease may be 2 to 10 times more common.[5,6] Because incidence increases with age, prevalence also increases with age, as shown in Table 4.1. Data from a San Diego population study[5] and from Rotterdam[6] provide comparable estimates by age both for IC and for noninvasive disease. Weighted data on IC alone, published in the TransAtlantic Inter-Society Consensus (TASC) and reported to be from "large population studies," offer somewhat higher prevalence estimates in the older age groups.[7] The male–female

TABLE 4.1
Prevalence Estimates of Peripheral Arterial Disease and Intermittent Claudication by Age

Age (yr)	Pooled Analysis,[7] IC (%)	Rotterdam[6] PAD by ABI <0.90 (%)	Rotterdam[6] IC (%)	San Diego Population Study[5] PAD by NI Tests (%)	San Diego Population Study[5] IC (%)
30–34	0.8				
35–39	0.8				
40–45	1.3				
46–49	1.3			2.5	0.0
50–54	2.0				
55–59	2.3	9	1.0		
60–64	3.1	11	1.2	8.3	2.4
65–69	5.8	15	1.7		
70–74	6.8	17	2.3	18.8	2.7
75–79		23	3.2		
80–84		40	4.0		
85–89		57	5.0		

ABI = ankle-brachial index; IC = intermittent claudication; NI = noninvasive; PAD = peripheral arterial disease.

ratio for all PAD has been reported to be about 1.3, which is lower than that for coronary disease.[5] However, for more severe, symptomatic disease, the gender ratio was more than that for PAD as a whole—approximately 2.7.[5] The recent PAD Awareness, Risk, and Treatment: New Resources for Survival (PARTNERS) Study examined the prevalence of PAD in nearly 7,000 patients in medical practices across the United States.[8] The target population was all patients 70 years of age or greater, and those 50 to 69 years of age with diabetes mellitus or at least 10 pack-years of cigarette smoking. Preliminary data indicated that 25% of all patients screened had PAD, 15% with PAD alone, and another 10% with PAD plus a history of CAD or CBVD. The PAD prevalence in women (24%) was nearly as high as in men (26%).

Symptomatic disease represents a modest fraction of all clinically important PAD, as those without symptoms are also at risk for cardiovascular events (just as many with asymptomatic CAD are at risk for cardiovascular disease [CVD] events). Prevalence rates increase when more liberal criteria for symptomatic disease are used, such as criteria that accept atypical symptoms as well as classic Rose criteria claudication;[5] rates increase again when PAD is defined by objective noninvasive criteria, typically an ankle–brachial index (ABI) less than 0.9 (a ratio of ankle to brachial systolic blood pressure values, signifying at least 10% lower blood pressure at the ankle than at the arm). Reported IC prevalence has varied from 1.6% to 12%, whereas rates of noninvasively defined disease have ranged from 3.8% to 33%.[5–7,9–12] Prevalence estimates depend strongly on the age of the examined population, both for IC and for noninvasively defined disease.[5,6] Perhaps surprisingly, fewer than half of all patients with PAD assessed by ABI less than 0.9 have IC.

It should be emphasized that IC per se is not only an insensitive indicator of PAD but may also fail to have good predictive value for PAD as ascertained by noninvasive objective measures. Only 6.3% of those with ABI less than 0.9 had classic IC (8.7% of men and 4.9% of women), demonstrating poor sensitivity of IC for PAD. Moreover, in a study based in Rotterdam,[6] only 69% of those with IC had ABI less than 0.9, indicating rather poor positive predictive value (PPV) of IC for noninvasively defined PAD; a similar PPV (63%) was seen in the Edinburgh artery study.[9] Assessment of the sensitivity, specificity, PPV, and negative predictive value (NPV) of IC for noninvasively defined disease was undertaken in a San Diego population study, which confirmed poor sensitivity and PPV. Rose claudication was associated with a sensitivity of 9.2%, specificity of 99%, PPV of 55%, and NPV of 90%.[13] Inclusion of "possible claudication" as part of IC led sensitivity to rise to 20% and specificity to decline to 96%, with lower PPV (38%) and NPV of 90%.

The San Diego Claudication Questionnaire[2] was adapted from the original Rose questionnaire,[1] the preferred questionnaire for assessing the pain of IC because it allows complete lateralization (right versus left) of all reported symptoms.[2] Tables 4.2 and 4.3, respectively, present the interviewer-administered and self-administered versions of this questionnaire. The scoring system is given in the footnote to Table 4.2. Each leg is separately classified into one of five categories, starting with the first question.

Assessment of peripheral pulses, particularly the dorsalis pedis and posterior tibial pulses, is often performed in the diagnostic assessment for PAD; however, neither peripheral pulses nor femoral bruits have sufficient sensitivity, specificity, or predictive value to be reliable markers for PAD.[13]

4.2 RISK FACTORS FOR PERIPHERAL ARTERIAL DISEASE

Because PAD, CAD, and CBVD each represent manifestations of atherosclerotic arterial disease (albeit each in a different vascular bed), it comes as no surprise that risk factors for PAD overlap those for CAD and CBVD. Nonetheless, the prognostic potency of these risk factors varies according to the site of atherosclerotic disease portended: thus, diabetes, smoking, and age, which are risk factors for CAD and CBVD, are particularly potent risk factors for PAD.[14–17] Hypertension is frequently present in patients with PAD. A recent review of cross-sectional, prospective, experimental evidence concluded that elevated blood pressure is likely to be a causal factor in PAD, although all

TABLE 4.2
San Diego Claudication Questionnaire: Interviewer Administered Version

	Right	Left
1) Do you get pain or discomfort in either leg or either buttock on walking? (If no, stop)		
No	1	1
Yes	2	2
2) Does this pain ever begin when you are standing still or sitting?		
No	1	1
Yes	2	2
3) In what part of the leg or buttock do you feel it?		
a) Pain includes calf/calves		
No	1	1
Yes	2	2
b) Pain includes thigh/thighs		
No	1	1
Yes	2	2
c) Pain includes buttock/buttocks		
No	1	1
Yes	2	2
4) Do you get it when you walk uphill or hurry?		
No	1	1
Yes	2	2
Never walks uphill/hurries	3	

5) Do you get it when you walk at an ordinary pace on the level?	No	1
	Yes	2
6) Does the pain ever disappear while you are walking?	No	1
	Yes	2
7) What do you do if you get it when you are walking?	Stop or slow down	1
	Continue on	2
8) What happens to it if you stand still?	Lessened or relieved	1
(If unchanged, stop)	Unchanged	2
9) How soon?	10 minutes or less	1
	More than 10 minutes	2

Scoring system:

1) No Pain: 1 = 1

2) Pain at rest: 1 = 2 and 2 = 2

3) Non-calf: 1 = 2 and 2 = 1 and 3a = 1 and 3b = 2 or 3c = 2

4) Non-Rose calf: 1 = 2 and 2 = 1 and 3a = 2, and not Rose

5) Rose: 1 = 2 and 2 = 1 and 3a = 2 and 4 = 2 or 3 (and if 4 = 3, then 5 = 2), and 6 = 1 and 7 = 1 and 8 = 1 and 9 = 1

From Criqui, M.H., Denenberg, J.O., Bird, C.E., Fronek, A., Klauber, M.R., and Langer, R.D., *Vasc. Med.*, 1,65, 1996.[2] With permission.

TABLE 4.3
San Diego Claudication Questionnaire: Self-Administered Version

	Circle Answer
1) Do you get pain or discomfort in either leg or either buttock on walking? (If no, stop)	Right leg Yes No Left leg Yes No
2) Does this pain ever begin when you are standing still or sitting?	Right leg Yes No Left leg Yes No
3) In what part of the leg or buttock do you feel it?	
a) Pain includes calf/calves	Right leg Yes No Left leg Yes No
b) Pain includes thigh/thighs	Right leg Yes No Left leg Yes No
c) Pain includes buttock/buttocks	Right leg Yes No Left leg Yes No

4) Do you get it when you walk uphill or hurry?

Right leg Yes No
Left leg Yes No
Never walk uphill / hurry

5) Do you get it when you walk at an ordinary pace on the level?

Right leg Yes No
Left leg Yes No

6) Does the pain ever disappear while you are walking?

Right leg Yes No
Left leg Yes No

7) What do you do if you get it when you are walking?

Right leg
Stop or slow down
Continue on
Left leg Stop or slow down
Continue on

8) What happens to it if you stand still?

Right leg
Lessened or relieved
Unchanged
Left leg
Lessened or relieved
Unchanged

9) If lessened or relieved, how soon?

Right leg <10 min >10 min
Left leg <10 min >10 min

From Criqui, M.H., Denenberg, J.O., Bird, C.E., Fronek, A., Klauber, M.R., and Langer, R.D., *Vasc. Med.*, 1, 65, 1996.[2] With permission.

available evidence is not concordant.[18] Additional shared risk factors include dyslipidemia—primarily the high triglyceride/low high-density lipoprotein (HDL) complex (see below), homocysteine, fibrinogen, and blood viscosity.[14,15,19,20] Of note, although high triglycerides (a key element of syndrome X, or insulin resistance profile) are linked to PAD and were found in one analysis to be the single factor most predictive of PAD progression,[16] other studies have shown the prognostic power of triglycerides to be reduced or lost after adjustment for other syndrome X-type characteristics.[14] Low levels of HDL cholesterol (HDL-C), often associated with high triglycerides as well as cigarette smoking and low levels of exercise (discussed below), have also been linked to PAD.[14,21,22] Moreover, although subjects with hypercholesterolemia may have high rates of PAD,[23] and although cholesterol-lowering treatments have been shown to reduce PAD,[24–26] elevated low-density lipoprotein cholesterol (LDL-C), a traditional risk factor for CAD but not for CBVD, has not been a consistent risk factor for PAD.[15] Indeed, in an analysis conducted by TASC, hypercholesterolemia per se was not clearly a risk factor for progression of disease in the legs, with odds ratios squarely centered around 1.[7] Table 4.4 shows data from the Physicians' Health Study, and illustrates the particularly strong associations of current and even past cigarette smoking and diabetes with subsequent surgery for PAD.[27] Table 4.5 shows comparative contributions by traditional risk factors to PAD compared with CAD and CBVD. The scoring system (+ to ++++) represents the authors' synthesis of an extensive literature. Important differences include the dominance of diabetes and cigarette smoking in PAD, the dominance of hypertension in CBVD, and the emerging importance of highly sensitive C-reactive protein in CAD.

Recent studies suggest that a number of the "emerging risk factors" for CAD also predict risk of PAD, including lipoprotein (a), C-reactive protein, circulating soluble intracellular adhesion molecule–1, vascular cell adhesion molecule–1, thrombin–antithrombin III complex, and von Willebrand factor, among others.[28–32] Lifestyle factors that might confer protection against PAD reportedly include physical exercise,[33] moderate alcohol ingestion,[34,35] and dietary vitamin C and E intake.[34,36]

TABLE 4.4
Multivariable Analysis of Risk Factors for Peripheral Artery Surgery

Factor	Multivariate RR[a] (95% CI)	P-Value
Aspirin[b]	0.51 (0.28–0.93)	0.03
Alcohol weekly[b]	0.88 (0.41–1.87)	0.74
Alcohol daily[b]	0.97 (0.45–2.06)	0.93
Diabetes[c]	3.62 (1.49–8.78)	0.005
High cholesterol[c]	2.26 (1.05–4.88)	0.04
Hypertension[c]	1.05 (0.52–2.10)	0.90
Obesity[c]	0.86 (0.36–2.05)	0.73
Past smoking[b]	3.80 (1.62–8.92)	<0.001
Current smoking[b]	10.28 (4.12–25.64)	<0.001

CI = confidence interval; RR = relative risk.

[a] RR includes control for every variable listed, as well as age.
[b] Referent for aspirin analysis is placebo assignment; for alcohol analysis is alcohol consumption less than once per month; for obesity is body mass index <27.8; and for smoking is never smoking.
[c] Referent is those without specified cardiovascular risk factor.

From Goldhaber, S.Z., Manson, J.E., Stampfer, M.J., et al., *Lancet*, 340, 143, 1992.[27] With permission.

4.3 VASCULAR RISK IN PERIPHERAL ARTERIAL DISEASE PATIENTS

Most existing evidence suggests that PAD confers independent increased risk for CAD and CBVD in addition to that expected by concomitant major coronary risk factors. PAD may confer this increased risk by serving as a proxy for the actions of unmeasured or unadjusted risk

TABLE 4.5
Contribution of Cardiovascular Disease Risk Factors to Peripheral Arterial Disease, Coronary Artery Disease, and Cerebrovascular Disease

	PAD	CAD	CBVD
Diabetes mellitus	++++	+++	+
Smoking	++++	+++	+
Advanced age	++++	+++	++++
Hypertension	++	++	++++
LDL-C	+	++	+
Low HDL-C	+++	++	+
Triglycerides	+++	++	+
Male sex	+	++	+
Homocysteine	+++	++	++
hs-CRP	+++	++++	+?

hs-CRP = highly sensitive C-reactive protein.

factors and as a marker of ongoing disease. Moreover, PAD has similar prognostic implications, predicting increased risk of CAD and CBVD events for those with and without previously identified CAD and CBVD.

4.3.1 PERIPHERAL ARTERIAL DISEASE RISK

Although PAD complications are strikingly higher in those with baseline PAD than those without, in PAD patients they are nonetheless overshadowed by other atherosclerotic events. In terms of mortal outcomes, among subjects with IC in the Framingham Study, 50% of deaths were due to CAD, 10% due to CBVD, and 13% due to "other vascular" causes, including more direct PAD causes.[3,37] However, the impact of PAD morbidity should not be underplayed. In a study from Edinburgh, among those with IC at baseline, 8.2% underwent vascular surgery or amputation and 1.4% developed leg ulceration after 5 years.[4]

In another study, among IC patients without other clinical indicators, 7.5% progressed to rest pain, ulcers, or gangrene in the first year, with 2.2% converting annually thereafter over 6.5 years' follow-up.[38]

4.3.2 CORONARY ARTERY DISEASE RISK

New angina, nonfatal myocardial infarction (MI), congestive heart failure (CHF), and fatal MI or CAD death are all increased in those diagnosed with PAD.[4,10–12,39,40] Whether PAD is symptomatic or silent, studies have shown 20% to 40% increased risk for nonfatal MI,[4] 60% increased risk of progression to CHF even after multivariable adjustment (in those without previously identified CVD),[12] and 90% to 500% increased risk of fatal MI and CAD death.[4,10,11,40] The increase in risk was greatest in a population-based study with a somewhat more stringent PAD definition (e.g., ABI cutoff less than 0.8) and 10-year follow-up. Although full multivariate adjustment was performed, data from this study suggested that limited adjustment (e.g., for age and sex) yields risk ratios similar to those obtained with full adjustment.[39] Data from this population study confirm a relation of PAD severity to CAD mortality risk. Among men, 11% of those with normal lower extremities in this population (aged 38 to 82 years; mean age, 66 years) experienced CAD death on 10-year follow-up, compared with nearly 40% of those with moderate PAD (defined as ABI between 0.6 and 0.9) and more than 60% of those with severe PAD (ABI less than 0.6). Mortality figures for women in each cohort group were just over half the rate for men but showed the same gradient with PAD.[41]

4.3.3 CEREBROVASCULAR DISEASE RISK

ABI less than 0.90 was associated with increased nonfatal stroke (although not with fatal stroke) in one study,[40] whereas in another, increasing PAD severity was correlated with the combined outcome of transient ischemic attack and definite and possible stroke.[4] An analysis of Spanish subjects showed that PAD was correlated with hemorrhagic as well as with ischemic stroke.[42] PAD has been linked to worse outcomes in patients who experience a stroke.[43]

4.3.4 OVERALL CARDIOVASCULAR RISK

Because PAD is linked to increased CAD and CBVD events and mortality, one might expect it to be linked to increased overall cardiovascular morbidity and mortality. Indeed, both combined CVD morbidity and mortality and CVD mortality itself are increased in those with PAD, by all definitions of PAD, with risk ratios on the order of 2 to 6.[4,10–12,39,40] More stringent PAD criteria (signifying more severe PAD) are again linked to greater risk. Thus, the San Diego study,[39] which used ABI cutoffs of 0.8 among the criteria, showed higher risk ratios than did studies using ABI cutoffs of 0.9.

4.3.5 OVERALL MORTALITY RISK

Some major risk factors for CVD predict CVD mortality but not overall mortality, and produce risks that are attenuated in women or the elderly. PAD, in contrast, is a powerful predictor not only of CVD outcomes but also of overall mortality; this is true for women as well as men, for the elderly as well as for the middle aged, with 50% to 400% increases in risk.[4,10–12,17,38,40,44] PAD severity is linked to the magnitude of increased overall mortality risk. In subjects with an average age of 66 years, mortalities were 15% in those free of PAD, 45% with asymptomatic PAD, and 75% with severe symptomatic PAD on 10-year follow-up in a San Diego population-based study.[39] Moreover, the increased relative risk of all-cause mortality associated with PAD appears to be unaffected by the presence of baseline CBVD.[39] Two vascular laboratory-based studies also showed a marked gradient in overall mortality as a function of PAD severity.[45,46] PAD has also been shown to predict increased mortality in special populations of high-risk subjects, such as those with acute MI[47] and those undergoing CABG.[48,49] In the latter group, both in-hospital survival and longer-term mortality in those who survive to discharge are predicted by PAD.

The increased risk of CAD mortality, total CVD mortality, and overall mortality associated with noninvasively defined PAD are illustrated in Table 4.6, which presents risk ratios and 95% confidence intervals (adjusted for multiple covariates) for these outcomes, using 10-year follow-up data from the San Diego population-based study.[39]

4.4 DISCUSSION

PAD represents atherosclerotic arterial disease in the vascular territory supplying the legs, which may be asymptomatic, symptomatic with exertion (IC, which can be considered "leg angina"), or symptomatic at rest. PAD shares many risk factors with CAD and CBVD,

TABLE 4.6
Prediction of Coronary Artery Disease, Coronary Vascular Disease, and Overall Mortality by Peripheral Arterial Disease

		Risk Ratio[a]	95% CI
CAD mortality	All	6.6	2.9–14.9
	No prior CVD	4.3	1.4–12.8
CVD mortality[b]	All	5.9	3.0–11.4
	No prior CVD	6.3	2.6–15.0
Overall mortality	All	3.1	1.9–4.9
	No prior CVD	3.1	1.8–5.3

CI = confidence interval.

[a] Risk ratios adjusted for age, body mass index, cigarettes per day, fasting glucose, log plasma triglycerides, LDL-C, HDL-C, and systolic blood pressure.

[b] Includes CAD, CBVD, and other CVD mortality.

From Criqui, M.H., Langer, R.D., Fronek, A., et al., Mortality over a period of 10 years in patients with peripheral arterial disease, *N. Engl. J. Med.*, 326, 381, 1992.[39] With permission.

as might be anticipated from the common atherosclerotic nature of the disease; the latter conditions reflect atherosclerotic arterial disease to vascular territories supplying the heart and brain, respectively. Nonetheless, selected risk factors such as advanced age, diabetes (or insulin resistance profile), and smoking are even more striking predictors of PAD than of CAD. Other risk factors, like LDL-C, are important for CAD but less important as independent risk markers for PAD. Because risk factors for PAD are shared with CAD and CBVD, and because all three conditions represent atherosclerotic disease manifested in different vascular beds, PAD is associated with a high prevalence of comorbid CAD and CBVD. Moreover, PAD is a strong predictor of CAD and CBVD morbidity and mortality, whether or not prior CAD or CBVD has been diagnosed. This predictive power appears to be independent of conventional risk factors for CVD.

The wide-reaching implications of PAD stretch beyond its association with CVD. Exercise, particularly walking, has been shown to potentially protect against a host of conditions that impact on the elderly including CVD,[50] PAD itself, insulin resistance,[51] depression,[52] cognitive decline,[53] osteoporosis (or fracture frequency),[54] and perhaps some forms of cancer.[55] Because PAD restricts exercise, and most notably limits ambulation, it could promote development of these untoward conditions, which may amplify the total morbidity (and mortality) burden associated with PAD. Of note, recent unpublished data from the PARTNERS Study showed that PAD was more specifically and strongly associated with restriction of ambulation than were CAD or CBVD.[8]

In symptomatic PAD patients, the clinician must always keep in mind two related but different goals of therapy. The obvious goal is to improve ambulation. Cigarette smoking cessation and supervised exercise have proven efficacy. Available medications in the United States are currently limited to cilostazol (effective) and pentoxifylline (marginally effective), although numerous others are under active study. A more important, and unfortunately often overlooked goal is to prevent the risk of CAD and CVBD events, including death, in both symptomatic and asymptomatic PAD patients. A multifactoral approach, which may include lifestyle modifications (e.g., cigarette smoking cessation, diet, and exercise) and medications (including antiplatelet, lipid-lowering, and antihypertensive agents, and therapies for diabetes and nicotine addiction) is necessary. Clinical trials evaluating the benefit of homocysteine reduction are under way.

4.5. CONCLUSIONS

PAD merits increased attention not only to prevent and mitigate PAD morbidity and mortality, but also (1) to more accurately gauge risk of CAD and CBVD, permitting aggressive use of preventive treatments, guided by risk of disease, in accordance with the existing paradigm[56,57]; and (2) to retard the indirect contribution by PAD in advancing other conditions that afflict the elderly—and that ambulation helps to prevent—such as depression, cognitive decline, osteoporosis, and possibly cancer.

To date, despite the potency of PAD as a risk predictor, PAD assessment has generally not figured in published risk factor analyses for CAD and CBVD. Moreover, although PAD may be an even stronger predictor of survival in CAD patients than is prior MI, those with prior MI (or identified CAD) are likely to receive more-intensive treatment and advice regarding lifestyle factors than those with PAD.[47,58] Of course, the body of evidence directly addressing benefits of treatment in those with PAD is more sparse than that regarding treatment of those with prior MI, but this, in turn, is a result of the lesser research attention historically paid to PAD. Clinically, too, PAD appears to be assessed and diagnosed less systematically than CAD and CBVD; this represents an error in strategy even if the goal were simply to predict future CAD and CBVD risk, because PAD is such a strong predictor. Clearly, increased clinical and research attention is due this powerful prognostic factor.

In short, PAD is a strong and independent predictor of risk—or, otherwise conceptualized, a predictor of the combined impact of unmeasured risk factors and ongoing disease processes—for CAD and CBVD, and should be assessed and incorporated in risk analysis for these conditions. Several additional factors converge to create a mandate for PAD as a focus for redoubled research efforts. First, PAD prevalence increases steeply with age in the elderly; the overall population is aging, with sharply increased numbers of elderly individuals. Second, PAD is potently associated with CAD risk, the leading cause of death in the elderly age group. Third, PAD is potently associated with risk of stroke, the leading cause of serious disability. Finally, by restricting ambulation, PAD plays an indirect role in promoting a host of other conditions that burden the elderly. Therefore, PAD must become a more prominent focus of future research and clinical efforts.

REFERENCES

1. Rose, G.A., The diagnosis of ischaemic heart pain and intermittent claudication in field surveys, *Bull. World. Health. Org.*, 27, 645, 1962.

2. Criqui, M.H., Denenberg, J.O., Bird, C.E., et al..,The correlation between symptoms and non-invasive test results in patients referred for peripheral arterial disease testing. *Vasc. Med.*, 1, 65, 1996.

3. Kannel, W. B., Skinner, J., Jr., Schwartz, M.J., et al.., Intermittent claudication: incidence in the Framingham Study, *Circulation*, 41, 875,1970.

4. Leng, G.C., Lee, A.J., Fowkes, F.G., et al., Incidence, natural history and cardiovascular events in symptomatic and asymptomatic peripheral arterial disease in the general population, *Int. J. Epidemiol.*, 25, 1172, 1996.

5. Criqui, M.H., Fronek, A., Barrett-Connor, E., et al., The prevalence of peripheral arterial disease in a defined population, *Circulation*, 71, 510, 1985.

6. Meijer, W.T., Hoes, A.W., Rutgers, D., et al., Peripheral arterial disease in the elderly: the Rotterdam Study, *Arterioscler. Thromb. Vasc. Biol.*, 18, 185, 1998.

7. Dormandy, J.A. and Rutherford, R.B., Management of peripheral arterial disease, TASC (TransAtlantic Inter-Society Consensus) Working Group, *J. Vasc. Surg.*, 31, S1, 2000.

8. Criqui, M.H., Preliminary data from the PARTNERS Study, presented at Peripheral Arterial Disease Awareness, Risk, and Treatment: New Resources for Survival, Round-up Meeting, Phoenix, January 15, 2000.

9. Fowkes, F.G., Housley, E., Cawood, E.H., et al., Edinburgh Artery Study: prevalence of asymptomatic and symptomatic peripheral arterial disease in the general population, *Int. J. Epidemiol.*, 20, 384, 1991.

10. Newman, A.B., Sutton-Tyrrell, K., Vogt, M.T., et al., Morbidity and mortality in hypertensive adults with a low ankle–arm blood pressure index, *JAMA*, 270, 487, 1993.

11. Kornitzer, M., Dramaix, M., Sobolski, J., et al., Ankle–arm pressure index in asymptomatic middle-aged males: an independent predictor of 10-year coronary heart disease mortality, *Angiology*, 46, 211, 1995.

12. Newman, A.B., Shemanski, L., Manolio, T.A., et al., Ankle–arm index as a predictor of cardiovascular disease and mortality in the Cardiovascular Health Study. *Arterioscler. Thromb. Vasc. Biol.*, 19, 538, 1999.

13. Criqui, M.H., Fronek, A., Klauber, M.R., et al., The sensitivity, specificity, and predictive value of traditional clinical evaluation of peripheral arterial disease: results from noninvasive testing in a defined population, *Circulation*, 71, 516, 1985.

14. Fowkes, F.G., Housley, E., Riemersma, R.A., et al., Smoking, lipids, glucose intolerance, and blood pressure as risk factors for peripheral atherosclerosis compared with ischemic heart disease in the Edinburgh Artery Study, *Am. J. Epidemiol.*, 135, 331, 1992.

15. Criqui, M.H., Langer, R.D., Fronek, A., et al., Large vessel and isolated small vessel disease, in *Epidemiology of Peripheral Vascular Disease*, Fowkes F, Ed., Springer-Verlag, London, 1991, 85 (Chap. 7).

16. Al Zahrani, H.A., Al Bar, H.M., Bahnassi, A., et al., The distribution of peripheral arterial disease in a defined population of elderly high-risk Saudi patients, *Int. Angiol.*, 16, 123, 1997.

17. Criqui, M.H., Denenberg, J.O., Langer, R.D., et al., The epidemiology of peripheral arterial disease: importance of identifying the population at risk, *Vasc. Med.*, 2, 221, 1997.

18. Criqui, M.H., Denenberg, J.O., Langer, R.D., et al., Peripheral arterial disease and hypertension. In *Hypertension Primer. The Essentials of High Blood Pressure*, Izzo, J., and Black, H., Eds., American Heart Association, New York, 1998, 215.

19. Taylor, L.M., Jr., DeFrang, R.D., Harris, E.J.,et al., The association of elevated plasma homocyst(e)ine with progression of symptomatic peripheral arterial disease, *J. Vasc. Surg.*, 13, 128, 1991.

20. Lowe, G.D., Fowkes, F.G., Dawes, J., et al., Blood viscosity, fibrinogen, and activation of coagulation and leukocytes in peripheral arterial disease and the normal population in the Edinburgh Artery Study, *Circulation*, 87, 1915, 1993.

21. Seeger, J.M., Silverman, S.H., Flynn, T.C., et al., Lipid risk factors in patients requiring arterial reconstruction, *J. Vasc. Surg.*, 10, 418, 1989.

22. Hensley, W.J. and Mansfield, C.H., Lipoproteins, atherogenicity, age, and risk of myocardial infarction, *Aust. N. Z. J. Public Health*, 23, 174, 1999.

23. Kroon, A.A., Ajubi, N., van Asten, W.N., et al., The prevalence of peripheral vascular disease in familial hypercholesterolaemia, *J. Intern. Med.*, 238, 451, 1995.

24. The Lipid Research Clinics Coronary Primary Prevention Trial results, I., Reduction in incidence of coronary heart disease, *JAMA*, 25, 351, 1984.

25. Buchwald, H., Bourdages, H.R., Campos, C.T., et al., Impact of cholesterol reduction on peripheral arterial disease in the Program on the Surgical Control of the Hyperlipidemias (POSCH), *Surgery*, 120, 672, 1996.

26. Pedersen, T.T., Kjekshus, J., Pyorala, K., et al., Effect of simvastatin on ischemic signs and symptoms in the Scandinavian Simvastatin Survival Study (4S), *Am. J. Cardiol.* 81, 333, 1998.

27. Goldhaber, S.Z., Manson, J.E., Stampfer, M.J., et al., Low-dose aspirin and subsequent peripheral arterial surgery in the Physicians' Health Study, *Lancet*, 340, 143, 1992.

28. Rosc, D., Kotschy, M., Rewakovicz, M., and Listopadzk, D., Thrombin/antithrombin III complex in patients with peripheral occlusive arterial disease, *Folia. Haematol. Int. Mag. Klin. Morphol. Blutforsch.*, 117, 405, 1990.

29. Tyrrell, J., Cooke, T., Reilly, M., et al., Lipoprotein [Lp(a)] and peripheral vascular disease, *J. Intern. Med.*, 232, 349, 1992.

30. Blann, A.D., Seigneur, M., Steiner, M., et al., Circulating ICAM-1 and VCAM-1 in peripheral artery disease and hypercholesterolaemia: relationship to the location of atherosclerotic disease, smoking, and in the prediction of adverse events, *Thromb. Haemost.*, 79, 1080, 1998.

31. Smith, F.B., Lowe, G.D., Lee, A.J., et al., Smoking, hemorheologic factors, and progression of peripheral arterial disease in patients with claudication, *J. Vasc. Surg.*, 29, 129, 1998.

32. Ridker, P.M., Cushman, M., Stampfer, M.J., et al., Plasma concentration of C-reactive protein and risk of developing peripheral vascular disease, *Circulation*, 97, 425, 1998.

33. Housley, E., Leng, G.C., Donnan, P.T., et al., Physical activity and risk of peripheral arterial disease in the general population: Edinburgh Artery Study, *J. Epidemiol. Community Health*, 47, 475, 1993.

34. Donnan, P.T., Thomson, M., Fowkes, F.G., et al., Diet as a risk factor for peripheral arterial disease in the general population: the Edinburgh Artery Study, *Am. J. Clin. Nutr.*, 57, 917, 1993.

35. Camargo, C.A., Jr., Stampfer, M.J., Glynn, R.J., et al., Prospective study of moderate alcohol consumption and risk of peripheral arterial disease in U.S. male physicians, *Circulation*, 95, 577, 1997.

36. Katsouyanni, K., Skalkidis, Y., Petridou, E., et al., Diet and peripheral arterial occlusive disease: the role of poly-, mono-, and saturated fatty acids, *Am. J. Epidemiol.*, 133, 24, 1991.

37. Dormandy, J., Mahir, M., Ascady, et al., M., Fate of the patient with chronic leg ischemia, *J. Cardiovasc. Surg.*, 30, 50, 1989.

38. Jelnes, R., Gaardsting, O., Hougaard Jensen, K., et al., Fate in intermittent claudication: outcome and risk factors, *BMJ*, 293, 1137, 1986.

39. Criqui, M.H., Langer, R.D., Fronek, A., et al., Mortality over a period of 10 years in patients with peripheral arterial disease, *N. Engl. J. Med.*, 326, 381, 1992.

40. Leng, G.C., Fowkes, F.G., Lee, A.J., et al., Use of ankle brachial pressure index to predict cardiovascular events and death: a cohort study, *BMJ*, 313, 1440, 1996.

41. Criqui, M.H. and Denenberg, J.O., The generalized nature of atherosclerosis: how peripheral arterial disease may predict adverse events from coronary artery disease, *Vasc. Med.*, 3, 241, 1998.

42. Caicoya, G.M., Corrales, C.C., Lasheras, M.C., et al., The association between a cerebrovascular accident and peripheral arterial disease: a case-control study in Asturias, Spain, *Rev. Clin. Esp.*, 195, 830, 1995.

43. Tonelli, C., Finzi, G., Catamo, A., et al., Prevalence and prognostic value of peripheral arterial disease in stroke patients, *Int. Angiol.*, 12, 342, 1993.

44. Kannel, W.B. and McGee, D.L., Update on some epidemiologic features of intermittent claudication, *J. Am. Geriatr. Soc.*, 33, 13, 1985.

45. McKenna, M., Wolfson, S., and Kuller, L., The ratio of ankle and arm arterial pressure as an independent predictor of mortality, *Atherosclerosis*, 87, 119, 1991.

46. McDermott, M.M., Feinglass, J., Slavensky, R., et al., The ankle-brachial index as a predictor of survival in patients with peripheral vascular disease, *J. Gen. Intern. Med.*, 9, 445, 1994.

47. Pardaens, J., Lesaffre, E., Willems, J.L., et al., Multivariate survival analysis for the assessment of prognostic factors and risk categories after recovery from acute myocardial infarction: the Belgian situation, *Am. J. Epidemiol.*, 122, 805, 1985.

48. Birkmeyer, J.D., O'Connor, G.T., Quinton, H.B., et al., The effect of peripheral vascular disease on in-hospital mortality rates with coronary artery bypass surgery, Northern New England Cardiovascular Disease Study Group, *J. Vasc. Surg.*, 21, 445, 1995.

49. Birkmeyer, J.D., Quinton, H.B., O'Connor, N.J., et al., The effect of peripheral vascular disease on long-term mortality after coronary artery bypass surgery, Northern New England Cardiovascular Disease Study Group, *Arch. Surg.* 131, 316, 1996.

50. Manson, J.E., Hu, F.B., Rich-Edwards, J.W., et al., A prospective study of walking as compared with vigorous exercise in the prevention of coronary heart disease in women, *N. Engl. J. Med.*, 341, 650, 1999.

51. Pan, X.R., Li, G.W., Hu, Y.H., et al., Effects of diet and exercise in preventing NIDDM in people with impaired glucose tolerance, The Da Qing IGT and Diabetes Study, *Diabetes Care*, 20, 537, 1997.

52. Blumenthal, J.A., Babyak, M.A., Moore, K.A., Craighead, W.E., Herman, S., Khatri, P., Waugh, R., Napolitano, M.A., Forman, L.M., Appelbaum, M., Doraiswamy, P.M., and Krishnan, K.R., Effects of exercise training on older patients with major depression, *Arch. Intern. Med.*, 159, 2349, 1999.

53. Williams, P., Lord, S.R., Moore, K.A., Effects of group exercise on cognitive functioning and mood in older women, *Aust. N. Z. J. Public Health*, 21, 45, 1997.

54. Ernst, E., Exercise for female osteoporosis: a systematic review of randomized clinical trials, *Sports Med.*, 25, 359, 1998.

55. Moore, M.A., Park, C.B., and Tsuda, H., Physical exercise: a pillar for cancer prevention?, *Eur. J. Cancer Prev.*, 7, 177, 1998.

56. Expert Panel on Detection Evaluation and Treatment of High Blood Cholesterol in Adults, Summary of the Second Report of the National Cholesterol Education Program (NCEP) Expert Panel on Detection, Evaluation, and Treatment of High Blood Cholesterol in Adults (Adult Treatment Panel II), *JAMA*, 269, 3015, 1993.

57. Stein, J.H. and McBride, P.E., Benefits of cholesterol screening and therapy for primary prevention of cardiovascular disease: a new paradigm, *J. Am. Board Fam. Pract.*, 11, 72, 1998.

58. McDermott, M.M., Mehta, S., Ahn, H., et al., Atherosclerotic risk factors are less intensively treated in patients with peripheral arterial disease than in patients with coronary artery disease, *J. Gen. Intern. Med.*, 12, 209, 1997.

5 Clinical and Vascular Laboratory Evaluation of Peripheral Arterial Disease

Michael R. Jaff and William R. Hiatt

CONTENTS

5.1 Introduction...81
5.2 Clinical Evaluation 82
    5.2.1 History..82
    5.2.2 Physical Examination...82
    5.2.3 Differential Diagnosis..83
5.3 Ankle–Brachial Index..84
5.4 Vascular Laboratory..87
5.5 Conclusions...93
References..93

5.1 INTRODUCTION

The noninvasive evaluation of patients with peripheral arterial disease (PAD) begins in the primary care physician's office. Patients considered at risk for PAD are older (aged 50 years or more), have cardiovascular risk factors of smoking or diabetes, or have exercise-induced leg symptoms. The initial evaluation includes a thorough vascular history and physical examination, followed by measurement of the ankle–brachial index (ABI).

0-8493-8413-3/01/$0.00+$1.50

5.2   CLINICAL EVALUATION

5.2.1   HISTORY

PAD of the lower extremity causes two characteristic pain syndromes: intermittent claudication (IC) and ischemic rest pain. Claudication is derived from the Latin word meaning "to limp," which accurately describes the walking pattern of the patient. Depending on the level and extent of the arterial occlusive disease, claudication may affect the buttock, thigh, calf, and, rarely, the foot. The discomfort develops only during exercise and steadily increases during walking activity to a point where the patient must stop because of intolerable pain. Rest relieves the discomfort within 10 minutes. Ischemic (or nocturnal) rest pain is a severe form of pain that involves the distal foot and may be most severe in the vicinity of an ischemic ulcer or gangrenous digit. The pain typically occurs at night when the patient assumes the horizontal position, and is relieved by dependency of the foot to improve gravitational effects on blood flow. Progression from claudication to rest pain indicates the presence of severe arterial occlusive disease.

The historical evaluation of patients with suspected PAD must also include symptoms suggestive of atherosclerosis elsewhere. Questions aimed at uncovering symptoms of transient cerebral ischemia, angina pectoris, and findings implying secondary causes of hypertension are important during the initial history.

5.2.2   PHYSICAL EXAMINATION

A complete physical examination should be performed to evaluate the patient for systemic hypertension, carotid bruits, or an abdominal aortic aneurysm. The skin of the legs, especially the feet, should be inspected for color changes, ulceration, infection, or trauma due to ill-fitting shoes. Palpation of all arterial pulses, including the brachial, femoral, and pedal arteries, should be performed. The location of the posterior tibial pulse is behind the medial malleolus, and the dorsal pedis pulse runs along the dorsum of the foot between the first and second metatarsal bones. Pulses are graded as normally present (easily palpable), diminished (difficult to palpate), or absent. Patients with a palpable femoral pulse but absent pedal pulses will have disease confined to the leg vessels, whereas a diminished or absent femoral pulse indicates disease of the aorta or iliac arteries (the inflow). Finally, all patients should have auscultation of the aorta and femoral vessels for bruits. Any patient with a femoral bruit or absent pedal pulses should be suspected of having PAD, which would subsequently need to be confirmed by measurement of the systolic ankle blood pressure.

With chronic limb ischemia, the physician may observe atrophy of the calf muscles. However, aside from absent limb pulses and the auscultation of bruits, the most reliable physical examination findings of PAD include pallor on elevation due to inadequate arterial pressure and flow to overcome gravity. Dependent rubor occurs with severe restriction in arterial inflow and chronic dilatation of the peripheral vascular bed. Severe chronic leg ischemia can cause ulceration initially affecting the most distal aspect of the toes or over bony prominences. These ulcers are painful, do not bleed when manipulated, and often have a dark necrotic base. At this advanced stage of ischemia, the foot may be edematous from being continually held in the dependent position in an attempt to relieve the ischemic pain.

5.2.3 DIFFERENTIAL DIAGNOSIS

IC should be differentiated from other causes of discomfort in the lower extremity. Pain from arthritis of the hip or knee is often present at rest and exacerbated by exercise. Claudication-like symptoms may also arise from spinal stenosis that is due to narrowing of the lumbar spinal canal. These symptoms often include numbness and weakness in the lower extremity that are produced by standing or bending backward at the hips rather than just ambulating. The symptoms are relieved, not simply by rest, but also by sitting down or leaning forward to straighten out the lumbar spine. Peripheral neuropathies are common in the elderly, but are associated with a continuous burning sensation in the feet that is unaffected by exercise. A history of diabetes or alcoholism is common. Older individuals also complain of nocturnal cramps in the calf that are not vascular in origin.

5.3 ANKLE–BRACHIAL INDEX

The first vascular laboratory test that must be performed in patients either at risk for PAD, or with symptoms and physical findings of PAD, is the ABI. Figure 5.1 is an algorithm presenting several common criteria that would indicate the need to measure the ABI, which is a safe, simple, highly accurate, and reproducible method of determining the presence and severity of PAD. Thus, in patients with signs or symptoms of arterial vascular disease in the leg, or in patients with leg pain on exertion, the ABI will reliably include or exclude the diagnosis of PAD. The ABI also provides additional information regarding the risk of myocardial infarction, stroke, and vascular death.[1–3] Arteriography is not necessary to make the diagnosis of PAD or to judge the severity and segmental locations of the occlusive disease process. Thus, an arteriogram should be reserved for patients who have failed medical therapy, where invasive therapy—namely surgical bypass or endovascular intervention—is being contemplated.

The ABI should be performed in the physician's office. It requires a routine sphygmomanometer, a handheld continuous-wave Doppler, and acoustic gel. Figure 5.2 is a schematic drawing of the locations for taking systolic pressure measurements in the arms and ankles. A sphygmomanometer cuff is placed on the left upper arm, whereupon the cuff is inflated above the systolic pressure and then gradually deflated. When the arterial Doppler signal returns, the resulting value represents the systolic pressure in the left arm. This process is then repeated on the right upper arm. The higher of the two systolic brachial pressures is used as the denominator of the ABI calculation. Following this, the sphygmomanometer cuff is placed on the right lower leg, just above the ankle. Again using the handheld Doppler, an arterial Doppler signal is obtained in the dorsalis pedis artery. The cuff is inflated until the arterial Doppler signal disappears, and then the cuff is gradually deflated. When the arterial Doppler signal returns, this represents the

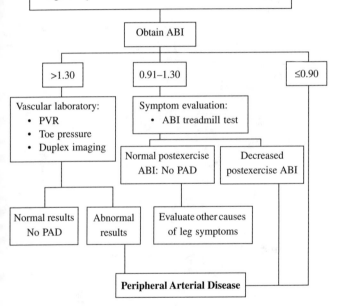

- Leg symptoms with exertion suggesting claudication
- Abnormal pulse exam in the lower extremity
- Coronary/carotid/renal arterial disease
- Age 50–69 yr and smoking, diabetes, or other risk factors
- Age ≥70 yr

Obtain ABI

>1.30 | 0.91–1.30 | ≤0.90

Vascular laboratory:
- PVR
- Toe pressure
- Duplex imaging

Symptom evaluation:
- ABI treadmill test

Normal postexercise ABI: No PAD | Decreased postexercise ABI

Normal results No PAD | Abnormal results | Evaluate other causes of leg symptoms

Peripheral Arterial Disease

FIGURE 5.1 Diagnostic algorithm for performance and interpretation of the ankle–brachial index (ABI). PAD = peripheral arterial disease; PVR = pulse volume recording. (Hiatt, W.R., Treatment of Peripheral Arterial diseaes and Claudication. *N. Eng. J. Med.*, in press. With permission.)

systolic pressure in the dorsalis pedis artery. The Doppler device is then positioned posterior to the medial malleolus and the arterial Doppler signal of the posterior tibial artery is obtained; the systolic pressure is then recorded as described above. The higher of the two right-ankle pressures (either the dorsalis pedis or posterior tibial artery)

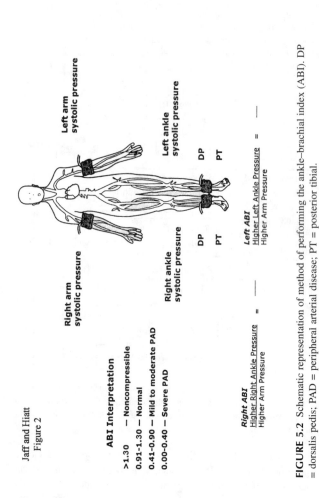

Jaff and Hiatt
Figure 2

ABI Interpretation

>1.30 — Noncompressible
0.91–1.30 — Normal
0.41–0.90 — Mild to moderate PAD
0.00–0.40 — Severe PAD

Right arm systolic pressure

Left arm systolic pressure

Right ankle systolic pressure

Left ankle systolic pressure

DP
PT

DP
PT

Right ABI
$$\text{Right ABI} = \frac{\text{Higher Right Ankle Pressure}}{\text{Higher Arm Pressure}}$$

Left ABI
$$\text{Left ABI} = \frac{\text{Higher Left Ankle Pressure}}{\text{Higher Arm Pressure}}$$

FIGURE 5.2 Schematic representation of method of performing the ankle–brachial index (ABI). DP = dorsalis pedis; PAD = peripheral arterial disease; PT = posterior tibial.

is used as the numerator of the ABI calculation for the right leg. Finally, a similar method is used in the left leg to obtain the left ABI.

A normal ABI is defined as a resting measurement greater than 0.90. Any value of 0.90 or less indicates the presence of PAD. Obviously, the lower the ABI, the more severe the PAD. Patients with ABI values of 0.70 to 0.90 may be asymptomatic or have very mild symptoms of IC. ABI values between 0.40 and 0.70 represent patients with more severe PAD, and values less than 0.40 suggest the most advanced stages of PAD, with ischemic rest pain, nonhealing ulcerations, and gangrene occurring with frequency.

5.4 VASCULAR LABORATORY

The ABI is a highly accurate method of determining the presence and severity of PAD. However, if the ankle vessel is calcified, as is occasionally seen in patients with diabetes mellitus or end-stage renal disease, an accurate ankle pressure cannot be obtained. The pressure in these calcified arteries is often more than 200 to 250 mm Hg, leading to an ABI value greater than 1.30. If not recognized as artificially high, the physician may falsely conclude that arterial circulation is adequate, or even normal, in these patients.[4] In this scenario, other tests available in the vascular diagnostic laboratory are necessary, including photoplethysmography,[5] digital pressures, arterial duplex ultrasonography,[6] and even assessments of wound-healing potential using transcutaneous oximetry.

Patients with classic historical symptoms of PAD may have a normal physical examination and ABI. In this scenario, the astute clinician must perform an exercise physiologic study in the vascular diagnostic laboratory. Patients have resting pressures measured, and are then placed on a treadmill at a constant speed and constant grade of incline. The patient is asked to report initial symptoms of limb discomfort and to terminate the exercise when the discomfort is limiting, or after 5 minutes. After exercise, ankle and arm pressures are again measured. A significant decrease in post-exercise pressures and ABI confirms the diagnosis of PAD (Table 5.1).

TABLE 5.1
Noninvasive Diagnostic Testing for Peripheral Arterial Disease

Vascular Laboratory Examination	Information Obtained	Clinical Indication	Limitations
Segmental limb pressures	•Localizes disease to specific segments of the lower extremity arteries •May aid in predicting wound healing potential	•Moderate to severe claudication or limb ischemia with consideration to revascularization	•Inaccurate in patients with noncompressible arteries •Requires special BP cuffs •Proximal thigh cuff occasionally uncomfortable for patient
PVRs	•Localizes disease to specific segments of the lower extremity arteries •May aid in predicting wound healing potential	•Moderate to severe claudication or limb ischemia with consideration to revascularization •Useful in calcified arteries	•Requires a skilled and meticulous technologist •Mainly qualitative information

Segmental Doppler waveforms	•Localizes disease to specific segments of the lower extremity arteries •Easy to perform and interpret	•Moderate to severe claudication or limb ischemia with consideration to revascularization	•Not accurate in calcified arteries •Less accurate in selected centers than PVRs
Exercise ABI	•Confirms diagnosis of PAD when resting ABI is >0.90	•Atypical symptoms of exertional limb discomfort •Serial examinations to demonstrate clinical effects of intervention	•Requires calibrated treadmill and close observation •Many patients may not be able to complete exercise study •Technologist must be competent to rapidly perform post-exercise arterial pressures

(continued)

TABLE 5.1 (CONTINUED)
Noninvasive Diagnostic Testing for Peripheral Arterial Disease

Vascular Laboratory Examination	Information Obtained	Clinical Indication	Limitations
Arterial duplex ultrasonography	•Specific identification of sites of atherosclerotic disease: stenosis, occlusion •Can accurately clarify options for invasive therapy: endovascular procedures or bypass surgery	•Advanced IC or CLI with need for revascularization •Postcatheterization access site complication (e.g., pseudoaneurysm, hematoma, arteriovenous fistula)	•Requires expensive equipment •Requires skilled technologist •Prolonged examination time •Calcified arteries cause acoustic shadowing/inability to obtain Doppler velocities •Gives only anatomic information; does not describe functional limitation

ABI = ankle–brachial index; CLI = critical limb ischemia; IC = intermittent claudication; PAD = peripheral arterial disease; PVR = pulsed volume recording.

The ABI provides information about the presence or absence of PAD, along with the severity and risk of comorbid atherosclerotic events. However, if the clinician desires more detailed information concerning the location of arterial occlusive disease, whether disease is represented by stenoses or occlusions, the length of atherosclerotic disease, and the status of the runoff arteries, other diagnostic tests are required. Segmental limb pressures,[7] pulse volume recordings, Doppler segmental waveforms, and arterial duplex ultrasonography are among the tests that should be considered (Table 5.1).

With the use of sequential limb blood pressure cuffs and commercially available equipment, segmental limb arterial blood pressures can be obtained in the thigh, calf, ankle, foot, and digit. Each pressure measurement is compared with the other pressures in the limb and the contralateral limb. For example, the pressure obtained in the proximal thigh cuff is normally at least 30 mm Hg higher than the brachial pressure. Lower pressures suggest the presence of inflow aortoiliac artery disease. Each cuff pressure should be no more than 20 mm Hg lower than the pressure cuff proximal to that level. Disease localization occurs in the segment proximal to the cuff with the lower pressure. Therefore, if the pressure in the lower thigh cuff is 40 mm Hg below that of the higher thigh cuff, this would suggest superficial femoral artery occlusive disease.

Pulse volume recordings (PVRs) are plethysmographic tests that provide qualitative information. Simply put, a blood pressure cuff is inflated to a level that does not interrupt arterial flow (approximately 40 to 65 mm Hg). As each arterial pulse passes through the segment of artery beneath the cuff, the volume of blood causes distention of the artery. This is sensed by the cuff, which then transmits the volume change to a recorder, providing a waveform. In the normal setting, this waveform is similar in appearance to an intra-arterial pressure waveform. As the arterial circulation worsens, the PVR looses the dicrotic notch, lowers in amplitude, and widens. These tests require a highly trained technologist, as well as a physician who understands the subtleties of waveform interpretation.

Segmental arterial Doppler waveforms can also be performed and are easier to interpret. Using a bidirectional Doppler probe, Doppler waveforms are obtained at each arterial level. Normal Doppler waveforms are triphasic. Mild to moderate PAD is represented by biphasic Doppler waveforms. Severe PAD results in monophasic and, ultimately, flat waveforms. Segmental Doppler waveforms are easy to perform, and require little training to interpret. However, in the scenario of noncompressible arteries, Doppler waveforms lose accuracy.

Arterial duplex ultrasonography is a highly accurate examination that can be performed from the aortic bifurcation to the ankles.[8] Using currently available Duplex ultrasound scanners, arteries are visualized, often with color imaging, and Doppler velocities are obtained. A doubling in the peak systolic velocity within a diseased arterial segment suggests a 50% to 99% stenosis.[9] Arterial duplex ultrasonography requires a highly skilled technologist. In addition, a complete examination of both lower extremities is time-consuming. In patients who are in need of revascularization, this examination is as accurate as arteriography in predicting the optimal revascularization method.[10]

Arterial duplex scanning is the ideal method of identifying and treating iatrogenic arterial pseudoaneurysms. This complication of arteriography and angioplasty occurs in 0.4% to 5.0% of all cases.[11] Although surgical repair of the defect is the classic method of therapy for pseudoaneurysms, ultrasound-guided compression repair and the recent refinement of the technique of ultrasound-guided bovine thrombin injection is rapidly becoming the therapy of choice. Using real-time duplex ultrasonography, the neck of the pseudoaneurysm is identified and direct manual compression is applied until arterial flow within the sac of the pseudoaneurysm has ceased. Compression is maintained for 20 to 60 minutes. Using this technique, more than 80% of pseudoaneurysms can be effectively treated.[12] However, this procedure is uncomfortable for the patient and the technologist. With the use of dilute bovine thrombin and real-time duplex ultrasonography, a needle can be placed in the sac of the pseudoaneurysm and small amounts of thrombin can be injected. This results in prompt thrombosis of the pseudoaneurysm sac. The procedure is effective in more than 90% of pseudoaneurysms and takes only minutes to complete.[13]

5.5 CONCLUSIONS

The initial evaluation of patients with suspected PAD begins with a thorough history and physical examination. This includes an evaluation of the entire cardiovascular system. Once this aspect of the evaluation has been completed, an ABI is performed. This simple, noninvasive, accurate, and reproducible examination not only describes the severity of PAD but also identifies overall cardiovascular morbidity and mortality.

If more information concerning the location, severity, and revascularization options is required for patients with advanced PAD, other tests should be considered. Segmental limb pressures, PVRs, segmental Doppler waveforms, digital pressures, photoplethysmography, transcutaneous oximetry, and arterial duplex ultrasonography can be used. Finally, in the event of an iatrogenic pseudoaneurysm, ultrasound-guided compression therapy and, more recently, thrombin injection, are exciting new methods of treating these arterial injuries without surgery.

REFERENCES

1. Kornitzer, M., Dramaix, M., Sobolski, J., et al., Ankle/arm pressure index in asymptomatic middle-aged males: an independent predictor of ten-year coronary heart disease mortality, *Angiology*, 46, 211, 1995.
2. McKenna, M., Wolfson, S., and Kuller, L., The ratio of ankle and arm arterial pressure as an independent predictor of mortality, *Atherosclerosis*, 87, 119, 1991.
3. Vogt, M.T., McKenna, M., Wolfson, S.K., et al., The relationship between ankle brachial index, other atherosclerotic disease, diabetes, smoking and mortality in older men and women, *Atherosclerosis*, 101, 191, 1993.

4. Fisher, C.M., Burnett, A., Makeham, V., et al., Variation in measurement of ankle-brachial pressure index in routine clinical practice, *J. Vasc. Surg.*, 24, 871, 1996.

5. Carter, S.A. and Tate, R.B., Value of toe pulse waves in addition to systolic pressures in the assessment of the severity of peripheral arterial disease and critical limb ischemia, *J. Vasc. Surg.*, 24, 258, 1996.

6. Jaff, M.R. and Dorros, G., The vascular laboratory: a critical component required for successful management of peripheral arterial occlusive disease, *J. Endovasc. Surg.*, 5, 146, 1998.

7. Gale, S.S., Scissons, R.P., Salles-Cunha, S.X., et al., Lower extremity arterial evaluation: are segmental arterial blood pressures worthwhile?, *J. Vasc. Surg.* 27, 831, 1998.

8. deSmet, A.A.E.A., Ermers, E.J.M., and Kitslaar, P.J.E.H.M., Duplex velocity characteristics of aortoiliac stenoses, *J. Vasc. Surg.*, 23, 628, 1996.

9. Whelan, J.F., Barry, M.H., and Moir, J.D., Color flow Doppler ultrasonography: comparison with peripheral arteriography for the investigation of peripheral vascular disease, *J. Clin. Ultrasound*, 20, 369, 1992.

10. Kohler, T.R., Nance, D.R., Cramer, M.M., et al., Duplex scanning for diagnosis of aortoiliac and femoropopliteal disease: a prospective study, *Circulation*, 76, 1074, 1987.

11. Cox, G.S., Young, J.R., Grubb, M.W., et al., Ultrasound-guided compression repair of post-catheterization pseudoaneurysms: results of treatment in one hundred cases, *J. Vasc. Surg.*, 19, 683, 1994.

12. Hajarizadeh, H., LaRosa, C.R., Cardullo, P., et al., Ultrasound-guided compression of iatrogenic femoral pseudoaneurysms: failure, recurrence, and long-term results, *J. Vasc. Surg.*, 22, 425, 1995.

13. Kang, S.S., Labropoulos, N., Mansour, A., et al., Expanded indications for ultrasound-guided thrombin injections of pseudoaneurysms, *J. Vasc. Surg.*, 31, 289, 2000.

6 Claudication: The Primary Symptom of Peripheral Arterial Disease

Judith G. Regensteiner and Alan T. Hirsch

CONTENTS

6.1 Intermittent Claudication: Definition, Epidemiology,
and Natural History 96
6.2 Treatment of Cardiovascular Risk in Peripheral
Arterial Disease 96
    6.2.1 Identification and Modification of Risk Factors 96
6.3 Assessment of Claudication 99
    6.3.1 Clinical, Office-Based Evaluation of the Patient
    with Claudication...99
        6.3.1.1 Diagnosis of Peripheral Arterial Disease
        and Claudication...100
    6.3.2 Objective Evaluation of Claudication Severity 102
        6.3.2.1 Measurement of Exercise Performance 103
        6.3.2.2 Functional Status Measurements: The
        Claudication Questionnaire as Clinical Tool.104
6.4 Treatment of Claudication...104
    6.4.1 Impact of Claudication on Functional Status...............104
    6.4.2 Goals of Treatment 105
    6.4.3 Treatments..105
        6.4.3.1 Exercise Rehabilitation 105

0-8493-8413-3/01/$0.00+$1.50
© 2001 by CRC Press LLC

            6.4.3.2 Pharmacologic Therapies 108
            6.4.3.3 Limb Bypass Surgery or Percutaneous
                     Transluminal Angioplasty 110
6.5 Conclusions...112
References..113

6.1 INTERMITTENT CLAUDICATION: DEFINITION, EPIDEMIOLOGY, AND NATURAL HISTORY

Peripheral arterial disease (PAD) is a prevalent disease estimated to be present in about 12% of the US population or about 8 to10 million persons.[1,2] The most common symptom of atherosclerotic PAD is intermittent claudication (IC). Defined as cramping, aching, fatigue, or discomfort that occurs in the muscles of the calves, thighs, or buttocks, IC is reproducibly elicited by walking and consistently relieved by rest. The symptom of IC is estimated to be present in 4 to 5 million persons in the United States.

As reported above, the prevalence of IC is not equal to the prevalence of PAD itself. On the contrary, over half of patients with PAD do not have typical limb exertional symptoms on routine medical history or by use of current epidemiologic survey tools. However, these patients, often referred to as asymptomatic, still experience some degree of functional impairment, as demonstrated in a recent nationwide screening study.[3]

This chapter will focus on the diagnosis and management of the patient with IC. A brief discussion of risk reduction is included, as it is imperative that all patients with PAD be treated to reduce the cardiovascular ischemic risk at the same time that IC is being assessed and treated.

6.2 TREATMENT OF CARDIOVASCULAR RISK IN PERIPHERAL ARTERIAL DISEASE

6.2.1 IDENTIFICATION AND MODIFICATION OF RISK FACTORS

PAD is an atherosclerotic syndrome, and therefore its incidence is dependent on the classic atherosclerotic risk factors that predict arterial disease in the coronary or cerebrovascular circulations. Cigarette smoking and diabetes mellitus are the risk factors with the greatest positive predictive value, followed by hypertension, hyperlipidemia (particularly a reduced high-density lipoprotein [HDL] cholesterol level), and abnormalities of homocysteine metabolism.[4–9] The role of these risk factors in the pathogenesis of PAD and of specific interventions is discussed more extensively in Chapters 1 and 4. Few prospective clinical trials have evaluated the efficacy of risk-factor interventions in large PAD populations, and thus, most therapeutic recommendations have been developed from coronary disease interventional studies.[10,11] A national consensus that patients with PAD of any severity should undergo intensive risk-factor reduction interventions to the same degree as patients with other forms of atherosclerotic disease has emerged from the power of these trials.[4] Specifically, patients with PAD should stop smoking, undergo lifestyle and pharmacologic interventions to achieve tight control of their diabetes (hemoglobin [Hb]A_{1C} < 7.0%), be treated to meet Joint National Committee on Prevention, Detection, Evaluation, and Treatment of High Blood Pressure guidelines for blood pressure control (<130/85 mm Hg) (12), and achieve National Cholesterol Education Program Guidelines for cholesterol normalization (low-density lipoprotein [LDL] cholesterol <100 mg/dL).[13] Guidelines have not yet been established for the treatment of elevations in plasma homocysteine levels. Thus, the degree to which assessment of this variable should be performed in any individual patient is left to the discretion of the treating clinician in the context of the age of the patient, the magnitude of the homocysteine abnormality, and the severity of the PAD. There is some evidence that modifying certain risk factors may improve the symptom of IC. For instance, simvistatin was found to reduce the incidence of new-onset IC.[14] In addition, data suggest that progression of disease and risk of IC can be improved by risk factor modification.[15]

The Antiplatelet Trialists' Collaboration (ATC) provided a comprehensive overview of the efficacy and safety of antiplatelet agents in the prevention of ischemic events in high-risk patients.[16] The study was performed via a meta-analysis that included 145 randomized trials that enrolled more than 100,000 patients at risk of vascular events. Of this total patient group, more than 75,000 were considered at high risk (i.e., had clinically evident atherosclerosis). The ATC analysis showed that aspirin was associated with a 25% reduction in events compared with placebo, and ticlopidine was 33% more effective than placebo for reducing events. Moreover, ticlopidine was approximately 10% more effective than aspirin for reducing vascular events. Unfortunately, few patients with PAD were included in the ATC analysis. Thus, conclusive evidence is missing on the efficacy of aspirin in preventing ischemic events in patients specifically affected with PAD.

However, robust data confirm the importance of antiplatelet therapy for reducing myocardial infarction (MI) and stroke in the PAD population. The Clopidogrel Versus Aspirin for the Prevention of Ischemic Events (CAPRIE) trial was a large, randomized, controlled trial conducted in 16 countries, including the United States, to compare the benefits of aspirin (325 mg/day) with clopidogrel (75 mg/day) in the prevention of ischemic events.[17] A total of 19,185 patients with recent ischemic stroke, recent MI, or symptomatic PAD were entered and observed for 1 to 3 years. The results showed that 5.83% of the aspirin-treated group per year and 5.32% of the clopidogrel-treated group per year (relative risk reduction in favor of clopidogrel, 8.7%; $P = 0.043$) suffered an MI, stroke or other vascular death in the total study population. *Post-hoc* analysis revealed that the 6000-plus patients with PAD experienced a significantly improved outcome, with a 23.8% cardiovascular risk reduction for the group treated with clopidogrel compared with aspirin alone. The study was designed with the power to detect significant differences between treatments in the entire study population, because it was presumed that coronary, cerebral, and limb arterial atherosclerosis would serve as clinical markers of a common systemic "atherothrombotic" disease. Thus the "amplified" effect in PAD patients was surprising. Mechanisms for this effect are unknown.

Importantly, patients with PAD are often undertreated with anti-platelet agents.[18] Given that PAD is a systemic atherosclerotic disease and that these patients have a strong and independent risk of cardio-vascular morbidity and mortality, PAD patients should be treated with antiplatelet agents unless contraindicated.

6.3   ASSESSMENT OF CLAUDICATION

6.3.1   CLINICAL, OFFICE-BASED EVALUATION OF THE PATIENT WITH CLAUDICATION

A critical step toward establishing the diagnosis of IC is recognition of the prevalence of limb symptoms in defined at-risk populations. Because PAD is relatively common among adults over 50 years of age, clinicians and healthcare professionals should consider adding directed questions about walking limitations and claudication symptoms to the routine review of physiological systems of these individuals. In the recent national PAD Awareness, Risk, and Treatment: New Resources for Survival (PARTNERS) study, patients at increased risk for PAD were screened for presence of the disease.[3] According to the PARTNERS criteria, a history of IC should be obtained in persons in whom PAD is likely to be present. These include individuals with other atherosclerotic syndromes (e.g., coronary or carotid arterial disease or their clinical sequelae), those who are over 70 years of age, or those over 50 years of age with a history of smoking or diabetes.[3] In this study, for which nearly 7,000 individuals were surveyed for PAD in diverse office practices, classic claudication symptoms, as narrowly defined by the Rose questionnaire, were present in only 6% to 10% of those with PAD. In contrast, as many as 25% of subjects had a "history of claudication" as recorded by the physician. Importantly, fewer than half of the subjects in this at-risk population were without any limb symptoms.[3] These data support the concept that a "walking impairment history" and specific claudication history should be considered part of the "review of systems" in populations who are "at risk."

Health professionals should be aware that patient descriptions of symptoms of IC may not always meet the criteria described above. For some patients, IC will meet the classic definition, whereas for others it will be reported as an exertional fatigue or even numbness. "Leg pain" is often accepted by patients in Western societies as an inevitable consequence of growing older, and the symptoms may be attributed by both patient and physician alike to nonvascular etiologies, such as degenerative joint disease, diabetic neuropathy, or simple deconditioning. Physicians should consider the possibility of IC in their patients with leg pain, even if they do not demonstrate classic symptoms of IC.

6.3.1.1 Diagnosis of Peripheral Arterial Disease and Claudication

To most sensitively assess the presence of PAD and its severity, the ankle–brachial index (ABI) should be performed (see Chapter 5). This measure is easily conducted in any office setting. An ABI value less than 0.90 establishes the diagnosis of PAD.[19] Whereas it has been noted by many vascular practitioners that ABI values between 0.50 and 0.90 are common in patients with IC, the relation between ABI values and the severity of IC is generally poor.[20] Some individuals may experience moderate to severe symptoms despite mild decrements in the ABI (as with aortoiliac stenoses), whereas others may experience (or complain of) few symptoms with much more severe decreases in the ABI value.

Claudication should be considered in patients who present with an absent pulse in the leg or in patients with any exertional leg symptoms. In these patients, and in those meeting the PARTNERS criteria,[3] an evaluation should take place to determine the severity of the disease and the degree of impairment imposed by it (see Figure 6.1).

The diagnosis of IC is occasionally clouded by the presence of comorbid medical conditions that can mimic the walking impairment caused by PAD. Examples of these conditions include pseudoclaudication (typically caused by spinal stenosis), degenerative joint disease,

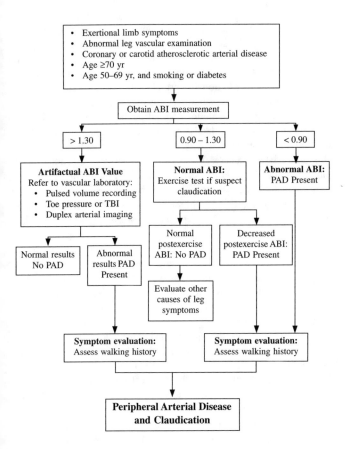

FIGURE 6.1 Peripheral arterial disease and claudication diagnosis algorithm. ABI = ankle–brachial index; PAD = peripheral arterial disease; TBI = toe–brachial index; Walking history = limitation in walking imposed by claudication. (Adapted from Hiatt, W.R., Medical treatment of peripheral arterial disease and claudication, *N. Engl. J. Med.* [in press]).

and peripheral neuropathy. These disorders may impair walking ability and can produce claudication-like symptoms. For such patients, the description of limb symptoms may offer clues that suggest a neural etiology, as patients may describe a "shooting" or "burning" quality to the discomfort. Additionally, pseudoclaudication is more likely to be induced by prolonged standing, or by extension of the lumbar spine. These patients may be able to "walk through" their nonvascular limb pain, which is much less likely in patients with ischemic claudication. In contrast, a correct diagnosis of vascular claudication requires an abnormal ABI and a careful history. If the history of exertional symptoms does not adequately differentiate the cause of the limb symptoms, or if the history is consistent with PAD but the resting ABI is normal (greater than 0.90), then the clinician can improve diagnostic accuracy by use of the exercise Doppler (also known as the "exercise ABI") stress test (see Chapter 5).

PAD-associated IC should elicit exertional muscle symptoms that are associated with a fall in the post-exercise ABI, whereas pseudoclaudication may elicit similar symptoms but with preservation of the ankle blood pressure measured after exercise. If there is no fall in the ABI after exercise, then alternative causes of the leg symptoms should be considered.

To summarize, for the patient who has leg pain on exertion, an ABI should be determined and questions should be utilized to assess the differential diagnosis (see Figure 6.1). Symptoms typical of IC, including leg discomfort (most typically in the calf), are reproducibly present with walking but consistently resolve with rest. It also is important to evaluate the limitations imposed by IC. This is because the perceived effect of these limitations as an impediment to the patient's functional goals will help direct the therapeutic approach to each patient's care.

6.3.2 OBJECTIVE EVALUATION OF CLAUDICATION SEVERITY

As with all cardiovascular illnesses, patient care can be enhanced by objective assessment of the severity of the primary disease symptom and of the disease itself. Just as care strategies for patients with coronary artery disease (CAD) are appropriately modified based on both the magnitude of the anginal symptoms and the extent of the anatomic CAD, so too PAD care should be prescribed in response to objective measures of the claudication symptom and PAD severity. Within this framework, treatments to improve functional status in patients with IC may be best used within the context of validated assessments of exercise performance and functional status. The primary tools that can be used for this purpose include exercise treadmill measurements and questionnaires.

6.3.2.1 Measurement of Exercise Performance

Most recent studies have used treadmill testing as the primary objective measure of changes in performance from a treatment for PAD. The typical treadmill protocol for persons with PAD differs from the protocols used to test normal subjects or persons with CAD. For normal subjects, the treadmill speed and grade are sequentially raised to provide a stepwise, but rapid, increase in workload so as to best assess central (cardiac and pulmonary) limitations to exercise. For patients with CAD, the exercise workload also increases in stages (by either increasing speed or grade) to symptom-limited maximal exertion but typically with lesser or more gradual increases of grade and speed. In contrast to the protocols used for healthy persons and for persons with CAD, PAD protocols do not call for increases in speed for the duration of the treadmill test. One widely used treadmill assessment for persons with PAD is also a "graded protocol," but the speed is fixed, as the grade increases every 2 or 3 minutes to a symptom-limited maximal (or "peak") performance.[21] This is because patients are often very limited as to speed of walking. Another widely used type of PAD exercise protocol is the "constant load" protocol, where both speed and grade are fixed. The primary endpoint of a treadmill test for the PAD patient is typically "peak walking time" (also called "absolute claudication distance"). This measure represents the maximum time a patient can walk on the treadmill. Often a secondary endpoint is the "pain-free walking time" (or "initial claudication distance"), which is the amount of time a patient can walk on the treadmill before the onset of IC.

6.3.2.2 Functional Status Measurements: The Claudication Questionnaire as Clinical Tool

To perform a comprehensive evaluation of functional status of the PAD population, standardized questionnaires can be incorporated in addition or as an alternative to treadmill tests. These questionnaires can be used to evaluate walking ability as well as broader areas such as health-related quality of life.[22,23] As with treadmill testing, it is recommended that standardized tools be used, and any PAD outcome questionnaire must be valid, reliable, and sensitive to change, as well as easy to use by both interviewer and patient. Several of the questionnaires used to assess function in persons with IC have been validated against treadmill walking performance. In the busy office setting, where treadmill testing for patients may not be available, valid questionnaires can be used as an effective surrogate tool for evaluating functional status. One example, the Walking Impairment Questionnaire (WIQ), has been validated against treadmill walking to assess walking impairment due to IC.[22,24] Another questionnaire, the Medical Outcomes Study Short Form-36 (SF-36), has been validated for use in all populations and has been widely used to evaluate health-related quality of life in individuals with IC.[23]

Thus, functional status and health-related quality of life questionnaires have been evaluated, validated, and utilized in the PAD population. These two questionnaires can provide additional and alternative ways of evaluating functional status.

6.4 TREATMENT OF CLAUDICATION

6.4.1 IMPACT OF CLAUDICATION ON FUNCTIONAL STATUS

Persons with IC often experience extreme disability in the absence of therapy. It has been observed that their walking ability is severely limited. Measurement of oxygen consumption, the "gold standard" measurement of cardiopulmonary functioning, reveals an approximate 50% decrement in individuals who present for treatment when compared with age-matched healthy controls (comparable to New York Heart Association [NYHA] class III heart failure).[20] In addition, questionnaire-based measures of walking ability, physical functioning, and health-related quality of life are decreased as well.[22–24] As a whole, the data confirm that IC has adverse effects on both functional status and quality of life. A limited ability to ambulate represents a life-altering disability such that individuals are often unable to perform their normal personal activities of daily living, satisfy their social obligations, or gainfully pursue their occupational activities. Individuals who experience IC usually suffer more or less the same level of walking impairment for the remainder of their lives. Although the claudication symptom is often relatively stable over a 5-year period,[25] deterioration may continue after initial diagnosis in as many as 10% to 20% of individuals.[26]

6.4.2   GOALS OF TREATMENT

For most patients with PAD, recognition of IC is a first step toward initiation of comprehensive medical therapies. Overall, the primary goal of treating IC should be to improve functional status and relieve disability. Thus, the clinician should strive to provide effective palliation or complete relief from the claudication symptom, thereby improving walking ability, community-based functional status, and maintaining patient autonomy and quality of life (see Figure 6.2).

6.4.3   TREATMENTS

6.4.3.1   Exercise Rehabilitation

A walking exercise program as a treatment for IC has been recommended for more than 50 years. There have been numerous reports on the efficacy and benefits of exercise training on walking ability for persons with PAD. [20,27–32]

Studies of exercise training are generally conducted in a supervised (usually hospital) setting, with the walking exercise performed on a treadmill.[20,32] Bouts of exercise are intermittent, the length of time for each bout being limited by the presence of moderate IC. Each bout is followed by a rest period to allow the claudication pain to subside.

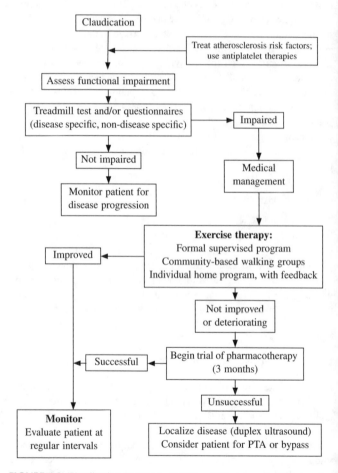

FIGURE 6.2 Claudication treatment algorithm. PTA = percutaneous transluminal angioplasty.

These exercise and rest sessions are repeated for 30 to 60 minutes, 2 to 3 times a week, for a total duration of 3 to 6 months, although some programs have been carried out for up to 1 year.

All studies of exercise conditioning in persons with PAD have reported an increase in graded treadmill exercise performance and a lessening of claudication pain severity during exercise.[20,27–32] Improvement in pain-free walking time ranged from 44% to 300%, while maximum walking time increased from 25% to 442% in the above studies. Thus, exercise training improves the ability to walk without claudication for longer periods and also for longer absolute periods of time. The consistency of these findings suggests that exercise training programs have a clinically important impact on functional capacity in PAD patients.

Of the randomized trials carried out to evaluate the efficacy of exercise rehabilitation, several assessed change in functional status using questionnaires.[22,24] These trials have uniformly shown that exercise rehabilitation improves functional status significantly in patients with PAD.

The relative efficacy of hospital-based versus home-based rehabilitation has been controversial, as the data now available are less clear for home-based programs. Some studies, particularly in Europe, have shown good results from a home-based program.[33,34] However, other studies have shown little benefit for this type of program.[35,36] In contrast, a hospital-based or supervised exercise rehabilitation program has provided consistent clinical improvement in almost every study. When such a supervised claudication rehabilitation program is possible, it is the preferred option. If a patient does not have access to such a program but is very motivated to exercise and will do so on a regular basis, a home-based program may provide some benefit. It is likely, however, in either type of program, that the degree of benefit will only approximate the degree of compliance.

Effective PAD exercise rehabilitation, as for all rehabilitative interventions that alter a patient's lifestyle, benefits from a system of social support.[37] For PAD rehabilitation to be succeed, it helps to be mindful of how other successful cost-effective rehabilitative interventions have succeeded in American medicine. For example, patients with acute or chronic lumbar pain might be effectively treated by physical therapy, medications, or laminectomy. Such patients are usually encouraged to first choose a non-operative approach in recognition of the high rates of clinical success that are thus often achieved. To accomplish these non-operative therapies, such patients are encouraged by their families, may be permitted time off work by their employer, are reimbursed for the cost of therapy by health-care insurers, and are permitted adequate time for a return to functional status. It is hoped that patients with IC would similarly be encouraged by physicians, employers, and health-care systems to enjoy the benefits of PAD claudication rehabilitation.

To summarize, exercise rehabilitation is a highly efficacious treatment for patients with PAD. There is no question that the great majority of patients who participate in such a program will improve walking ability. However, the role of PAD exercise rehabilitation will be determined to some extent by the rate of its acceptance by clinicians and PAD patients alike.

6.4.3.2   Pharmacologic Therapies

Numerous medications have been historically proposed for the treatment of IC; however, the current range of clinically relevant medications remains limited. The symptom of claudication has seemed, until recently, to be an elusive target for successful pharmacologic treatment. This is perhaps because targets for therapeutic intervention cover a wide range of possible mechanisms. The following discussion is not meant to be exhaustive, but to provide an assessment of the currently approved agents and a brief review of other medications being evaluated for the treatment of IC.

6.4.3.2.1   Pentoxifylline
Patients with PAD have been shown to have hemorheologic defects including non-deformable red cells, elevated fibrinogen levels, and increased platelet aggregation leading to increased blood viscosity.[38] The magnitude of effects of these phenomena on limb

blood flow during exercise are unknown. However, it has been reported that pentoxifylline, an agent that improves red cell deformability, lowers fibrinogen levels, and decreases platelet aggregation, increases walking distance in patients with PAD. In one trial, pentoxifylline produced a 22% improvement over placebo in walking distance before the onset of claudication and a 12% improvement in the maximum walking distance in controlled trials.[39]

6.4.3.2.2   Cilostazol

Cilostazol is the first new medication to gain U.S. Food and Drug Administration approval for the treatment of IC since the approval of pentoxifylline in 1984. Cilostazol belongs to the class of drugs called phosphodiesterase III inhibitors. Thus, the primary mechanism by which cilostazol alters vascular function is via increases in cyclic adenosine monophosphate, both in vascular smooth muscle cells and in platelets. This drug has both antiplatelet and vasodilatory properties.[40] In addition, cilostazol has antiproliferative properties, inhibiting vascular smooth muscle cell proliferation *in vitro*.[41]

The modest improvements in IC that can be obtained by pentoxifylline treatment, as described above, have limited the utility of this medication in the view of many vascular clinicians, especially as alternative therapies become increasingly available. Recently, the results were reported of a trial comparing cilostazol 100 mg twice daily with pentoxifylline 400 mg three times daily or placebo.[42] It was found that PAD patients taking cilostazol experienced a significant improvement in maximum walking distance on the treadmill of approximately 54% compared with baseline. In contrast, pentoxifylline improved walking distance by 30% and placebo improved walking distance by 34% compared with baseline. The improvement observed in walking distance with cilostazol was greater than that observed with either pentoxifylline or placebo.[42]

In other randomized, controlled, clinical trials, [43,44] cilostazol (100 mg bid) has also been shown to be efficacious for increasing pain-free walking time by 30% to 50% and maximum walking time by 50% to 80%. This improvement in pain-free and maximum walking ability requires that patients use the medication for at least 2 to 3 months.

Although this medication is well tolerated, the prescribing clinician should monitor the patient for any adverse effects, including headache, palpitations, nausea, or loose stools. The significant clinical benefits, as compared with adverse effects, were documented in the prospective trials of this medication. Cilostazol use was associated with significant improvements in functional status and quality of life, as measured by the SF-36 and WIQ. As mentioned above, in a single prospective trial reported to date, cilostazol was more effective than pentoxifylline in improving claudication symptoms.[42] Cilostazol also serves as the only claudication medication that, like exercise training, can elicit small improvements in the patient's lipid profile. The usual prescribed dose causes increases in HDL cholesterol concentration and decreases in fasting triglyceride levels. Thus, cilostazol appears to be an effective medication to ameliorate symptoms for patients with IC. Cilostazol should not be prescribed in patients with any clinical history of heart failure (specifically left ventricular systolic dysfunction, usually confirmed by an ejection fraction less than 0.40) because long-term use of other phosphodiesterase III inhibitors, as a class, has been associated with increased mortality in patients with severe heart failure.[45] For the practitioner, suspicion of underlying heart failure in a patient with PAD and IC should cause exclusion of this drug.

6.4.3.2.3   Other Potential Claudication Medications
Other pharmacotherapeutic medications are currently under active investigation for use in decreasing symptoms in patients with IC. These include metabolic agents (such as propionyl-L-carnitine), vasodilators (serotonin antagonists and arginine supplementation), orally active prostaglandins, and angiogenic growth factors (such as basic fibroblast growth factor and vascular endothelial growth factor). Information about these newer investigational drugs is outside the scope of this chapter and can be reviewed elsewhere.[46]

6.4.3.3   Limb Bypass Surgery or Percutaneous Transluminal Angioplasty

Patients with severe IC that is unresponsive to a reasonable trial of other medical treatments, and limits their home, leisure, or occupational activities, should be considered candidates for limb revascularization. Operative bypass procedures for IC are associated with a proven ability to improve functional status, [47,48] and these interventions may be particularly appropriate for patients with high-grade aortoiliac PAD, in which aortobifemoral bypass or femoral-femoral bypass may be associated with excellent long-term durability. However, all operative procedures in patients with PAD are associated with a procedure-derived cardiovascular ischemic risk, small perioperative mortality rate, and significant financial expense. Femoral-distal bypass may not always be associated with long-term patency or adequate improvement in symptoms, and not all patients present with limb arterial anatomy that permits adequate surgical revascularization. Thus, although surgical bypass should always be considered for selected individuals, other therapeutic interventions may be more appropriate in the treatment of IC and the majority of individuals with IC can be effectively managed without a surgical procedure.

Thus, the risk–benefit ratio should be carefully evaluated for patients who are considered for operative bypass for IC. Although limb bypass is less frequently used in the claudicating population, a functional benefit may be obtained, as suggested above. A study evaluating exercise performance and functional status in patients with IC who received peripheral bypass surgery revealed that these measures were substantially improved by the surgery.[48] Patient improvements in treadmill walking time of 100% were accompanied by a 200% improvement in the ability to walk distances and 100% in the ability to walk at faster speeds (by the WIQ) as well as improvements in claudication symptoms.[48]

Endovascular therapy with percutaneous transluminal angioplasty (PTA) is generally believed to be less invasive than surgical interventions and to be associated with lower morbidity. Thus, in theory, percutaneous revascularization could potentially be offered to more patients than might traditionally have been treated by surgical therapies. Although percutaneous revascularization procedures are quite safe, and can be effective, they are still associated with small rates of adverse effects (bleeding, hematomas, arterial dissection, contrast nephropathy, atheroembolism, and thrombosis), and rare severe complications may arise during such treatment and require an open surgical procedure. With such cautions, appropriate patient selection may also permit this endovascular approach to be applied with both great efficacy and reasonable durability. A detailed review of the indications and benefits of limb angioplasty, with or without stent placement, is beyond the scope of this chapter. However, patients with proximal aortoiliac PAD have been shown to receive particular benefit from such endovascular procedures.[49] In addition, a patient with IC and a femoropopliteal stenosis may also benefit from angioplasty.[50]

A randomized study comparing medical treatment in patients with IC showed that PTA improved treadmill walking more than conventional treatment.[51] However, of the 600 patients considered to be candidates for PTA, only 62 were found to have suitable lesions for this treatment. Another study used questionnaire assessment to evaluate functional status and quality of life in 29 patients with IC before and after PTA.[52] This study found that after PTA, perceived health state, mobility, usual activities, pain, and mood all improved significantly.

6.5   CONCLUSIONS

PAD is a marker of systemic atherosclerosis, and therefore is associated with an increased rate of cardiovascular ischemic events and increased mortality. Claudication is both the most common and easily recognized symptom of PAD and is associated with decreased functional status and quality of life. Although large vessel arterial stenoses represent the initial lesion responsible for exertional limb ischemia and discomfort, a series of complex pathophysiologic consequences to leg muscles and nerves also contribute to the development of IC. Therapies for IC, therefore, can target the stenosis, the collateral microvessels, or the working skeletal muscles themselves, and each potential therapeutic target is associated with potential efficacy. Although past treatments of IC have relied on revascularization, these invasive strategies are feasible in only a subset of patients, are associated with a finite procedural risk of both cardio-vascular ischemic events and limb loss, and have limited durability. Angioplasty, with or without stent placement, may be effective. Proximal (above-knee) surgical limb bypass may be feasible, but is not indicated in the great majority of patients. The benefits of a supervised walking exercise program have been consistently demonstrated in persons with PAD, and exercise rehabilitation constitutes a hallmark of care for individuals who experience IC and who are motivated to participate in supervised programs of therapeutic exercise. Pharmacologic therapy with cilostazol should also be considered for patients with IC in the absence of symptoms of heart failure or evidence of left ventricular systolic dysfunction. In the next few years, newer "second-generation" claudication pharmacotherapies are likely to become available. All therapies that are used to treat claudication should ideally incorporate objective measures of functional status, quality of life, and treadmill walking to ascertain the benefit of the treatment for the individual patient.

REFERENCES

1. Criqui, M.H., Fronek, A., Barrett-Connor, E., et al., The prevalence of peripheral arterial disease in a defined population, *Circulation*, 71, 510, 1985.
2. Hiatt, W.R., Hoag, S., and Hamman, R.F., Effect of diagnostic criteria on the prevalence of peripheral arterial disease, The San Luis Valley diabetes study, *Circulation*, 91,1472, 1995.
3. Hirsch, A.T., Criqui, M.H., Treat-Jacobson, D., et al., The PARTNERS Program: A National Survey of Peripheral Arterial Disease Prevalence, Awareness, and Ischemic Risk. *Circulation*, in press.
4. Hirsch, A.T., Treat-Jacobson, D., Lando, H.A., et al., The role of tobacco cessation, antiplatelet and lipid-lowering therapies in the treatment of peripheral arterial disease, *Vasc. Med.*, 1997, 2, 243.
5. Kannel, W.B., Shurtleff, D., National Heart and Lung Institute, National Institutes of Health, The Framingham study: cigarettes and the development of intermittent claudication, *Geriatrics*, 28, 61, 1973.

6. Kannel, W.B. and McGee, D.L., Update on some epidemiologic features of intermittent claudication: the Framingham Study, *J. Am. Geriatr. Soc.*, 33, 3, 1985.

7. Johansson, J., Egberg, N., Hohnsson, H., et al., Serum lipoproteins and hemostatic function in intermittent claudication, *Arterioscler. Thromb.*, 13, 1441, 1993.

8. Murabito, J.M., D'Agostino, R.B., Silbershatz, H., et al., Intermittent claudication: a risk profile from The Framingham Heart Study, *Circulation*, 96, 44, 1997.

9. Taylor, L.M., DeFrang, R.D., Harris, E.J., et al., The association of elevated plasma homocyst(e)ine with progression of symptomatic peripheral arterial disease, *J. Vasc. Surg.*, 13,128, 1991.

10. Shepherd, J., Cobbe, S.M., Ford, I., et al., Prevention of coronary heart disease with pravastatin in men with hypercholesterolemia, West of Scotland Coronary Prevention Study Group, *N. Engl. J. Med.*,333,1301, 1995.

11. Randomised trial of cholesterol lowering in 4444 patients with coronary heart disease: the Scandinavian Simvastatin Survival Study (4S), *Lancet*, 344,1383, 1994.

12. Sheps, S.G., Overview of JNC VI: new directions in the management of hypertension and cardiovascular risk, *Am. J. Hypertens.*, 12, 65S, 1999.

13. Report of the National Cholesterol Education Program Expert Panel on Detection, Evaluation, and Treatment of High Blood Cholesterol in Adults, The Expert Panel, *Arch. Intern. Med.*, 148, 36, 988.

14. Pedersen, T.R., Kjekshus, J., Pyorala, K., et al., Effect of simvastatin on ischemic signs and symptoms in the Scandinavian simvastatin survival study (4S), *Am. J. Cardiol.*, 81, 333, 1998.

15. Blankenhorn, D.H., Azen, S.P., Crawford, D.W., et al., Effects of colestipol-niacin therapy on human femoral atherosclerosis, *Circulation*, 83, 438, 1991.

16. Antiplatelet Trialists' Collaboration, Collaborative overview of randomised trials of antiplatelet therapy–I: prevention of death, myocardial infarction, and stroke by prolonged antiplatelet therapy in various categories of patients, *BMJ*, 308, 81, 1994.

17. CAPRIE Steering Committee, A randomised blinded trial of clopidogrel versus aspirin in patients at risk of ischaemic events (CAPRIE), *Lancet*, 348,1329, 1996.

18. McDermott, M.M., Mehta, S., Ahn, H., et al., Atherosclerotic risk factors are less intensively treated in patients with peripheral arterial disease than in patients with coronary artery disease, *J. Gen. Intern. Med.*, 12, 209, 1997.

19. Hiatt, W.R., Hoag, S., and Hamman, R.F., Effect of diagnostic criteria on the prevalence of peripheral arterial disease, The San Luis Valley diabetes study, *Circulation*, 91,1472, 1995.

20. Hiatt, W.R., Regensteiner, J.G., Hargarten, M.E., et al., Benefit of exercise conditioning for patients with peripheral arterial disease, *Circulation*, 81, 602, 1990.

21. Hiatt, W.R., Nawaz, D., Regensteiner, J.G., et al., The evaluation of exercise performance in patients with peripheral vascular disease, *J. Cardiopulm. Rehabil.*, 12, 525, 1988.

22. Regensteiner, J.G., Steiner, J.F., Panzer, R.J., and Hiatt, W.R., Evaluation of walking impairment by questionnaire in patients with peripheral arterial disease, *J. Vasc. Med. Biol.*, 2,142, 1990.

23. Tarlov, A.R., Ware, J.E., Jr., Greenfield, S., et al., The medical outcomes study, an application of methods for monitoring the results of medical care, *JAMA* 262, 925, 1989.

24. Regensteiner, J.G., Steiner, J.F., and Hiatt, W.R., Exercise training improves functional status in patients with peripheral arterial disease (PAD), *J. Vasc. Surg.*, 23,104,1996.

25. Lassila, R., Lepantalo, M., and Lindfors, O., Peripheral arterial disease—natural outcome, *Acta Med. Scand.*, 220, 295, 1986.

26. Weitz, H.H., Cardiac risk stratification prior to vascular surgery, *Med. Clin. North Am.*, 77, 377, 1993.

27. Larsen, O.A. and Lassen, N.A., Effect of daily muscular exercise in patients with intermittent claudication, *Lancet*, 2,1093, 1966.

28. Skinner, J.S. and Strandness, D.E., Exercise and intermittent claudication. II. Effect of physical training, *Circulation*, 36, 23, 1967.

29. Zetterquist, S., The effect of active training on the nutritive blood flow in exercising ischemic legs, *Scand. J. Clin. Lab. Invest.*, 25, 101, 1970.

30. Alpert, J.S., Larsen, O.A., and Lassen, N.A., Exercise and intermittent claudication. Blood flow in the calf muscle during walking studied by the xenon-133 clearance method, *Circulation*, 39, 353,1969.

31. Lepantalo, M., Sundberg, S., and Gordin, A., The effects of physical training and flunarizine on walking capacity in intermittent claudication, *Scand. J. Rehab. Med.*, 16,159, 1984.

32. Mannarino, E., Pasqualini, L., Innocente, S., et al., Physical training and antiplatelet treatment in stage II peripheral arterial occlusive disease: alone or combined? *Angiology*, 42, 513, 1991.

33. Hiatt, W.R., Wolfel, E.E., Meier, R.H., and Regensteiner, J.G., Superiority of treadmill walking exercise vs. strength training for patients with peripheral arterial disease: implications for the mechanism of the training response, *Circulation*, 90, 1866, 1994.

34. Jonason, T., Ringqvist, I., and Oman-Rydberg, A., Home-training of patients with intermittent claudication, *Scand. J. Rehabil. Med.*, 13,137, 1981.

35. Neilsen, S.L., Larsen, B., Prahl, M., et al., Hospitalstraening contra hjemmetraening af patienter med claudicatio intermittens, *Ugeskrift for Laeger*, 139, 2733, 1977.

36. Regensteiner, J.G., Meyer, T., Krupski, W., et al., Hospital vs. home-based exercise rehabilitation for patients with peripheral arterial occlusive disease, *Angiology*, 48, 291, 1997.

37. Hirsch, A.T. and Ekers, M.A., A comprehensive vascular medical therapeutic approach to peripheral arterial disease: the foundation of effective vascular rehabilitation, in *Vascular Nursing*, 3rd edition, Fahey, V. A., Ed., W.B. Saunders, Philadelphia, 1999.

38. Smith, F.B., Lowe, G.D., Rumley, A., et al., Smoking, hemorheologic factors and progression of peripheral arterial disease in patients with claudication, *J. Vasc. Surg.*, 28, 129, 1998.

39. Porter, J.M., Cutler, B.S., Lee, B.Y., et al., Pentoxifylline efficacy in the treatment of intermittent claudication: multicenter controlled double-blind trial with objective assessment of chronic occlusive arterial disease patients, *Am. Heart J.*, 104, 66, 1982.

40. Ikeda, Y., Kikuchi, M., Murakami, H., et al., Comparison of the inhibitory effects of cilostazol, acetylsalicylic acid, and ticlopidine on platelet functions *ex vivo*, randomized, double-blind cross-over study, *Arzneimittelforschung*, 37, 563, 1987.

41. Ikeda, Y., Matsumata, T., Takenaka, K., et al., Effects of doxorubicin and/or cilostazol on cancer cells during liver regeneration after two-thirds hepatectomy in rats, *Oncology*, 55, 354, 1998.

42. Dawson, D.L., Cutler, B.S., Hiatt, W.R., et al., A comparison of cilostazol and pentoxifylline for treating intermittent claudication, *Am. J. Med.*, in press.

43. Beebe, H.G., Dawson, D.L., Cutler, B.S., et al., A new pharmacological treatment for intermittent claudication: results of a randomized, multicenter trial, *Arch. Intern. Med.*, 159, 2041, 1999.

44. Money, S.R., Herd, J. A., Isaacsohn, J.L., et al., Effect of cilostazol on walking distances in patients with intermittent claudication caused by peripheral vascular disease, *J. Vasc. Surg.*, 27, 267, 1998.

45. Cohn, J.N., Goldstein, S.O., Greenberg, B.H., et al., A dose-dependent increase in mortality with vesnarinone among patients with severe heart failure, Vesnarinone Trial Investigators, *N. Engl. J. Med.*, 339, 1810, 1998.

46. Hiatt, W.R., Medical treatment of peripheral arterial disease and claudication, *N. Engl. J. Med.*, in press.

47. Lundgren, F., Dahllof, A.G., Lundholm, K., et al., Intermittent claudication—surgical reconstruction or physical training? A prospective randomized trial of treatment efficiency, *Ann. Surg.*, 209, 346, 1989.

48. Regensteiner, J.G., Hargarten, M.E., Rutherford, R.B., and Hiatt, W.R., Functional benefits of peripheral vascular bypass surgery for patients with intermittent claudication, *Angiology*, 44, 1, 1993.

49. Becker, G.J., Katzen, B.T., and Dake, M.D., Noncoronary angioplasty, *Radiology*, 170, 921, 1989.

50. Hunink, M.G., Wong, J.B., Donaldson, M.C., et al., Revascularization for femoropopliteal disease: a decision and cost-effectiveness analysis, *JAMA*, 274,165, 1995.

51. Whyman, M.R., Fowkes, F.G., Kerracher, E.M., et al., Randomized controlled trial of percutaneous transluminal angioplasty for intermittent claudication, *Eur. J. Vasc. Endovasc. Surg.*, 12,167, 1996.

52. Cook, T.A., O'Regan, M., and Galland, R.B., Quality of life following percutaneous transluminal angioplasty for claudication, *Eur. J. Vasc. Endovasc. Surg.*, 11, 191, 1996.

7 Critical Limb Ischemia

Helen L. Moore and John V. White

CONTENTS

7.1 Introduction..120
7.2 Epidemiology...121
    7.2.1 Incidence 121
7.3. Natural History 121
7.4 Pathophysiology...123
7.5 Diagnosis and Evaluation 124
    7.5.1 Clinical Evaluation..124
        7.5.1.1 History 124
        7.5.1.2 Signs and Symptoms...125
        7.5.1.3 Physical Examination 126
7.6 Investigations 127
    7.6.1 Macrocirculatory Investigations.......................................127
        7.6.1.1 Ankle–Brachial Index 127
        7.6.1.2 Segmental Limb Systolic
                    Pressure Measurement.....................................127
        7.6.1.3 Segmental Plethysmography
                    or Pulse Volume Recordings...........................128
        7.6.1.4 Doppler Velocity Waveform.............................128
        7.6.1.5 Evaluation of Atherosclerosis
                    in the General Circulatory System 128
    7.6.2 Basic Hematological and Biochemical Tests 129
    7.6.3 Microcirculatory Investigations 129

0-8493-8413-3/01/$0.00+$1.50
© 2001 by CRC Press LLC

	7.6.4	Imaging	130
		7.6.4.1 Angiography	130
		7.6.4.2 Other Imaging Modalities	130
	7.6.5	Differential Diagnosis	131
7.7	Treatment		133
	7.7.1	Immediate Treatment	133
	7.7.2	Longer Term Treatment	135
	7.7.3	Nonoperative Treatment	136
		7.7.3.1 Pharmacotherapy	136
	7.7.4	Operative Intervention	136
		7.7.4.1 General Principles of Revascularization	136
		7.7.4.2 Aortoiliac Disease	137
		7.7.4.3 Infrainguinal Disease	138
	7.7.5	Alternative Therapies	138
	7.7.6	Amputation	138
	7.7.7	Surveillance after Interventional Therapy	139
References			141

7.1 INTRODUCTION

Critical limb ischemia (CLI) can be defined as chronic ischemic rest pain, ulcers, or gangrene due to objectively proven arterial occlusive disease.[1] Objective proof is normally obtained by recording ankle–brachial (ABI) or toe–brachial pressure indices. Patients falling within this definition equate to Fontaine stages III and IV or Rutherford categories 4, 5, and 6.[2,3] These patients range from those with mild rest pain that is controllable with analgesia to those with extensive gangrene, where major amputation is the only therapeutic option available. Although this may seem too simple a definition, alternatives such as hemodynamic criteria and the terms "limb-threatening ischemia" and "limb salvage" have proven to be too restrictive when applied to everyday clinical practice.

7.2 EPIDEMIOLOGY

7.2.1 INCIDENCE

Figures extrapolated from studies of intermittent claudication (IC) or based on hospitalizations and major amputations for CLI give an incidence ranging from 400 to 1,000 per million per year.[1] This figure equates to approximately one new patient developing CLI for every patient with IC in the population. Recent studies in which arterial disease was determined objectively have reported the proportion of patients with IC who progress to CLI as varying anywhere from 9% to 12.5%[4,5] up to 34% to 41%.[6,7]

7.3. NATURAL HISTORY

Data on the natural history of CLI comes from those patients who do not undergo intervention. However, because these patients have severe unreconstructable disease or failed primary intervention, this group is not truly representative of the natural history of the disease.

Smoking has been widely accepted as the most important modifiable risk factor for development of CLI. Jonason and colleagues found that, in patients with IC, 21% of those who smoked or who stopped smoking more than 1 year after initial evaluation went on to develop CLI compared with only 8% of patients who were nonsmokers or who stopped within 1 year of initial evaluation.[4]

Diabetes mellitus is also an important modifiable risk factor for progression to CLI. McDaniel and associates reported that, of patients with IC, 21% of those with coexisting diabetes went on to develop CLI requiring major amputation compared with just 3% of nondiabetics.[8] This finding was similar to those reported in other studies,[9,10] although two further investigations did not find diabetes to be a significant variable for progression of IC to CLI.[6,11] Hypertriglyceridemia[5] has been reported to be a risk factor and ABI [6,7,11] to be a predictor for progression from IC to CLI. Figure 7.1 shows the approximate magnitude of the increase in risk for developing CLI with each of the independent major risk factors.

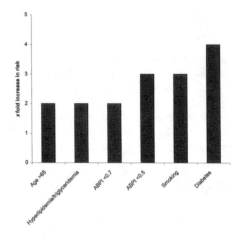

FIGURE 7.1   Increase in risk of developing CLI with each independent risk factor.

In the control or placebo arm of clinical trials, 30% to 49% of ulcers healed or reduced in size,[12–14] whereas 23% of patients had a reduction in rest pain.[15] However, these studies enrolled small numbers of patients and the maximum follow-up period was only 2 months. Overall, the prognosis for patients with untreated or untreatable CLI remains poor, with a 40% amputation rate,[16,17] a 27% mortality rate at 6 to 12 months,[15–17] and a mortality rate of 40% to 70% at 5 years.[18] Multicenter studies have reported rates from surgical series of approximately 20% amputation and 25% mortality at 1 to 2 years.[19,20] Single-center, large surgical series have reported mortality rates of 28% to 52% at 2 to 5 years.[21,22] In these series, approximately 50% of patients underwent revascularization, 25% underwent primary amputation, and 25% had either medical treatment, minor surgical treatment, or no treatment.[19,21,22] Studies have investigated whether the same risk factors for the progression of IC to CLI also influence patient outcome. One large, prospective study of patients with CLI found no association between mortality and sex, smoking, hypertension, diabetes, hypercholesterolemia, or ABI.[19] However, other studies have reported smoking,[23,24] diabetes,[24] age,[24] and the presence of gangrene, ulceration, or bilateral CLI[16,23] to be significantly associated with a poorer prognosis.

ABI has been suggested to be predictive of amputation risk by some studies,[25,26] although other studies found it to have little predictive value.[20,27] Approximately the same number of below-knee amputations are performed as above-knee amputations. However, full mobility is achieved in two to three times as many below-knee as above-knee amputees, and early hospital mortality ranges from 3% to 10% after below-knee amputation and almost 20% after above-knee amputation.[28] Despite favorable results for below-knee compared with above-knee amputations, the prognosis for below-knee amputees is still poor, with 50% dead and only 20% alive with one intact leg at 5 years. Table 7.1 summarizes the outcome of patients with critical limb ischemia for different treatment groups.

7.4   PATHOPHYSIOLOGY

The underlying disease process in CLI is progressive atherosclerosis. In the macrocirculation this causes severe narrowing or occlusion of the proximal arteries, thus reducing blood flow and perfusion pressure to the distal circulation. This condition is often complicated by thrombosis. Increased tissue pressure from venous insufficiency, emboli from other sites, and decreased cardiac output may all contribute to further reduction in the capillary perfusion.

The overlap of ankle or toe pressures found in patients with and without CLI illustrates the importance of the microcirculation in CLI. Capillary collapse due to low transmural pressure and interstitial edema, arteriolar vasospasm, microthrombosis, abnormal vasomotion, platelet aggregates, adhesive leukocytes, and local activation of the immune system are some of the processes that contribute to decreased capillary perfusion. Compensatory mechanisms,

TABLE 7.1
Outcome of Patients with Critical Limb Ischemia

Treatment[a] Group	Operative Mortality (%)	Mortality (%) 6-12 mo	2–5 yr
Revascularization	0–6	20–25	28–52
Primary amputation			
Below knee	3–10		
Above knee	20	50[b]	70[b]
Medical, minor surgical, or no treatment	44[c]	27	40–70

[a] At initial presentation.
[b] Mortality data beyond 30 days are not segregated by amputation type.
[c] Mortality during initial hospitalization.

Adapted from Lepantalo, M. and Matzke, S., *Eur. J. Vasc. Endovasc. Surg.*, 11, 153, 1996;[16] Criqui, M.H., et al., *N. Engl. J. Med.*, 1992, 326, 381;[18] ICAI Group, *Eur J. Vasc. Surg.*, 14, 91, 1997;[19] Wolfe, J.N., *Br. J. Surg.*, 73, 318, 1986[20]; Veith, F.J., et al., *Ann. Surg.*, 194, 386, 1981.[22]

such as collateral formation in the macrocirculation and arteriolar vasodilation in the microcirculation, attempt to maintain nutritive flow. CLI results when decreased macrocirculatory blood flow, maldistribution of skin microcirculation, and insufficient compensatory mechanisms combine.

7.5 DIAGNOSIS AND EVALUATION

7.5.1 CLINICAL EVALUATION

7.5.1.1 History

Patients with CLI present with symptoms that range from mild rest pain that can be relieved with analgesia to extensive gangrene. The main presenting symptom is usually pain that typically occurs at night. The pain is often localized in the distal part of the foot, unlike IC, where the pain is experienced in a muscle group. The patient will often complain of being awakened by the pain at night and of gaining partial relief by hanging the affected limb down over the side of the bed, sleeping in a reclining chair, or taking a short walk around the room. The tendency to keep the limb dependent can be counterproductive because it leads to edema, which further compromises tissue perfusion. The presence of paresthesia, muscle paresis, and contracture of the knee or ankle joint contribute to the reduced limb function. Strong analgesia is usually required in large regular doses. In cases where the blood flow has fallen below the level required to maintain normal resting tissue metabolism, the patient presents with tissue necrosis. At the time of ulcer formation, patients may experience temporary relief from ischemic pain, but this pain usually increases again if inflammation and local infection are present. In the most severe cases, pain only diminishes or totally disappears when complete gangrene of the ischemic limb has developed.

Documentation of patient history should include any family history of cardiovascular disease plus the onset and duration of other risk factors, i.e., cigarette usage, diabetes mellitus, hypertension, and hyperlipidemia. Current treatment for coexisting conditions and any previous arterial interventions should be noted.

7.5.1.2   Signs and Symptoms

The skin of the affected limb is often atrophied and appears shiny and scaly with loss of hair growth. The skin feels cool, although it may be warmer surrounding an area of infection or inflammation. Toenails are often thickened by delayed growth. Skin color is usually pale or cyanotic, but there may be rubor on dependency where even slight application of pressure produces pallor. Capillary refill may occur so quickly that it might be mistaken for an indication of hyperemia rather than chronic dilatation of the pre- and postcapillary vessels caused by chronic ischemia.

Trophic lesions usually form on the pressure points of the foot, such as the ends of toes or the heel, or where trauma is caused (e.g., while cutting toenails). Ulcers due to arterial disease usually have irregular margins. The base of the ulcer can be either pale or inflamed and, if present, local infection may cause production of exudate or pus. Gangrene often develops in the digits, but, in more severe cases, involves the whole forefoot. If local infection is not present, gangrenous tissue tends to shrink, develop a clear demarcation line between viable and nonviable tissue, mummify, and autoamputate the affected tissue.

7.5.1.3 Physical Examination

The skin of the legs and feet and the nails should be examined for the signs and symptoms detailed above. Skin color and changes in temperature, plus any other abnormalities such as edema or scarring from previous ulceration should be noted. The femoral, popliteal, dorsalis pedis, and posterior tibial artery pulses should be palpated, remembering that one or the other of the two pedal pulses is not palpable in a small number of normal cases.[18] Pulses are graded as 0 = absent, 1 = diminished, and 2 = normal. An especially prominent pulse might indicate an aneurysm and should be investigated further. Additional useful information is gained by auscultation of proximal vessels for bruits, especially over the iliofemoral segment. The finding of decreased amplitude of femoral pulse, for example, in conjunction with a loud bruit proximally over the iliac artery usually indicates the presence of a significant iliac lesion. In cases of complete occlusion, bruits will not be present, but an absent pulse distal to the occlusion would be a consistent physical finding.

CLI is often coexistent with other arterial disease. Therefore, the physical examination should assess the circulatory system as a whole for incidental findings of systemic hypertension, carotid bruits, cardiac murmur or arrhythmia, or abdominal aortic aneurysm.

7.6   INVESTIGATIONS

7.6.1   MACROCIRCULATORY INVESTIGATIONS

7.6.1.1   Ankle–Brachial Index

Ankle pressure should be recorded in all patients. A sphygmomanometer cuff is placed above the ankle, and the Doppler probe
detects the systolic pressure in the posterior tibial and then the
dorsalis pedis artery on deflating the cuff. Ankle pressure is standardized against the highest brachial pressure to give the ABI. The
ABI varies between observers such that a change in ABI of less
than 0.15 is not considered to be clinically significant (or 0.10 if
there is a change in clinical status).[3] Patients with calcified arteries,
such as diabetics, may have falsely high ankle pressures due to their
incompressible arteries. In these patients, toe pressure can be
recorded instead because the more distal pedal vessels are usually
preserved and not calcified. A small digital cuff is placed on the
hallux or second toe, while a flow sensor, such as a plethysmograph
with a light-emitting diode, detects the systolic pressure as the cuff
is deflated. Ischemic rest pain most often occurs below an ankle
pressure of 40 mm Hg or a toe pressure of 30 mm Hg (which
corresponds to Society for Vascular Surgery / International Society
for Cardiovascular Surgery[3] category 4).

7.6.1.2   Segmental Limb Systolic Pressure Measurement

The ankle (see above) is the most commonly used level to record
systolic pressure, but measurements can be obtained at other levels
on the leg to accurately detect and localize hemodynamically significant lesions. Segmental limb systolic pressure measurement (SLP)
is obtained in the same way as described above. A sphygmomanometer cuff is placed at the desired level on the leg while a Doppler
probe held over one of the pedal arteries will detect the systolic
pressure in the major arteries underneath the cuff. The location of
arterial lesions becomes apparent from the pressure gradients

between the different levels. Using a normal-width cuff on the upper and lower thigh allows differentiation between proximal and distal disease, although this gives rise to pressures that are artifactually higher by approximately 25%. Using a larger-width thigh cuff gives a low false positive rate but does not distinguish well between proximal and distal disease.

7.6.1.3   Segmental Plethysmography or Pulse Volume Recordings

When taking segmental plethysmography or pulse volume recording (PVR), a mercury-in-silastic tube strain gauge or calibrated air-filled cuff is placed around the limb at the selected level. It is then connected to a plethysmograph, which produces a PVR. The presence of a significant lesion at a particular level can be determined by comparing the magnitude and contour of the PVRs of the proximal and distal cuffs. Using PVR in conjunction with SLP has been shown to be 95% accurate compared with angiography in detecting hemodynamically significant lesions.

7.6.1.4   Doppler Velocity Waveform

Doppler velocity waveform (VWF) can be used instead of PVR but is highly operator dependent. The arterial VWF is recorded using a continuous-wave Doppler. Qualitative differences in the magnitude and contour of the VWF between adjacent recording levels detect the presence of a hemodynamically significant lesion.

7.6.1.5   Evaluation of Atherosclerosis in the General Circulatory System

Almost 30% of patients with peripheral arterial disease (PAD) have clinically significant coronary atherosclerosis. However, because as many as 90% have anatomically significant coronary vessel disease, all patients with PAD should be considered at high risk for myocardial infarction.[29] Therefore, a resting electrocardiogram should be obtained in all patients with CLI when a recent report is not available. Patients at risk for peripheral embolization often have atrial fibrillation; therefore, an echocardiogram should be performed when embolization is suspected. Further investigations of the coronary circulation and referral to a cardiologist may be indicated.

Approximately 10% to 15% of patients with PAD have clinically evident cerebrovascular disease, but, as with coronary disease, the anatomic prevalence is much higher. Studies have revealed anatomically significant carotid disease in up to 57% of patients with PAD.[30] These patients should also be considered at high risk for stroke. For patients with any history suggestive of carotid disease or with a carotid bruit, a duplex Doppler scan of the carotid bifurcation is justified. The cost-effectiveness of performing duplex scans on all patients with CLI has not been established. In addition, a chest radiogram, computed tomography, or ultrasound of the abdominal aorta may be indicated in selected patients.

7.6.2   BASIC HEMATOLOGICAL AND BIOCHEMICAL TESTS

In all patients presenting with CLI, the following basic laboratory tests should be carried out:

- Complete blood count
- Platelet count
- Blood glucose or hemoglobin A_{1c}
- Urea, creatinine
- Lipid profile

In atypical patients, such as those with early-age onset, atypical distribution of lesions, history of thrombotic events, or lack of common risk factors, homocysteine levels and a hypercoagulability screen are additional laboratory tests that should be conducted.

7.6.3   MICROCIRCULATORY INVESTIGATIONS

Various techniques, such as transcutaneous partial pressure of oxygen ($TcPO_2$), laser Doppler flowmetry, and capillary microscopy, have been used to investigate microcirculation in CLI. While these techniques are useful complements to the macrocirculatory investigations and imaging studies, intervention in patients with CLI should not be delayed in order to perform these tests. TcPO$_2$ has a positive predictive value of 77% to 87% for classifying severe ischemia,[31] and it is generally accepted that a reading of 30 mm Hg (±10 mm Hg) predicts nonhealing.[32] Capillary microscopy visualizes the nutritive skin capillaries directly and allows tissue ischemia to be estimated.[33] Capillary morphology can reveal underlying conditions such as systemic collagen disease. Recording the peak red blood cell velocity during reactive hyperemia yields additional data useful for detecting CLI.[33]

7.6.4 IMAGING

7.6.4.1 Angiography

Because detailed anatomy of the arterial tree is required to plan intervention, angiography remains the imaging of choice in most cases of CLI. A complete angiogram from the level of the renal arteries to the pedal arch should be performed. Angiography carries minimal risk of contrast reaction, severe complications, risk, and mortality.[34] Nevertheless, cost considerations and patient discomfort mean that other imaging modalities are being increasingly used in place of, or before, angiography.

7.6.4.2 Other Imaging Modalities

Duplex imaging is noninvasive, carries no risk, and is relatively inexpensive. Most of the anatomical and functional information needed in the management of CLI can be obtained with duplex scanning, but there is the disadvantage of its being highly operator dependent. Contrast-enhanced magnetic resonance angiography (MRA) has been reported to be comparable to conventional angiography[35] but is not available in all centers. Further studies will be needed to determine to what extent these alternative imaging modalities can replace conventional angiography.

7.6.5   DIFFERENTIAL DIAGNOSIS

Causes of foot pain can be differentiated from ischemic pain as follows:

- Diabetic sensory neuropathy can be differentiated from ischemic pain in that the former is usually symmetrically distributed in both legs and is associated with cutaneous hypersensitivity, failure to gain relief by dependency, and decreased reflexes.[36] Vibratory assessment with a tuning fork is a simple, reliable test that can be included in the physical examination of these patients to detect diabetic neuropathy. Less common causes of sensory neuropathy include vitamin B12 deficiency,[37] alcohol intake,[38] and certain drugs.[39]

- Reflex sympathetic dystrophy usually results from trauma and features pain that is often burning, hypersensitivity along a dermatome, and autonomic imbalance (usually hyperhidrosis and mottling cyanosis).

- Nerve root compression is typically associated with backache, pain along the course of a dermatome, and limited straight-leg raising.

- Night cramps are common but may be differentiated from ischemic pain because they are usually associated with muscle spasm and involve the calf as well as the foot.

- Other conditions that should be considered when a patient presents with foot pain include gout, rheumatoid arthritis, tarsal tunnel nerve compression, or plantar fasciitis. Table 7.2 summarizes the characteristics that allow differentiation between common foot and leg ulcers. Figure 7.2 presents an algorithm for evaluating patients presenting with foot pain with or without ulcers or gangrene.

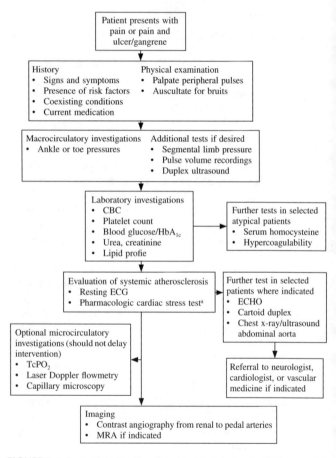

FIGURE 7.2 Evaluation algorithm for critical limb ischemia. CBC = complete blood count; ECG = electrocardiogram; ECHO = echocardiogram; HbA₁c = hemoglobin A₁c; MRA = magnetic resonance angiography; TcPO₂ = transcutaneous oxygen. [a]May be considered in high-risk patients, those with angina or other cardiac symptoms

7.7 TREATMENT

7.7.1 Immediate Treatment

While investigations and imaging are being performed to plan intervention, the immediate treatment of patients also includes controlling pain, wound care, prevention of thrombosis or progression of existing thrombosis, and treatment of coexisting conditions that may be contributing to the ischemia.

Pain control can be monitored using simple pain scales. Regular administration of analgesics gives better control than analgesia on demand. For mild to moderate pain, nonsteroidal anti-inflammatory drugs, or acetaminophen, are usually prescribed; more-severe pain requires treatment with narcotics. Use of a tilting bed or reclining chair may give additional relief by allowing dependency of the limb.

Topical antibiotics have not been shown to be of benefit in CLI. Systemic antibiotics can be used when infection or cellulitis is evident. Debridement of ischemic ulcers should be kept to minimum. Saline-soaked dressings should be used to help remove pus and tissue debris, and dry dressings can be used once the ulcer is dry. There are insufficient data to recommend seaweed and hydrophilic dressings in the treatment of ischemic ulcers. If an ischemic ulcer is on the weight-bearing area of the foot, mobilization should be limited; otherwise, walking should be promoted.

Thromboembolism or progression of existing thrombosis in the hospitalized patient is prevented by administration of subcutaneous heparin. Coexisting conditions that may influence the CLI should be treated. For example, improving poor cardiac function may improve peripheral perfusion. Nonselective β-adrenergic blockers for treatment of hypertension or angina may aggravate ischemic symptoms, although there is evidence that pretreatment with β-blockers reduces the risk of postoperative cardiac events in patients undergoing major vascular surgery.[40]

TABLE 7.2
Characteristics of Common Ulcers

Origin	Cause	Location	Pain	Appearance
Main arteries	PAD, Buerger's, acute occlusion	Toes, foot	Severe	Irregular, pale base
Venous	Venous disease	Malleolar	Mild	Irregular pink base
Skin infarct	Systemic disease, embolism, hypertension	Lower third of leg	Severe	Small, often multiple
Neurotrophic	Neuropathy	Sole and pressure points of foot	None	Often deep, infected

PAD = peripheral arterial disease. (From TransAtlantic Inter-Society Consensus (TASC), *J. Vasc. Surg.,* 31, S1, 2000.[1] With permission.)

7.7.2 LONGER TERM TREATMENT

The priorities of patient management in CLI are to treat the symptoms and carry out prompt intervention as discussed. In addition, patients with CLI are at high risk for cardiovascular disease, so aggressive systemic risk factor control is warranted in the overall management plan, despite the end-stage nature of CLI. Risk factor control should include the following (see also Natural History):

- *Smoking cessation* should be strongly encouraged. Amputation rates have been reported as 11% to 23% in those patients who continue to smoke compared with 0% to 10% in those who cease smoking.[41] Patient survival at 1, 3, and 5 years is also highly correlated with smoking; therefore, even for patients with end-stage disease, smoking cessation is still highly beneficial. Birkenstock and associates found that 85% of patients who stopped smoking had improvement in symptoms of lower leg ischemia compared with only 20% of those who continued to smoke.[42]
- *Diabetes mellitus* parameters should be tightly controlled at target levels: fasting blood sugar less than 120 mg/dL, postprandial sugar less than 180 mg/dL, and glycohemoglobin levels less than 7.0%.
- *Hyperlipidemia* control should follow the same National Cholesterol Education Program guidelines as for patients with IC, as both groups have the same lipid risk profile. Low-density lipoprotein cholesterol level should be less than 100 mg/dL.[43]
- *Hypertension* is a risk factor for all cardiovascular diseases and should be controlled. Nonselective β-blockers should be avoided where possible because of their vasoconstrictive effect. If used, CLI patients should be monitored for worsening of ischemic ulcers.

7.7.3   NONOPERATIVE TREATMENT

7.7.3.1   Pharmacotherapy

Prostanoids have been tested extensively in patients with CLI. In recent randomized controlled studies, prostanoids were shown to significantly reduce ulcer size, rest pain, and use of analgesics.[17,44,45] As there is some evidence of efficacy, prostanoids may be used to treat patients with unreconstructable disease, where surgery has a small chance of success or has previously failed, and where the alternative is amputation. Further studies are needed to establish whether prostanoids have a role as adjunctive therapy to operative intervention.

Studies have clearly shown that antiplatelet agents significantly reduce the incidence of cardiovascular ischemic events in high-risk groups. Therefore, all patients with arterial disease should receive long-term treatment with aspirin, ticlopidine, or clopidogrel.[46] Evidence also suggests that antiplatelet therapy may be of benefit in slowing progression of atherosclerosis[47] and improving long-term outcome after revascularization,[48] although this needs to be fully investigated. The role of other pharmacotherapies including anticoagulants,[49] hemodilution, defibrinogenating agents,[50] L-arginine,[51] and pentoxifylline[52] has not yet been fully established. Initial clinical studies of gene-induced therapeutic angiogenesis have shown increased collateral vessel development and reduced rest pain but further studies are needed.

7.7.4   OPERATIVE INTERVENTION

7.7.4.1   General Principles of Revascularization

The choice of operative intervention depends on predicted success, mortality and morbidity risk, lesion morphology, comorbid risk factors, previous procedures, and patient's life expectancy. In a few patients, when all such factors have been considered, primary amputation (see section 7.6) or pharmacotherapy (see section 7.7.3.1) emerges as the preferred option but, with technological advances, most patients are currently offered revascularization. Furthermore, failure of a revascularization procedure does not adversely affect leg survival or predispose to a higher level of amputation, and initial attempts at reconstruction are warranted. Patients with graft occlusions at 6 to 12 months are often pain free at rest and maintain a better quality of life than those with an amputation and prosthesis. Moneta and colleagues suggested that, postoperatively, patients with rest pain will require an ABI of 0.55 for relief of pain, whereas patients with gangrene require a postoperative resting ABI of more than 0.80 for healing.[53] Alternatively, an increase in ABI of 0.15 (or an increase of 0.10 with resolution of rest pain) has been suggested as a measure of clinical success.[3]

Endovascular techniques have a lower mortality and morbidity risk than surgical revascularization, but long-term success results are less well-documented in published literature. However, it is not always necessary to choose exclusively either an endovascular or surgical intervention. Most patients with CLI have multilevel disease, for which a combination of endovascular and surgical procedures may provide the best outcome. When all lesions are of equal severity, the most proximal lesion should be treated first. When lesions are of differing severity, the more severe lesion should be treated first, assuming that there is adequate inflow.

7.7.4.2 Aortoiliac Disease

Aortobifemoral bypass is the preferred intervention for aortoiliac disease in CLI because diffuse disease, for which endovascular techniques are unsuitable, is often present. Primary patency rates for surgical revascularization in CLI are 80% at 5 years and 72% at 10 years, with overall operative mortality of 0% to 3.3% and systemic morbidity of 8.3%.[54] Endovascular techniques have lower morbidity and mortality rates than surgery for aortoiliac disease[54] but have lower long-term patency results. For endovascular procedures, the primary patency rates at 4 years, adjusted to include technical failures, are 53% after percutaneous transluminal angioplasty (PTA) and 67% after stent placement for aortoiliac stenoses.[55]

7.7.4.3   Infrainguinal Disease

For surgical revascularization of infrainguinal disease, the choice of conduit has a major influence on long-term outcome. A meta-analysis of surgical bypass grafts for femoral distal grafts revealed results clearly in favor of autogenous vein.[56] The 5-year primary patency rates for autogenous vein, above-knee polytetrafluoroethylene (PTFE), and below-knee PTFE were 66%, 47%, and 33%, respectively.[56] A second review of published data also found autogenous vein to be the conduit of choice for below-knee femoropopliteal grafts.[57] Primary patency rates at 4 years for reverse saphenous vein, *in situ* vein bypass, human umbilical vein, and PTFE were 77%, 68%, 60%, and 40%, respectively.[57] Mortality rates of up to 6% have been reported.[58]

For endovascular treatment of femoropopliteal lesions, the weighted average primary patency for PTA was calculated to be 51% at 3 years, 48% at 5 years, and for stents was 58% at 3 years.[1] However, the majority of data are from claudicants, so it is therefore difficult to make comparisons with the results of surgery. Wagner and Rager carried out a review of PTA for infrapopliteal lesions.[59] From studies including only patients with CLI, the technical success rate was 82% to100% and limb salvage was 52% to 86% during a follow-up period ranging from 8 to 24 months.[59] Stents of infrapopliteal lesions show limb salvage rates of 60% to 80% at 2 years and seem to be dependent on anatomical factors.

7.7.5   ALTERNATIVE THERAPIES

Alternatives to the therapies already discussed have been proposed, including epidural electrical stimulation and chelation. To date, there is insufficient evidence from prospective controlled randomized studies to recommend these forms of treatment.

7.7.6   AMPUTATION

For patients with severe unreconstructable CLI, primary amputation is indicated when there is also necrosis of significant portions of weight-bearing areas of the foot; fixed, unremediable flexion contracture of the leg; or significantly reduced life expectancy due to terminal illness or comorbid conditions. Secondary amputation may be necessary when vessels become unreconstructable due to advancing atherosclerosis or in cases of persistent infection unresponsive to aggressive treatment. The aim of amputation is relief of rest pain; removal of diseased, infected, or necrotic tissue; complete healing; and construction of a stump suitable for ambulation with a prosthesis. Amputation should be at the most distal level possible to achieve healing. Various investigations, such as $TcPO_2$, have been suggested to select the appropriate level of amputation, but, in clinical practice, this is usually determined by clinical examination alone. When made by experienced surgeons, clinical determination of the amputation level results in uninterrupted primary healing of the below-knee stump in 75% to 85% of cases and the above-knee stump in 85% to 93% of cases.[60]

7.7.7   SURVEILLANCE AFTER INTERVENTIONAL THERAPY

After revascularization, patients should be entered into a surveillance program. The program should consist of:

- History and physical examination
- Resting ABI or toe pressure index in patients with incompressible arteries
- Color flow duplex scanning. General guidelines on duplex criteria indicative of a failing graft are a peak systolic velocity increase to more than 150 cm/s, a peak systolic velocity ratio of greater than 2.0 across a stenosis, or a reduction of peak systolic velocity to less than 45 cm/s. Duplex scanning is less useful in synthetic grafts. Most centers obtain a postoperative scan at 1 week or before discharge. Common programs then scan at 1, 3, 6, 12, 18, and 24 months, and then yearly thereafter. Cost-effectiveness of frequent surveillance beyond 2 years is controversial because of reduced incidence of graft failure after this

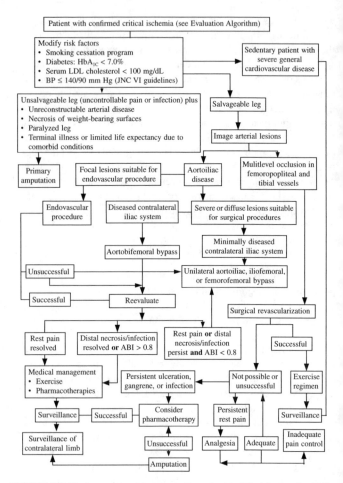

FIGURE 7.3 Treatment algorithm for confirmed critical limb ischemia. ABI= ankle–brachial index; BP = blood pressure; HbA_{1c} = hemoglobin a_{1c}; JNC VI = Joint National Committee on Prevention, Detection, Evaluation, and Treatment of High Blood Pressure; LDL = low-density lipoprotein.

time period.[61,62] Figure 7.3 depicts a treatment algorithm for patients with confirmed CLI.

REFERENCES

1. TransAtlantic Inter-Society Consensus (TASC), Management of peripheral arterial disease (PAD), *J. Vasc. Surg.*, 31, S1, 2000.
2. Fontaine, R., Kim, M., and Kieny, R., Die chirurgische Behandlung der peripheren Durch-blutungsstorungen, *Helv. Chir. Acta.*, 5/6, 199, 1954.
3. Rutherford, R.B., Baker, D., Ernst C., et al., Recommended standards for reports dealing with lower extremity ischemia, Revised version, *J. Vasc. Surg.*, 26, 517, 1997.
4. Jonason, T. and Ringqvist, I., Factors of prognostic importance for subsequent rest pain in patients with intermittent claudication, *Acta. Med. Scand.*, 218, 27, 1985.
5. Smith, I., Franks, P.J., Greenhalgh, R.M., et al., The influence of smoking cessation and hypertriglycerideaemia on the progression of peripheral arterial disease and the onset of critical ischaemia, *Eur. J. Vasc. Endovasc. Surg.*, 11, 402, 1996.
6. Rosenbloom, M.S., Flanigan, D.P., Schuler, J.J., et al., Risk factors affecting the natural history of intermittent claudication, *Arch. Surg.*, 123, 867, 1988.
7. Bowers, B.L., Valentine, R.J., Myers, S.I., et al., The natural history of patients with claudication with toe pressures of 40 mm Hg or less, *J. Vasc. Surg.*, 18, 506, 1993.
8. McDaniel, M.D. and Cronenwett, J.L., Basic data related to the natural history of intermittent claudication, *Ann. Vasc. Surg.*, 3, 273, 1989.
9. Dormandy, J.A. and Murray, G.D., The fate of the claudicant—a prospective study of 1969 claudicants, *Eur. J. Vasc. Surg.*, 5, 131, 1991.
10. Peabody, C.N., Kannel, W.B., and McNamara, P.M., Intermittent claudication: surgical significance, *Arch. Surg.*, 109, 693, 1974.
11. Jelnes, R., Gaardsting, O., and Hougaard Jensen, K., Fate in intermittent claudication: outcome and risk factors, *BMJ*, 293, 1137, 1986.

12. Telles, G.S., Campbell, W.B., Wood, R.F.M., et al., Prostaglandin E₁ in severe lower limb ischaemia: a double-blind controlled trial, *Br. J. Surg.*, 71, 506, 1984.

13. Schuler, J.J., Flanigan, D.P., Holcroft, J.W., et al., Efficacy of prostaglandin E₁ in the treatment of lower extremity ischemic ulcers secondary to peripheral vascular occlusive disease: results of a prospective randomized, double-blind, multicenter clinical trial, *J. Vasc. Surg.*, 1, 160, 1984.

14. Eklund, A.E., Eriksson, G., and Olsson, A.G., A controlled study showing significant short term effect of prostaglandin E₁ in healing of ischaemic ulcers of the lower limb in man, *Prostaglandin Leukot. Med.*, 8, 265, 1982.

15. Belch, J.J.F., McArdle, B., Pollock, J.G., et al., Epoprostenol (prostacyclin) and severe arterial disease: a double-blind trial, *Lancet*, 12, 315, 1983.

16. Lepantalo, M. and Matzke, S., Outcome of unreconstructed chronic critical leg ischaemia, *Eur. J. Vasc. Endovasc. Surg.*, 11, 153, 1996.

17. U.K. Severe Limb Ischaemia Study Group, Treatment of limb threatening ischaemia with intravenous iloprost: a randomized double-blind placebo controlled study, *Eur. J. Vasc. Endovasc. Surg.*, 5, 511, 1991.

18. Criqui, M.H., Langer, R.D., Fronek, A., et al., Mortality over a period of 10 years in patients with peripheral arterial disease, *N. Engl. J. Med.*, 326, 381, 1992.

19. ICAI Group [Gruppo di Studio dell'Ischemia Cronica degli Arti Inferiori], The Study Group of Critical Chronic Ischemia of the Lower Extremities, Long-term mortality and its predictors in patients with critical leg ischaemia, *Eur. J. Vasc. Endovasc. Surg.*, 14, 91, 1997.

20. Wolfe, J.N., Defining the outcome of critical ischemia: a 1-year prospective study, *Br. J. Surg.*, 73, 318, 1986.

21. Hickey, N.C., Thomson, I.A., Shearman, C.P., et al., Aggressive arterial reconstruction for critical lower limb ischaemia, *Br. J. Surg.*, 78, 1476, 1991.

22. Veith, F.J., Gupta, K.G., Samson, R.H., et al., Progress in limb salvage by reconstructive arterial surgery combined with new or improved adjunctive procedures, *Ann. Surg.*, 194, 386, 1981.

23. Juergans, J.L., Barker, N.W., and Hines, E.A., Arteriosclerosis obliterans: review of 520 cases with special reference to pathogenic and prognostic factors, *Circulation*, 21, 188, 1960.

24. Liedberg, E. and Persson, B.M., Age, diabetes, and smoking in lower limb amputation for arterial occlusive disease, *Acta. Orthop. Scand.*, 54, 383, 1983.

25. McDermott, M.M., Feinglass, J., Slavensky, R., et al., The ankle-brachial index as a predictor of survival in patients with peripheral vascular disease, *J. Gen. Intern. Med.*, 9, 445, 1994.

26. Belcher, G. Effects of iloprost and factors affecting outcome in patients with severe inoperable lower limb ischaemia, in *Prostaglandins in the Cardiovascular System*, Schror, K., Ed., Karger, Basel, 1992, 354.

27. Matzke, S., Ollgren, J., and Lepantalo, M., Predictive value of distal pressure measurements in critical leg ischaemia, *Ann. Chir. Gynaecol.*, 85, 315, 1996.

28. Gregg, R.O., Bypass or amputation? Concomitant view of bypass arterial grafting and major amputations, *Am. J. Surg.*, 149, 397, 1985.

29. Hertzer, N., Beven, E., Young, J., et al., Coronary artery disease in peripheral vascular patients: a classification of 1000 coronary angiograms and results of surgical management, *Ann. Surg.*, 199, 223, 1984.

30. Alexandrova, N., Gibson, W., Norris, J., et al., Carotid artery stenosis in peripheral vascular disease, *J. Vasc. Surg.*, 23, 645, 1996.

31. Ubbink, D.T., Jacobs, M.J., Tangelde, G.J.,et al., The usefulness of capillary microscopy, transcutaneous oximetry, and laser Doppler fluxmetry in the assessment of the severity of lower limb ischaemia, *Int. J. Microcirc. Clin. Exp.*, 14, 34, 1994.

32. Scheffler, A. and Rieger, H., A comparative analysis of transcutaneous oximetry (tcPO2) during oxygen inhalation and leg dependency in severe peripheral arterial occlusive disease, *J. Vasc. Surg.*, 16, 218, 1992.

33. Fagrell, B. and Lindberg, G., A simplified evaluation of vital capillary microscopy for predicting skin viability in patients with severe arterial insufficiency, *Clin. Physiol.*, 4, 403, 1984.

34. Spring, D.B., Bettmann, M.A., and Barkan, H.E., Nonfatal adverse reactions to iodinated contrast media: spontaneous reporting to the U.S. Food and Drug Administration, 1978-94, *Radiology*, 204, 325, 1997.

35. Cambria, R., Kaufman, J.A., L'Italien, G.J., et al., Magnetic resonance angiography in the management of lower extremity arterial occlusive disease: a prospective study, *J. Vasc. Surg.*, 25, 380, 1997.

36. Ross, M.A., Neuropathies associated with diabetes, *Med. Clin. North. Am.*, 77, 111, 1993.

37. Freeman, A.G., Vitamin B12 deficiency and diabetic neuropathy, *Lancet*, 2, 963, 1969.

38. Adler, A.I., Boyko, E.J., Ahroni, J.H., et al., Risk factors for diabetic peripheral sensory neuropathy: results of the Seattle Prospective Diabetic Foot Study, *Diabetes Care*, 20, 1162, 1997.

39. Windebank, A.J., Drug-induced neuropathies, *Baillieres Clin. Neurol.*, 4, 529, 1995.

40. Poldermans, D., Boersma, E., Bax, J.J., et al., The effect of bisoprolol on perioperative mortality and myocardial infarction in high-risk patients undergoing vascular surgery, *N. Engl. J. Med.*, 341, 1789, 1999.

41. Hirsch, A.T., Treat-Jacobson, D., Lando, H.A., et al., The role of tobacco cessation, antiplatelet and lipid-lowering therapies in the treatment of peripheral arterial disease, *Vasc. Med.*, 2, 243, 1997.

42. Birkenstock, W.E., Louw, J.H., Terblanche, J., et al., Smoking and other factors affecting the conservative management of peripheral vascular disease, *S. Afr. Med. J.*, 49, 1129, 1975.

43. National Cholesterol Education Program (NCEP) guidelines on detection, evaluation and treatment of high blood cholesterol in adults, *JAMA*, 269, 3015, 1993.

44. Trubestein, G., von Bary, S., Breddin, K., et al., Intravenous prostglandin E1 versus pentoxifylline therapy in chronic arterial occlusive disease—a controlled randomized multicenter study, *Vasa*, 28, 44, 1989.

45. Guilmot, J.L. and Diot, E., for the French Iloprost Study Group, Treatment of lower limb ischaemia due to atherosclerosis in diabetic and nondiabetic patients with iloprost, a stable analogue of prostacyclin: results of a French multicenter trial, *Drug. Invest.*, 3, 351, 1991.

46. CAPRIE Steering Committee, A randomized, blinded trial of clopidogrel versus aspirin in patients at risk of ischaemic events (CAPRIE), *Lancet*, 348, 1329, 1996.

47. Hess, H., Mietaschk, A., and Deichsel, G., Drug-induced inhibition of platelet function delays progression in peripheral occlusive arterial disease: a prospective double-blind arteriographically controlled trial, *Lancet*, 1, 415, 1985.

48. Nevelsteen, A., Mortelmans, L., van de Cruys, A., et al., Effect of ticlopidine on blood loss, platelet turnover, and platelet deposition on prosthetic surfaces in patients undergoing aorto-femoral bypass grafting, *Thromb. Res.*, 64, 363, 1991.

49. Kretschmer, G., Wenzl, E., Schemper, M., et al., Influence of postoperative anticoagulant treatment on patient survival after femoropopliteal vein bypass surgery, *Lancet*, 1, 797, 1988.

50. Lowe, G.D., Defibrination, blood flow and blood rheology, *Clin. Hemorheol.*, 4, 15, 1984.

51. Bode-Boger, S.M., Boger, R.H., Alfke, H., et al., L-Arginine induces nitric oxide-dependent vasodilatation in patients with critical limb ischemia: a randomized controlled study, *Circulation*, 93, 85, 1996.

52. Norwegian Pentoxifylline Multicenter Trial Group, Efficacy and clinical tolerance of parenteral pentoxifylline in the treatment of critical lower limb ischemia: a placebo controlled multicenter study, *Int. Angiol.*, 15, 75, 1996.

53. Moneta, G.L., Yeager, R.A., Taylor, L.M., et al., Hemodynamic assessment of combined aortoiliac/femoropopliteal occlusive disease and selection of single or multilevel revascularization, *Semin. Vasc. Surg.*, 7, 3, 1994.

54. De Vries, S.O. and Hunink, M.G., Results of aortic bifurcation grafts for aortoiliac occlusive disease: a meta-analysis, *J. Vasc. Surg.*, 26, 558, 1997.

55. Wolf, G.L., Wilson, S.E., Cross, A.P., et al., for the principal investigators and their associates of Veterans Administration Cooperative Study Number 199, Surgery or balloon angioplasty for peripheral vascular disease: a randomized clinical trial, *J. Vasc. Inter. Radiol.*, 4, 639, 1993.

56. Hunink, M.G., Wong, J.B., Donaldson, M.C., Meyerovitz, M.F., and Harrington, D.P., Patency results of percutaneous and surgical revascularization for femoropopliteal arterial disease, *Med. Decis. Making*, 14, 71, 1994.

57. Dalman, R.L. and Taylor, L.M., Basic data related to infrainguinal revascularization procedures, *Ann. Vasc. Surg.*, 4, 309, 1990.

58. Harris, R.W., Andros, G., Salles-Cunha, S.X., Dulawa, L.B., et al., Totally autogenous venovenous composite bypass grafts, *Arch. Surg.*, 121, 1128, 1986.

59. Wagner, H.J. and Rager, G., Infrapopliteal angioplasty: a forgotten region? [in German], *Rofo. Fortschr. Geb. Rontgenstr. Neuen. Bildgeb. Verfahr.*, 168, 415, 1998.

60. Lim, R.C., Jr., Blaisdell, F.W., Hall, A.D., et al., Below-knee amputation for ischemic gangrene, *Surg. Obstet. Gynecol.*, 125, 493, 1967.

61. Ho, G.H., Moll, F.L., Kuipers, M.M., et al., Long-term surveillance by duplex scanning of nonrevised infragenicular graft stenosis, *Ann. Vasc. Surg.*, 9, 547, 1995.

62. Machleder, H.I., Prognosis of the failed infrainguinal vascular graft, *Semin. Vasc. Surg.*, 3, 43, 1990.

8 Acute Arterial Ischemia

Kenneth A. Harris

CONTENTS

8.1 Introduction 148
8.2 Epidemiology 148
8.3 Natural History and Outcome 149
8.4 Pathophysiology 150
8.5 Diagnosis and Evaluation 151
    8.5.1 Categories of Acute Limb Ischemia 153
        8.5.1.1 Category I: Viable Limb 153
        8.5.1.2 Category IIa: Marginally Threatened
                Limb Viability 153
        8.5.1.3 Category IIb: Immediately Threatened
                Limb Viability 153
        8.5.1.4 Category III: Irreversible
                Ischemic Changes..154
8.6 Treatment 157
    8.6.1 Acute Limb Ischemia Due to Embolus 159
    8.6.2 Acute Limb Ischemia Due to Native
        Artery Thrombosis 161
    8.6.3 Acute Limb Ischemia Due to Graft Thrombosis 161
    8.6.4 Acute Limb Ischemia Due to Popliteal Artery
        Aneurysm Thromboembolism 163
    8.6.5 Thrombolysis..163
    8.6.6 Complications of Treatment 165
References..165

0-8493-8413-3/01/$0.00+$1.50
© 2001 by CRC Press LLC

8.1   INTRODUCTION

Acute arterial ischemia affecting the peripheral circulation can be defined as a sudden reduction of the perfusion of an extremity that may produce symptoms ranging from a worsening of preexisting symptoms to a dramatic threat to limb viability. In this chapter, only thromboembolic ischemic events involving the lower extremities will be considered.

8.2   EPIDEMIOLOGY

There are relatively few articles reporting on the epidemiology of acute limb ischemia (ALI). In a review of population-based studies it was estimated that the incidence of ALI ranges from four to17 per 100,000 population.[1] The age of affected individuals is usually older than 70 years. In large centers, it is estimated that ALI amounts to 10% to 20% of the vascular surgeon's practice. The etiology of ALI is shown in Table 8.1.

TABLE 8.1
Etiology of Acute Arterial Limb Ischemia

Intrinsic to Artery	Extrinsic to Artery
• Embolus	• Trauma
• Thrombus	• Extrinsic compression
• Native artery	• Neoplasm
• Bypass graft	
• Aortic/arterial dissection	
• Atheroemboli	
• Popliteal aneurysm	
• Traumatic injury	
• Penetrating	
• Blunt	

A review of a national database on ALI demonstrated a changing frequency distribution, with emboli representing 63% of episodes in the time period 1987 to 1990 and decreasing to 54% in the 1991 to1995 period.[2] In all, 20% of emboli enter the cerebral circulation, 10% the visceral circulation, and the remainder lodge in the peripheral circulation (distribution of peripheral emboli: aorta 16%, iliac artery 18%, femoral 43%, popliteal 15%, and upper extremity 8%).[3] Embolic material usually lodges at bifurcations where the caliber of the artery dramatically diminishes. An increasing number of acute ischemic events are related to bypass graft thrombosis after arterial reconstruction for chronic arterial ischemia.

8.3   NATURAL HISTORY AND OUTCOME

In an acutely ischemic extremity of category IIa or greater, the risk of limb loss is very high or inevitable without intervention. The outcome of treatment of ALI should be considered with respect to the patient's life and the outcome of the limb. Survival after embolectomy or treatment for acute thrombosis is compromised with respect to the general population (for embolus, operative mortality is 16% to 17%, 5-year survival is 17%, and early amputation is 10%; for thrombosis, operative mortality is 13% to14%, 5-year survival is 44%, and early amputation is 26%).[4,5] A generally accepted concept is that thrombosis carries a worse prognosis for the extremity, and embolus a worse prognosis for life. Although morbidity and mortality remain high, there has been a gradual improvement in results over the past few decades. The risk of amputation after embolectomy is increased in patients with two or more myocardial infarcts, chronic lower limb ischemia, prolonged duration of ischemia (greater than 14 days) and postoperative congestive heart failure.[6] An increased risk of cardiac death after intervention for ALI can be predicted if any of the following are present: thigh ischemia, cardiac decompensation, mean blood pressure less than 90 mm Hg, or a history of myocardial infarction within 4 weeks.[7] Several other factors have been cited as important in the determination of outcome, including tolerance of tissue for ischemia,

duration of ischemia, prior sensitization of tissue to ischemia (precon-
ditioning or collateralization), degree of thrombus propagation,
response to circulatory restoration, and medical state of the patient.[8]

The situation of a popliteal aneurysm has been extensively studied.
Once symptoms have developed, the risk of limb loss is very high.
Patients presenting with an acutely thrombosed popliteal aneurysm
have an amputation rate of 33%.[9]

Although cardiac risks are also high, ALI presents a major threat
to the limb, necessitating treatment for both limb salvage and prolongation of life.

8.4   PATHOPHYSIOLOGY

An embolus can be defined as a substance foreign to the usual contents
of the vascular tree that travels from its site of origin to a distal site.
The most common embolus is thrombotic material arising in the heart.
The source of the embolus is the heart in 85% to 90% of cases (atherosclerotic heart disease, 65%; mitral valvular disease with atrial fibrillation, 35%).[10] Thrombosis of a native artery most commonly occurs when
there is a preexisting arterial occlusive lesion with endothelial disruption.
Any factor that induces a state of hypercoagulabilty, low flow, or worsening of the preocclusive plaque may lead to final thrombosis of the
artery. In these individuals, there has been time for collateral circulation
to develop, and therefore their presentation may be less dramatic when
compared with that of an embolus. Thrombosis of an arterial bypass
graft is usually secondary to progressive atherosclerosis in the proximal
or distal artery or pathology in the bypass graft itself. Prosthetic bypass
grafts may develop intimal hyperplasia at the distal anastomosis. In
addition, autogenous conduits may develop intimal hyperplasia or stenosis at the site of venous valves, which may lead to critical flow-limiting
lesions. All types of bypass grafts could be threatened in the case of
progression of distal or proximal atherosclerosis.

Distal to any acute arterial occlusion, there is a region of low/no
flow with a relative increase in clotting factors. This might lead to
distal propagation of a thrombus over a variable distance, often to the

next major branch that carries significant flow. There is also a risk of distal embolization from the initiating or propagated thrombus.

During the ischemic phase, skeletal muscle with a low resting metabolic rate will be less critically affected than the skin and nerves. Loss of aerobic metabolism results in a decreased level of high energy phosphates (adenosine triphosphate, adenosine diphosphate, adenosine monophosphate) and leads to cellular membrane dysfunction and release of potassium and acid from the cells. Myoglobin and protein breakdown products will be released into the extracellular space. At the time of reperfusion, oxygen free radicals and hydroxyl radicals may lead to increased injury and further damage resulting in cellular dysfunction and swelling (reperfusion injury). There will also be a release of metabolic products into the systemic circulation that might tax an already compromised heart and affect renal function as well as other organs (reperfusion syndrome). Further discussion of these events is beyond the scope of this chapter, but review articles are available.[11]

8.5 DIAGNOSIS AND EVALUATION

Figure 8.1 presents an evaluation algorithm for ALI. Patients may present at variable times after the onset of ALI depending on the severity of the symptoms. The classic "5 Ps"—pain, pallor, pulselessness, paralysis, and paresthesia—are still valid diagnostic criteria, with paralysis and paresthesia being the most predictive of long-term limb loss and the urgency of the situation.

The differential diagnosis includes acute nerve compression that can be distinguished from ALI by the distal presence of pulses, Doppler signals out of keeping with symptoms (including normal ankle brachial index, or ABI), a warm extremity, and location of pain centered on the nerve distribution. Deep venous thrombosis can be diagnosed by swelling (an unusual feature in ALI), cyanosis, and the presence of pulses (after the edema is milked away) or good arterial Doppler signals.

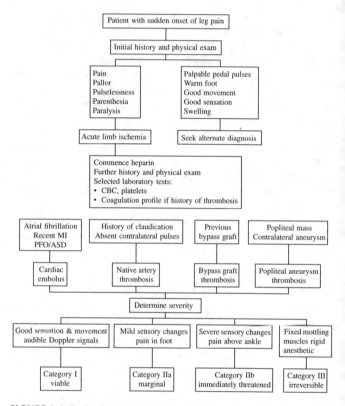

FIGURE 8.1 Evaluation algorithm for acute limb ischemia.

Because the treatment for the varying causes differs, attempts should be made to determine the etiology of ALI. Factors supporting the diagnosis of an embolus include a source of embolus (e.g., atrial fibrillation, recent myocardial infarction), no past history of intermittent claudication (IC), normal pulses in the contralateral extremity, and relatively dense ischemia. There may be tenderness over the site where the embolus has lodged. The diagnosis of thrombosis of an arterial stenosis is suggested by a preceding history of claudication, and the generalized nature of atherosclerosis may lead to an absence of pulses in the contralateral extremity. The prior stenosis will have led to the development of collateral circulation, thereby possibly lessening the degree of ischemia. The diagnosis of a popliteal aneurysm should be evident by the presence of either a pulsatile or nonpulsatile (thrombosed) popliteal mass and a 50% chance of a contralateral popliteal aneurysm. Venous filling or troughing on elevation, muscle consistency, and degree of motor and sensory dysfunction will help determine the degree of ischemia and viability of the limb.

For the purpose of determining treatment, the degree of ischemia should be categorized according to the TransAtlantic Inter-Society Consensus (TASC) group modification of the Society for Vascular Surgery/International Society for Cardiovascular Surgery (SVS/ISCVS) classification summarized below.[12]

8.5.1   CATEGORIES OF ACUTE LIMB ISCHEMIA

8.5.1.1   Category I: Viable Limb

The limb is not immediately threatened and presents with worsening IC or resolving symptoms of pain, numbness, and paresthesia. There will be no sensory or motor findings, and usually both arterial and venous Doppler signals will be audible.

8.5.1.2   Category IIa: Marginally Threatened Limb Viability

The limb may be salvaged if treated promptly. The limb has no or minimal sensory changes involving just the toes, with no associated motor signs. Doppler signals may be audible, and pain is usually mild and limited to the foot.

8.5.1.3   Category IIb: Immediately Threatened Limb Viability

The limb is salvageable but requires immediate treatment. Sensory changes will extend beyond the toes, and there will be decreased voluntary movement of the toes. Rest pain will be severe and there may be tenderness of the calf. Arterial Doppler signals are often inaudible but venous signals may be heard.

8.5.1.4 Category III: Irreversible Ischemic Changes

Major tissue loss or permanent nerve damage is inevitable. The limb is profoundly anesthetic and motor function is markedly reduced. Muscle rigidity may be present and neither arterial nor venous Doppler signals are audible. In the early presentation, there may be difficulty in differentiating category IIb from category III ischemia.

The spectrum of presentation will range from the viable extremity (category I) with minor symptoms that can be managed electively (usually in the same manner as patients presenting with chronic limb ischemia) to patients with category III ischemia and nonviable extremities. Between these two categories is a range of patients for whom the risks of delaying reperfusion must be balanced against the benefits of obtaining more complete information about their medical condition and the status of the arterial bed. As yet, there exists no validated objective test to determine the reversibility and viability of an ischemic extremity. Nonviability is suggested by marbled mottling, fixed cyanosis, prolonged and profound paralysis and paresthesia, myositis (as evidenced by calf pain, muscle rigidity, and a doughlike consistency to the palpated muscle), and the absence of arterial and venous Doppler signals. Laboratory findings such as low pH, hyperkalemia, increased creatine phosphate levels, and myoglobinuria indicate muscle damage but not an irretrievable extremity. The constellation of signs, symptoms, and laboratory data is necessary to facilitate clinical categorization and prediction of viability.

In the ideal situation, a complete investigation of the arterial system and concurrent medical diseases would be undertaken. A basic history of other medical conditions and a physical examination are mandatory in all patients. These should be complemented by basic blood work (hemoglobin, white blood cell count, platelets, international normalized ratio, activated partial thromboplastin time, serum electrolytes, creatinine, blood gases), electrocardiogram, and chest radiogram. Time factors related to viability of the extremity may limit the extent of investigations. Doppler assessment of the extremity could be of some value in the prediction of time available for investigation. Experience from the Vietnam War showed that the presence of arterial Doppler signals indicates that the limb and patient can survive evacuation for definitive treatment.[13] This has been validated in civilian investigations. The presence or absence of Doppler signals will augment, but does not replace, information gained during the clinical examination. Duplex scanning may be helpful in localizing the level of obstruction if this is not obvious from the clinical exam. It will also confirm the occlusion of a bypass graft.

Visualization of arterial inflow, outflow, and localization and character of the arterial obstruction should be undertaken if time permits. Angiography will outline the level of the occlusion and any occult lesions in the in-flow circulation as well as providing definition of the outflow tract. Complete angiography including the abdominal aorta and runoff beds is ideal. Patients with acute dense ischemia, usually secondary to an embolus, may have no distal peripheral vessels visualized on angiography because of lack of collateral flow. Differentiation between arterial thrombosis and embolus is presented in Table 8.2 and Figure 8.2.

TABLE 8.2
Differentiation Between Arterial Thrombosis and Embolus on Angiography

Diagnostic Criteria From Angiography	
Embolus	Thrombosis
• Meniscus sign or clot silhouette	• Shart cutoff
• Rest of circulation normal	• Diffuse atherosclerosis
• Few collateral vessels	• Collateral vessels present
• Multiple filling defects in multiple arterial beds	• Single long obstruction
• No distal circulation visualized	• Distal vessels seen

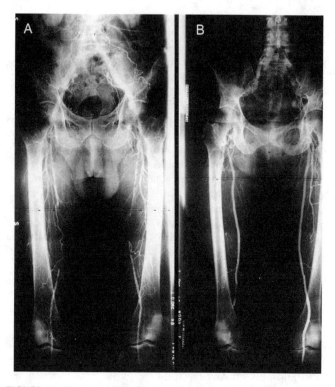

FIGURE 8.2 Transfemoral arteriogram of abdominal aorta and proximal run-off vessels. (A) Thrombosis of the superficial femoral artery (bilateral) with multiple collateral vessels and filling and visualization of the distal circulation. (B) Right distal superficial femoral artery embolus with minimal collateral vessel development and no visualizaiton of the distal circulation. Not appreciated in this picture is the clot silhouette.

At the time of angiography, it is important when considering the approach to be aware that thrombolysis might be a potential option. Appropriate puncture site and catheter placement should be considered.

When a popliteal artery aneurysm is suspected, ultrasound examination can be used to confirm the diagnosis. However, angiography is necessary to define the extent of aneurysmal disease and demonstrate the outflow arteries, which are frequently severely diseased.

Time factors may dictate that vascular imaging of the distal vessels be performed on the operating room table after initial revascularization. On-table angiography can be accomplished by injecting 15 to 20 mL of contrast medium through a catheter introduced into the distal artery through the arteriotomy.

8.6 TREATMENT

The goal of treatment of ALI is to achieve a viable, functional, pain-free extremity in a healthy patient. Many factors must be taken into account in the pursuit of this goal. Figure 8.3 presents a treatment algorithm for ALI. The therapeutic modality selected will depend on the etiology and length of time since the onset of ischemia, the clinical status of the leg, the degree of thrombus propagation, and the medical condition of the patient.

Standard teaching suggests that, in all cases of ALI, anticoagulation should be administered as soon as the diagnosis is made. Heparin (5,000 U to 10,000 U) should be given intravenously, provided there are no absolute contraindications. The purpose of anticoagulation is to prevent propagation of the thrombus and to prevent further embolization. This should only be delayed when operation under spinal anesthetic is contemplated. A randomized trial from Sweden has questioned the routine practice of postoperative anticoagulation, demonstrating no difference in survival of patient or limb.[14] However, the short postoperative follow-up period (1 month) has been criticized. Despite the debate, many believe that anticoagulation is of benefit.

Urgency of treatment depends on the degree of ischemia. Patients with category I ischemia, with a clearly viable extremity, can be treated similarly to patients presenting with chronic arterial ischemia or IC. The possible exception would be in the case of an embolus, where the circulation could be returned to normal with an embolectomy. Those

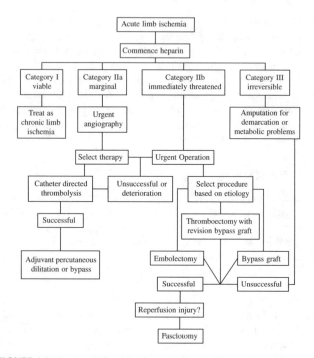

FIGURE 8.3 Treatment algorithm for acute limb ischemia. ASD = atrial septal defect; CBC = complete blood cell count; MI = myocardial infarction; PFO = patent foramen ovale.

patients with category III ischemia and clearly nonviable extremities should undergo primary amputation. At times, it may be difficult to differentiate advanced category IIb from category III ischemia. If presentation has been early, it is recommended that attempts at limb salvage be made if there remains a question of reversibility. Category IIa ischemia affords the opportunity for more extensive investigations before intervention, but category IIb frequently requires immediate intervention with minimal prior investigation.

If the etiology of ischemia is an embolus, an embolectomy and clearing of distal propagation of thrombus will return the arterial tree to its normal status. Further treatment revolves around addressing the underlying source and prevention of further embolization. Conversely, thrombosis will occur in vessels that already have diseased and stenotic segments. Native artery or graft thrombectomy alone will not reduce the predisposition of such vessels to thrombosis. Therefore, treatment of the underlying cause (usually by bypass grafting) will be required to achieve a better long-term result.

8.6.1 ACUTE LIMB ISCHEMIA DUE TO EMBOLUS

A great advance in the treatment of thromboembolic events was realized when Fogarty and associates introduced the concept of the embolectomy catheter.[15] Embolectomy, even in the medically compromised patient, can be conducted under local anesthesia or neurolept anesthesia. The most accessible lower extremity artery is the common femoral artery, which is exposed through an incision in the groin. After exposure and control of the common femoral artery bifurcation, either a longitudinal or a transverse arteriotomy can be made. A 5-French embolectomy catheter (see Figure 8.4) is passed proximally to clear the iliac inflow system. In the case of an aortic "saddle embolus," both common femoral arteries are exposed and simultaneous embolectomy is carried out to ensure bilateral arterial clearing. After assuring good inflow a small (3-French) embolectomy catheter is passed distally. This usually will enter the peroneal artery. Multiple simultaneous catheters may be passed to direct entry into other vessels. Correct inflation volumes in the balloon can be assessed by inflating only while the catheter is being moved. Overinflation should be avoided to prevent endothelial damage or stripping, or vessel rupture. If compromise of the lumen is a concern when closing the arteriotomy, an autogenous or synthetic patch is sutured in place. If the results of embolectomy are less than predicted or desired, an on-table angiogram should be obtained. Assessment of results is aided by placing the foot in a sterile plastic bag during the procedure so that color (reactive hyperemia)

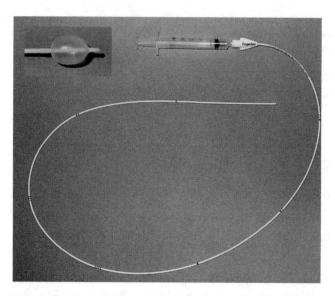

FIGURE 8.4 Balloon embolectomy catheter. After insertion the balloon is inflated (*inset*) to facilitate thrombus removal on withdrawal of the catheter.

and flow are more easily assessed. The rate of retained thrombus after embolectomy is reportedly as high as 40%.[16] If there is retained thrombus, reopening of the artery with repeat thrombectomy or intraoperative thrombolysis should be considered. For emboli lodged in distal arteries (e.g., popliteal), a direct approach under general anesthetic might permit more meticulous removal of thrombus from all the crural vessels. Most work on intraoperative thrombolysis has been done with urokinase infusion or bolus injection of 125,000 IU to 500,000 IU over 30 minutes. This has been shown to be effective in salvage of both limb and life.[17] Postoperative anticoagulation is necessary to prevent recurrence of embolization to any vascular bed. Pooled data suggest that the risk of recurrent embolization drops from 21% or more to 7% with the addition of systemic long-term anticoagulation.[3]

Investigations should be undertaken to detect the source of the embolus by two-dimensional echocardiography and abdominal ultrasound as indicated. These investigations can be done in the postoperative phase while the patient is recovering from intervention and is fully anticoagulated.

8.6.2 ACUTE LIMB ISCHEMIA DUE TO NATIVE ARTERY THROMBOSIS

In the case of a native-vessel arterial thrombosis, thrombectomy alone carries a risk of recurrent ischemia ranging from 21% to 53%.[12] In the case of arterial thrombosis, either balloon angioplasty or bypass grafting is necessary to improve the results and treat the underlying cause. Arterial imaging is essential to carry out optimal bypass grafting. In the case of acute aortic thrombosis, patients may present with densely ischemic extremities and in a condition of metabolic compromise that carries a mortality rate of more than 25%. If bilateral femoral thromboembolectomy is unsuccessful, extra-anatomic bypass grafting should be considered. Thrombosis of the infrainguinal native arteries frequently requires femoral distal bypass grafting. The long saphenous vein remains the conduit of choice, but time constraints may mandate the use of a prosthetic graft if outflow can be established to the popliteal artery.

It is very helpful to have full arteriography before embarking on a reconstruction of the lower extremity to ensure adequate inflow and outflow and optimal long-term patency of the graft.

8.6.3 ACUTE LIMB ISCHEMIA DUE TO GRAFT THROMBOSIS

Graft thrombosis is a problem seen with increasing frequency. Decisions regarding optimal treatment will depend on the type of graft in place and the time from the original procedure. The usual cause of graft thrombosis can be classified based on the time between insertion and thrombosis. Early (less than 30 days) occlusion is usually secondary to technical error and, in the case of vein grafting, intrinsic graft pathology. Later graft occlusion (up to 2 years) has been attributed to intimal hyperplasia at the distal anastomosis or stenosis at a valve cusp. Later occlusions may be secondary to progression of the atherosclerotic process in proximal or distal arteries. Patients with aortic graft occlusions are best managed with exploration of the vessels at the groin and patch angioplasty to improve outflow. In the case of extensive disease of the superficial femoral artery and profunda femoris, artery bypass grafting to distal vessels may be necessary to achieve adequate outflow. The surgeon must be alert to the fact that the distal anastomosis of the contralateral limb may have undergone a similar process. Angiography in the pre- or postoperative phase may permit assessment of this and allow elective repair of this lesion.

Infrainguinal grafts, either autogenous or prosthetic, are treated somewhat differently. Early graft occlusions are best managed operatively with correction of the inciting cause. The thrombus should be removed from the graft and technical and anastomotic errors corrected. Autogenous patch angioplasty or replacement of the affected segment of the graft might be required if there is intrinsic graft pathology (e.g., sclerotic vein from previous phlebitis or valvultome-related injury).

The usual cause of late prosthetic graft failure is progression of distal (or more rarely proximal) atherosclerotic disease or intimal hyperplasia at the distal anastomosis. Operative approach is usually at the distal anastomosis so that outflow can be assessed and corrected at the same time as graft clearing. The cause of late graft failure when autogenous vein has been used is either intimal hyperplasia or intrinsic graft problems that occur at the site of anastomosis or within the graft at the site of valves. Reports on thrombectomy of autogenous grafts indicate that success is limited. This has prompted interest in thrombolysis followed by correction of the underlying lesion with surgery or interventional radiology. If, after clearing the graft, there is a short segment stenosis within the graft, this can be treated with a local bypass or patch. However, if there is general deterioration or a long stenosis of the graft, replacement should be undertaken. Some investigators advocate routine graft replacement if failure occurs within the first 6 to 10 months after placement because this suggests intrinsic, diffuse graft problems.[18]

Liberal use of routine imaging has a role in reducing the risk of graft failure. On-table angiography or duplex imaging at the time of primary operation may demonstrate technical deficiencies and allow early correction. A protocol of postoperative follow-up duplex scans can identify grafts at risk with critical stenosis and permit correction in the preocclusion phase.

Newer techniques such as percutaneous mechanical thrombectomy and percutaneous aspiration thromboembolectomy require further assessment before they can be recommended for widespread use.

8.6.4 Acute Limb Ischemia Due to Popliteal Artery Aneurysm Thromboembolism

The treatment of a thrombosed popliteal artery aneurysm will depend on the presentation. If there is reasonable runoff visualized at the time of angiography, then autogenous bypass grafting with exclusion of the aneurysm is ideal. If there is poor infrapopliteal runoff, then intra-arterial thrombolysis or distal thrombectomy will be required before exclusion of the aneurysm and bypass.[19] Elective repair of popliteal artery aneurysms is the best method of preventing potentially devastating complications.

8.6.5 Thrombolysis

It is agreed that systemic intravenous administration of thrombolytic agents is not indicated because of low efficacy and high complication rates. If thrombolytic therapy is elected, the best method is the catheter-directed, intrathrombus infusion technique. If a guidewire cannot be passed across the occlusion at the time of angiography, then a short course of infusion through a catheter situated just proximal to the thrombus may be indicated.

A number of studies have been published on the use of catheter-directed thrombolysis in the treatment of ALI. None of the trials is directly comparable, due to differences in protocols and entry criteria as well as endpoints. The Rochester Study demonstrated no difference in limb salvage rates but a higher cardiopulmonary mortality

rate in the surgically treated group.[20] The Surgery or Thrombolysis
for the Ischemic Lower Extremity (STILE) trial was concluded when
interim analysis revealed poorer results with thrombolysis (based on
the endpoint "composite outcome index" score) mainly owing to
ongoing or recurrent ischemia in the nonoperated group.[21] A subgroup analysis of the STILE results also revealed that native artery
thrombosis responded poorly to thrombolysis. The Thrombolysis or
Peripheral Arterial Surgery (TOPAS) trial showed no difference in
amputation-free survival between groups treated with surgery or
catheter-directed thrombolysis. Thrombolysis did decrease the number and magnitude of surgical interventions.[22] The design of the
TOPAS trial and selection of patients allowed for few patients with
category II ischemia being entered, thus rendering the results not
universally applicable for patients presenting to the emergency room
with ALI. Another study examined the use of thrombolysis in the
management of occluded bypass grafts and demonstrated that if
catheter placement was successful (61% patients), autogenous
bypass grafts had a good chance of lysis with reduction in the
magnitude of the procedure required to prevent recurrent thrombosis.[23] The ideal patient for initial treatment with thrombolytic agents
is one with a recently occluded autogenous vascular bypass graft
that has been in place for more than 10 months and who has marginal
threat to limb viability. The surgeon must be prepared to operate on
any focal lesion uncovered once the graft is recanalized. The candidate best treated surgically is one with dense ischemia of the extremity caused by arterial thrombosis or embolus. Patients who fall elsewhere along the spectrum require individual assessment. The
consensus document on the use of thrombolysis in the management
of limb ischemia recommends that patients unable to tolerate a delay
in reperfusion because of the severity of the ischemia be given
surgical treatment and that thrombolysis be attempted in others.[24]

   It is clear that no single therapeutic modality will address all
situations. Therefore, thrombolysis and surgery should be considered
complementary therapies. To date, the cost-effectiveness of any single
therapy or combination has yet to be fully investigated.

8.6.6 COMPLICATIONS OF TREATMENT

After successful revascularization there is always a risk of developing a reperfusion syndrome. This might manifest itself as an acute myocardial depression related to an influx of acid and potassium ions into the systemic circulation at the time of revascularization. Communication with the anesthesiologist and anticipation of this problem will permit the institution of such measures as bicarbonate administration for prevention of acidosis and the treatment of hyperkalemia with insulin and glucose. Somewhat later, myonecrosis may lead to myoglobinuria with renal failure. Maintenance of renal function can be assisted by alkalization of the urine and forced diuresis. Some patients may go on to develop full-blown multiorgan failure with myocardial renal and liver failure.

Local reperfusion syndromes manifest as a compartment syndrome. Significant swelling within muscles deep to the fascial layer can result in capillary occlusion and myonecrosis. This must be treated with fasciotomy. Measurement of compartment pressures has been advocated, but there is disagreement about the threshold pressure. Some investigators recommend routine fasciotomy after a period of 8 hours of ischemia; others are selective, deciding whether to carry out fasciotomy based on clinical judgment or measurement of compartment pressures. The procedure should be performed at the same time as the primary procedure if ischemia has been prolonged or if there is evidence of increased compartment pressure. A full four-compartment fasciotomy should be carried out, decompressing the anterior and lateral compartment through an anterior incision two finger breadths lateral to the tibia, and the superficial and deep posterior compartments should be opened through a medial incision. Rarely, fasciotomy of the individual muscles of the thigh may be required. Wounds are left open for later closure.

REFERENCES

1. Dormady, J., Heeck, L., and Vig, S., Acute limb ischemia, *Semin. Vasc. Surg.*, 12, 148, 1999.

2. Bergqvist, D., Troeng, T., Elfstrom, J., et al., The Steering Committee of Swedvasc, Auditing surgical outcome: ten years with the Swedish Vascular Registry_ Swedvasc, *Eur. J. Surg.*, 164, 3, 1998.

3. Mills, J.L. and Porter, J.M., Basic data related to clinical decision making in acute limb ischemia, *Ann. Vasc. Surg.*, 5, 96, 1991.

4. Aune, S. and Trippesrad, A., Operative mortality and long term survival of patients operated on for acute lower limb ischemia, *Eur. J. Vasc. Surg.*, 15, 143,1998.

5. Kuukasjaarvi, P. and Salenius, J. P., Perioperative outcome of acute lower limb ischemia on the basis of the national vascular registry, The Finvasc Study Group, *Eur. J. Vasc. Surg.*, 8, 578, 1994.

6. Ljungman, C., Adami, H.O., Bergqvist, D., et al., Risk factors for early lower limb loss after embolectomy for acute lower arterial occlusion: a population-based case-controlled study, *Br. J. Surg.*, 78, 1482, 1991.

7. Jivegard, L., Bergqvist, D., Holm, J., et al., Preoperative assessment of the risk for cardiac death following thromboembolectomy for acute lower limb ischemia, *Eur. J. Vasc. Surg.*, 6, 83, 1992.

8. Ouriel, K. and Veith, F. J., Acute lower limb ischemia: determinants of outcome, *Surgery*, 124, 336, 1998.

9. Lowell, R.C., Gloviczki, P., Hallett, J.W., et al., Popliteal artery aneurysms: the risk of nonoperative management, *Ann. Vasc. Surg.*, 8, 14, 1994.

10. Elliott, J.P., Hageman, J.H., Szilagyi, D.E., et al., Arterial embolization: problems of source, multiplicity, recurrence, and delayed treatment, *Surgery*, 88, 833, 1980.

11. Rubin, B.B., Romaschin, A., Walker, P.M., et al., Mechanisms of postischemic injury in skeletal muscle: intervention strategies, *J. Appl. Physiol.*, 80, 369, 1996.

12. Dormandy, J.A. and Rutherford, R.B., Management of peripheral arterial disease (PAD), TASC Working Group, TransAtlantic Inter-Society Consensus (TASC), *J. Vasc. Surg.*, 31, S1, 2000.

13. Lavenson, G.S., Rich, N.M., and Strandness, D.E., Ultrasonic flow detector in combat vascular injuries, *Arch. Surg.*, 103, 644, 1971.

14. Jivegard, L., Holm, J., Bergqvist, D., et al., Acute limb ischemia: failure of anticoagulant treatment to improve one month results of arterial thromboembolectomy: a prospective randomised multicentre study, *Surgery*, 109, 610, 1991.

15. Fogarty, T.J., Daily, P.O., Shumway, N.E., Experience with balloon catheter technic for arterial embolectomy, *Am. J. Surg.*, 122, 231, 1979.

16. Pleacha, F. and Pories, W. J., Intraoperative angiography in the immediate assessment of arterial reconstruction, *Arch. Surg.*, 105, 902, 1972.

17. Comerota, A.J., Rao, K.A., Throm, R.C., et al., A prospective, randomized, blinded, and placebo controlled trial of intra-operative intra-arterial urokinase infusion during lower extremity revascularization: regional and systemic effects, *Ann. Surg.*, 218, 534, 1993.

18. Berkowitz, H.D. and Kee, J.C., Occluded infrainguinal grafts: when to choose lytic therapy versus a new bypass graft, *Am. J. Surg.*, 170, 289, 1995.

19. Varga, Z.A., Locke-Edmunds, J.C., and Baird, R.N., A multicenter study of popliteal aneurysms. Joint Vascular Research Group. *J. Vasc. Surg.*, 20, 171, 1994.

20. Ouriel, K., Shortell, C.K., De Weese, J.A., et al., A comparison of thrombolytic therapy with operative vascularization in the initial treatment of acute peripheral arterial ischemia, *J. Vasc. Surg.*, 19, 1021, 1994.

21. The STILE Investigators, Results of a prospective randomized trial evaluating surgery versus thrombolysis for ischemia of the lower extremity (The STILE trial), *Ann. Surg.* 220, 251, 1994.

22. Ouriel, K., Veith, F.J., and Sasahara, A.A., Thrombolysis or peripheral artery surgery: phase I results, *J. Vasc. Surg.*, 23, 64, 1996.

23. Comerota, A.J., Weaver, F.A., Hosking, J.D., et al., Results of a prospective, randomized trial of surgery versus thrombolysis for occluded lower extremity bypass grafts, *Am. J. Surg.*, 172, 105, 1996.

24. Working Party on Thrombolysis in the Management of Limb Ischemia, Thrombolysis in the management of lower limb peripheral arterial occlusion—a consensus document, *Am. J. Cardiol.*, 81, 207, 1998.

9 Extracranial Carotid Artery Disease

Anthony J. Comerota and Lori L. Cindrick

CONTENTS

9.1 Introduction...169
9.2 Pathology 172
9.3 Evaluation 173
9.4 Treatment 176
    9.4.1 Symptomatic Stenosis...176
    9.4.2 Asymptomatic Stenosis...178
    9.4.3 Special Considerations...181
    9.4.4 Carotid Angioplasty and Stenting...............................184
    9.4.5 Role of Platelet Inhibitors...185
    9.4.6 Risk Factor Modification 185
9.5 Conclusions...186
References..186

9.1 INTRODUCTION

Stroke is the third leading cause of death in the United States and the leading cause of disability in adults. There are more than 600,000 new or recurrent strokes each year with an initial mortality of 15% to 30%, and an overall 5-year mortality of 50%. Of stroke survivors, 30% will have a slight deficit or return to normal, and 24% to 53% will be partially or completely dependent on others for the activities of daily life.[1]

Survivors of stroke remain at high risk for a subsequent stroke, averaging 6% to12% per year.[2] Although the leading cause of death in patients with extracranial arterial occlusive disease is myocardial infarction (MI), the leading cause of death in stroke survivors is recurrent stroke. It is estimated that more than 80% of strokes could be prevented if those at risk were identified and treated appropriately.[3]

The two basic mechanisms of stroke are ischemic (embolism or thrombosis) and hemorrhagic (intraparenchymal or subarachnoid hemorrhage resulting from cerebral aneurysm rupture, bleeding from an arteriovenous malformation or a hypertensive bleed). This chapter focuses on the ischemic causes of stroke as they relate to extracranial carotid artery occlusive disease, which is responsible for 20% to 30% of strokes. [4]

The most common cause of an ischemic stroke is embolism, of which the heart is the major source. Typically, this occurs in the setting of atrial fibrillation (risk: 4% to 7% per year), MI, prosthetic valves, or valvular heart disease. The carotid arteries account for a large portion of embolic strokes' occurring as a consequence of morphologic change on the luminal surface, mainly in the setting of atherosclerosis. An irregular surface serves as a nidus for platelet activation and aggregation. Furthermore, atherosclerotic plaques can undergo central degeneration with sudden expansion and intimal rupture due to intraplaque hemorrhage (Figure 9.1). This may result in embolization of debris such as calcium, cholesterol crystals, or thrombotic material, producing a sudden focal event. Some smaller emboli may go initially unrecognized and may be detected on routine brain imaging studies obtained as part of the patient's evaluation.[5]

Carotid thrombosis is another cause for an ischemic stroke. When an atherosclerotic plaque progresses to produce a critical reduction in blood flow, thrombosis of the artery can occur. If this happens in the internal carotid artery, it may propagate to the origin of the ophthalmic artery. With adequate collateral circulation via the circle of Willis, the event may go unrecognized. However, if thrombus extends into the middle cerebral artery or if there is insufficient collateral perfusion, an ischemic infarct occurs.[5]

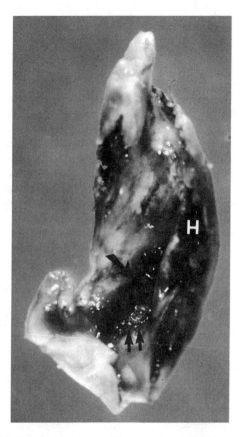

FIGURE 9.1 Carotid plaque removed from a patient who had an urgent carotid endarterectomy for crescendo transient ischemic attacks. This plaque has the typical characteristics of unstable atheroma, and illustrates how plaques can rapidly (and suddenly) progress from a mild or moderate asymptomatic stenosis to a severe symptomatic stenosis. Note: acute thrombus (*blood*) within the layers of the plaque indicating intraplaque hemorrhage (*H*), laminated luminal thrombus (double arrow), and plaque ulceration (single arrow).

9.2   PATHOLOGY

The pathology of carotid disease is divided into two categories: flow-restrictive lesions and lesions with embolic potential. The most common lesion affecting the extracranial carotid system is atherosclerotic plaque at the carotid bifurcation, which can cause both flow restriction and emboli. Several well-known risk factors for atherosclerosis include age, smoking, hypertension, hyperlipidemia, diabetes mellitus, elevated plasma homocysteine, and familial predisposition. A number of theories attempt to explain why the carotid bifurcation is particularly susceptible to the development of atherosclerotic plaque. The mechanical theory of low shear stress, boundary layer separation, and turbulent flow is one of the most popular. Regardless of the mechanism, once intimal injury occurs, platelet adhesion, smooth muscle cell proliferation, and accumulation of lipoproteins lead to plaque formation and progression. Of particular importance is the role of platelets. Platelets aggregate initiating thrombus formation, embolize, and are potent mediators of local effects, including vasospasm and smooth muscle cell proliferation. Atherosclerotic plaque is prone to intraplaque hemorrhage, which can rapidly reduce luminal diameter, often causing acute retinal or hemispheric symptoms.

Fibromuscular dysplasia (FMD) is a nonatherosclerotic lesion that affects medium-sized arteries such as the carotids, vertebrals, and renals. There are four histologic types; however, the most prevalent is medial fibroplasia. It can appear as alternating regions of narrowing and dilation, know as a "string of beads" (type I), tubular stenosis and webs (type II), and microaneurysms (type III). Embolism is the usual cause of symptoms in patients with FMD, rather than flow reduction from a stenosis. FMD usually affects the distal cervical carotid and vertebral arteries, and up to 30% of patients have an associated intracranial aneurysm. FMD is more common in women (92%) and usually affects those over age 50.

Other pathologic processes affecting the carotid arteries include coiling and kinking, aneurysm formation, Takayasu arteritis, and postoperative myointimal fibroplasia causing recurrent carotid stenosis after carotid intervention.

The clinical syndromes produced by cervical carotid disease are discussed in detail elsewhere in this book. In brief, carotid disease has two basic presentations, symptomatic and asymptomatic. Symptoms include transient ischemic attacks (TIA), amaurosis fugax (AF), or stroke. Patients who present with hemispheric or retinal symptoms should have a full evaluation of the cervical carotid arteries in addition to a cardiac evaluation to exclude arrhythmias, valvular disease, and other potential sources of cardiogenic emboli.

The asymptomatic patient with significant carotid disease often presents with a cervical bruit found during neck auscultation, although it is well known that the presence or absence of a bruit does not exclude significant disease. A bruit results from vessel wall vibration; it can exist in vessels without significant disease and be absent in arteries with a high-grade stenosis. Bruits with a musical character and those that extend into and through diastole are usually the result of significant disease of the internal carotid artery (ICA). Because the ICA normally has pandiastolic flow, bruits extending into or through diastole usually originate from a stenosis of the ICA. Patients at high risk of carotid disease are those with the common risk factors of atherosclerosis mentioned earlier, and patients with other systemic manifestations of atherosclerosis, such as cardiac and especially lower-extremity arterial occlusive disease.

9.3 EVALUATION

After a complete history and physical examination, the carotid arteries are objectively evaluated with a carotid duplex examination. "Duplex" refers to the combination of B-mode imaging and pulsed Doppler velocity spectrum analysis to evaluate the degree of luminal compromise (Figure 9.1). B-mode imaging defines the anatomy of the carotid bifurcation and the characteristics of the atherosclerotic plaque, and is used to guide the pulsed Doppler sample volume. The degree of stenosis is based on peak systolic and end-diastolic velocities generated by the pulsed Doppler spectral waveform. Blood flow in normal vessels is laminar. A stenosis produces turbulence, and when luminal

TABLE 9.1
**Criteria for Interpreting Carotid Duplex
Examination**[a]

ICA Stenosis (%)	B-Mode and Velocity Spectrum Analysis
0 –15	No plaque
	Peak systolic velocity <125–140 cm/s
	Normal spectral window
16 – 49	Mild plaque present
	Peak systolic velocity <125 –140 cm/s
	Turbulence obliterates spectral window
50 – 69	Moderate plaque present
	Peak systolic velocity >125 –140 cm/s
	No spectral window
70 – 99	Significant plaque present
	End-diastolic velocity >125 – 140 cm/s
	No spectral window
	ICA/CCA ratio >4.0
Occlusion	Transluminal plaque
	No Doppler signal in the ICA

CCA = common carotid artery; ICA = internal carotid artery.

[a] Criteria represent generally accepted guidelines for most vascular
laboratories. Specific threshold values should be established for each
laboratory based on review of arteriograms and constructing receiver-
operator characteristic curves.

obstruction approaches 50% (in the ICA), the systolic velocity begins
to rise (Table 9.1). Duplex scanning is reliable for identifying (or
eliminating) carotid disease (Figure 9.2). Its sensitivity may be
improved by calculating the common carotid to internal carotid peak
systolic velocity ratio, with a value greater than 4 suggesting high-
grade ICA stenosis.[6] In some cases, it may be difficult for the carotid

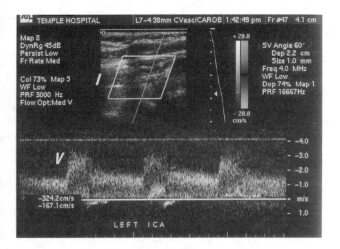

FIGURE 9.2 Carotid duplex scan of a patient with a high-grade stenosis of the left internal carotid artery (ICA). Image (*I*), shows a stenosis with turbulent flow. Velocity analysis (*V*) permits quantification of the stenosis. In this case, the peak systolic velocity is 324 cm/s and end-diastolic velocity is 167 cm/s, consistent with an 80% to 99% diameter reduction stenosis.

duplex to differentiate between internal carotid occlusion and a pre-occlusive (string sign) lesion. The stenosis may be so tight and the flow stream so narrow that it is missed by the scan probe. In these cases, careful evaluation of the distal cervical ICA is helpful.[7,8]

Magnetic resonance angiography (MRA) offers the advantages of being noninvasive, safe, and painless; it also can be performed without contrast. Unfortunately, motion artifact is present in approximately 20% of completed studies. MRA tends to overestimate the degree of stenosis and offers no information about the morphology of the plaque. It is not suitable for patients who are claustrophobic, unstable, or who have metallic implanted devices. It has been found to correlate reasonably well with duplex, but, in most cases, does not add appreciable information to a technically adequate duplex examination.[9]

Arteriography remains the "gold standard" for the confirmation of extracranial carotid disease. It is an invasive test, usually performed via femoral artery cannulation. The severity of the internal carotid stenosis is calculated by dividing the smallest residual lumen by the most normal internal luminal diameter distal to the stenosis. Arteriography should not be used as a screening test for disease, but rather as a selective preoperative study that confirms an accessible lesion and assists in planning the surgical procedure. In addition to the risk of contrast administration, arteriography carries a 0.6% to 1.2% risk of stroke. Preoperative arteriography is no longer routine in most treatment centers, because of its associated risk of stroke and the availability of improved noninvasive alternatives. However, when noninvasive studies are inconsistent or inconclusive or when multilevel disease is suspected, arteriography is valuable in making appropriate recommendations for care and planning operative revascularization.[10]

9.4 TREATMENT

Treatment of the patient with carotid artery disease is essentially prophylaxis. All treatment is intended to prevent subsequent cerebral ischemic events or to prevent a stenotic vessel from occluding. Similar to any other disease state, treatment should be evaluated by balancing risk versus benefit in known risk categories. In general, it is accepted that symptomatic patients are at higher risk than asymptomatic patients, risk increases with the severity of stenosis, and ulcerated lesions have a poorer prognosis than nonulcerated lesions.

9.4.1 SYMPTOMATIC STENOSIS

In the last decade, three major trials that randomly studied patients with symptomatic carotid disease have been reported. The first is the North American Symptomatic Carotid Endarterectomy Trial (NASCET).[11] The NASCET trial tested the hypothesis that carotid endarterectomy reduces stroke in patients with symptomatic carotid stenosis. This study randomized patients with symptomatic 30% to

99% carotid stenoses to best medical care or to best medical care plus carotid endarterectomy. The surgical group was further stratified into three categories according to the severity of their disease: severe stenosis (70% to 99%), moderate stenosis (50% to 69%), and mild stenosis (30% to 49%). Randomization of patients with a high-grade stenosis was halted by the data and safety monitoring committee because of a major benefit observed in patients randomized to carotid endarterectomy. The 2-year incidence of ipsilateral fatal and nonfatal strokes was 9% in the surgical group, including perioperative strokes, and 26% in the medical group ($P < 0.001$), which represents a relative risk reduction of 65% in favor of operative management. Subsequently, patients with a 50% to 69% stenosis were also found to have significantly fewer strokes with carotid endarterectomy compared with the best nonoperative management.[12] When the group randomized to best medical care was analyzed, it was found that the risk of stroke increased with the severity of stenosis and the presence of ulceration. Furthermore, the risk of subsequent stroke correlated with the number of risk factors present (Table 9.2). The NASCET study is a landmark trial demonstrating the benefit of endarterectomy in the prevention of stroke for patients with a 50% to 99% symptomatic stenosis.

The European Carotid Surgery Trial (ECST)[13] reported its results at approximately the same time as the NASCET study and confirmed the observation that carotid endarterectomy was beneficial for patients with moderate to severe symptomatic stenosis.

The Veterans Administration Cooperative (VA Co-op) Study of Symptomatic Carotid Stenosis[14] was terminated prematurely in February 1991 after the announcement of the initial results from the NASCET and ECST trials. The results from the VA Co-op trial complement the findings of the other studies by showing a reduction in the risk of stroke with carotid endarterectomy.

The presence of a plaque ulceration deserves special attention. As supported in the NASCET trial, the presence of an ulcerated plaque was associated with a more virulent course, as ulceration is a marker of an unstable plaque. Although carotid endarterectomy is not advocated for lesions of less than 50% stenosis, a patient with

TABLE 9.2
Relation Between Risk Factors[a] and Subsequent Stroke: NASCET Trial

Risk (No. of Risk Factors)	Medical Therapy (%)	Surgical Therapy (%)
Low (0 – 5)	17	9
Moderate (6)	23	9
High (≥7)	39	9

NASCET = North American Symptomatic Carotid Endarterectomy Trial.

[a] Risk factors include: age >70 years, hypertension, previous myocardial infarction, diabetes mellitus, tobacco abuse, congestive heart failure, claudication, hyperlipidemia, systolic pressure >160 mm Hg, diastolic pressure >90 mm Hg, degree of internal stenosis, and the presence of ulceration.

an ulcerated plaque and repetitive TIAs on maximal platelet inhibition should be considered for operation. Because this scenario is unusual, the numbers of patients are small. However, these patients can benefit significantly from carotid endarterectomy.

In summary, three prospective studies evaluating patients with symptomatic carotid stenosis demonstrated consistent benefit of carotid endarterectomy compared with best nonoperative care. A suggested algorithm for patients presenting with symptomatic carotid artery disease is found in Figure 9.3.

9.4.2 ASYMPTOMATIC STENOSIS

Three randomized trials have been performed to evaluate the benefit of carotid endarterectomy in patients with asymptomatic carotid stenosis. The Carotid Surgery Versus Medical Therapy in Asymptotic

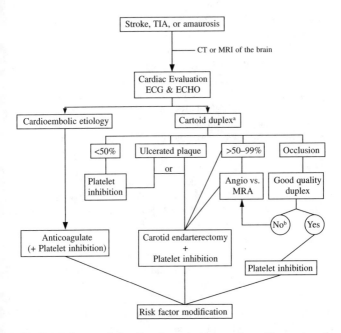

FIGURE 9.3 Suggested algorithm for patients presenting with symptomatic carotid disease. ANGIO = angiogram; AVM = arteriovenous malformation; CEA = carotid endarterectomy; CT = computed tomography; ECG = electrocardiogram; ECHO = echocardiogram; MRA = magnetic resonance angiography; MRI = magnetic resonance imaging; TIA = transient ischemic attack. ªTreatment on basis of duplex scan alone assumes a good-quality examination with conclusive findings. In other cases, ANGIO or MRA should be performed. ᵇANGIO or MRA confirmation of occlusion should receive platelet inhibition.

Carotid Stenosis (CASANOVA) trial was published in *Stroke* in 1991. This study compared medical therapy with aspirin to carotid endarterectomy for patients with a 50% to 90% stenosis. The study erroneously concluded that there was no benefit from prophylactic endarterectomy. There were major methodologic flaws in this trial. Patients with a greater than 90% stenosis were not randomized, but underwent carotid endarterectomy. This was also true for patients randomized to medical therapy who subsequently progressed to 90% stenosis, as well as those who developed TIAs. Unfortunately, progression to a critical stenosis and development of ischemic symptoms in patients assigned to medical therapy were not considered treatment failures. These flaws in the study design and data analysis invalidate the trial's conclusions.[15]

The second asymptomatic trial was the Veterans Administration Trial. This prospective randomized multicenter trial compared best medical therapy with aspirin to carotid endarterectomy for the combined endpoints of TIA, AF, or stroke in patients with 50% or more stenosis. The combined incidence of ipsilateral neurological events was 8.0% in the surgical arm and 20.6% in the medical group ($P < 0.001$). The incidence of ipsilateral stroke was 4.7% in the surgical group compared with 9.4% in the medical group ($P = 0.056$). Unfortunately, the trial sample size was too small to show a 50% reduction in ipsilateral stroke to achieve statistical significance.[16]

The most recently published trial is the Asymptomatic Carotid Atherosclerosis Study (ACAS), appearing in the *Journal of the American Medical Association* in 1995. This was a randomized multicenter trial comparing best medical management to carotid endarterectomy for asymptomatic carotid disease of 60% or more stenosis with outcome measures of stroke or death. The primary outcome of ipsilateral stroke at 5 years was 5.1% in the surgical group and 11% in the medically treated group ($P = 0.006$), a 54% relative risk reduction. All patients randomized to surgery underwent obligatory carotid arteriography. There was a 1.2% stroke complication rate of arteriography, and patients who had arteriographic strokes were assigned to the surgical group, although none actually underwent an operation. Of the patients who did, the combined neurologic morbidity and mortality was 1.5%.[17] A suggested algorithm for patients presenting with asymptomatic carotid is presented in Figure 9.4. Although carotid endarterectomy for an asymptomatic 60% stenosis is supported by the ACAS study, it is usually reserved for patients with a higher degree of stenosis, who are

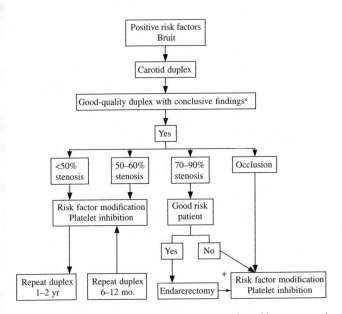

FIGURE 9.4 Suggested algorithm for patients presenting with asymptomatic carotid disease. [a]Confirmatory magnetic resonance angiogram or arteriogram required in patients with an inconclusive duplex scan.

good operative candidates. A summary of the clinical trials for symptomatic and asymptomatic carotid disease is presented in Table 9.3.

9.4.3 SPECIAL CONSIDERATIONS

Carotid endarterectomy in the setting of acute ischemic stroke is usually contraindicated; however, the old convention of waiting a minimum of 6 weeks before proceeding with an operation has recently been challenged. It is still thought inadvisable to operate if there is a dense neurologic deficit, a depressed level of consciousness, or cardiovascular instability. However, once a neurologic plateau has been

TABLE 9.3 (CONTINUED)
Summary of NASCET and ACAS Trials

Study (% Stenosis)	Medical, Surgical, n (%)	Surgical, n (%)	Relative Risk Reduction (%)	P-Value
NASCET (70 – 99)[a]				
Patients (n)	331	328		
Any ipsilateral stroke	61 (26)	26 (9.0)	65	<0.001
Major/fatal ipsilateral stroke	29 (13.1)	8 (2.5)	81	<0.001
Any stroke	64 (27.6)	34 (12.6)	54	<0.001
Any major stroke or death	38 (18.1)	19 (8.0)	56	<0.01
Any stroke or death	73 (32.3)	41 (15.8)	51	<0.001
NASCET (50 – 69)[b]				
Patients (n)	428	430		

Any ipsilateral stroke	80 (22.2)	57 (15.7)	29	<0.045
Any stroke	113 (32.3)	85 (23.9)	26	<0.026
Any stroke or death	156 (43.3)	120 (33.2)	23	<0.005
ACAS (60 – 99) [b]				
Patients (n)	834	825		
Any ipsilateral stroke	92 (11.0)	42 (5.1)	53	<0.004
Major/fatal ipsilateral stroke	50 (6.0)	28 (3.4)	43	0.12
Any major stroke or death	213 (25.5)	171 (20.7)	19	0.16
Any stroke or death	266 (31.9)	211 (25.6)	20	0.08

ACAS = Asymptomatic Carotid Atherosclerosis Study; NASCET = North American Symptomatic Carotid Endarterectomy Trial.

[a] 2-year follow-up.
[b] 5-year follow-up.

reached, which could take days to weeks, an endarterectomy can be considered.

If the patient's neurologic status is improving, we favor waiting for maximal improvement. Mentzer and colleagues[18] evaluated surgical outcomes in patients operated for crescendo TIAs and stroke-in-evolution. Although the operative risk of stroke and death was appreciable in these high-risk patients, the operated patients had significantly better outcomes than nonoperated patients. Indications for an urgent or emergent carotid endarterectomy include free-floating or propagating thrombus, crescendo TIA, asymptomatic preocclusive lesion, and selected patients with stroke-in-evolution and acute carotid occlusion.[19] Patients with symptomatic carotid lesions, and especially those with multiple symptoms, often have an unstable atheroma, as shown in Figure 9.2.

9.4.4 CAROTID ANGIOPLASTY AND STENTING

Carotid endarterectomy is the gold standard for treatment of patients with symptomatic and asymptomatic carotid atherosclerosis associated with moderate to severe stenoses. In the past several years, some centers have extended percutaneous balloon angioplasty to carotid bifurcation lesions. It appears to have gained premature popularity among the interventional radiology and cardiology specialties. Diethrich and colleagues recently reported a 13% rate of morbidity and mortality in 110 patients treated with carotid angioplasty. If asymptomatic stent thrombosis (occlusion) is included as morbidity, the adverse outcome event rate rises to 15%.[20] The North American cerebral percutaneous transluminal angioplasty register prospectively enrolled patients having carotid percutaneous transluminal angioplasty (PTA) by skilled interventionalists with an interest in endovascular techniques. The initial report showed a neurologic morbidity and mortality of 10%. An updated report recently demonstrated a combined morbidity and mortality of 9%.[21] In time, carotid PTA and stenting will have its role in patients with carotid atherosclerosis. However, it currently cannot achieve the results of carotid endarterectomy, and should be restricted to patients enrolled in randomized trials and perhaps a select subgroup of patients with carotid lesions who have an unacceptably high operative risk.

9.4.5 ROLE OF PLATELET INHIBITORS

The beneficial effects of platelet inhibitors in patients with atherosclerosis was shown by the Antiplatelet Trialists' Collaboration, in which a widespread meta-analysis of 142 trials demonstrated that antiplatelet agents reduced the incidence of ischemic stroke, MI, and vascular death, with a relative odds reduction of 27%. The Ticlopidine Aspirin Stroke Study (TASS) demonstrated an additional 12% benefit of ticlopidine compared with aspirin.[22] The most recent comparative analysis is the Clopidogrel Versus Aspirin in Patients at Risk of Ischemic Events (CAPRIE) trial, in which aspirin was compared with clopidogrel (Plavix®*), a recently introduced platelet inhibitor (clopidogrel and ticlopidine are chemically similar and both inhibit the adenosine diphosphate receptor on the platelet membrane). The randomized CAPRIE trial demonstrated a statistically significant relative risk reduction of 8.7% in favor of clopidogrel.

Most treatment algorithms recommend the use of an antiplatelet agent for carotid artery disease, and some recommend combination therapy with aspirin and clopidogrel.[23] The perioperative use of aspirin significantly reduces operative stroke after carotid endarterectomy and appears to reduce all neurologic events and mortality.[24] We believe that it is important for all patients with carotid disease to take platelet inhibitors, and we instruct patients undergoing carotid endarterectomy to continue their aspirin up to the day of their operation.

9.4.6 RISK FACTOR MODIFICATION

As stated previously, the risk factors for atherosclerosis and carotid disease have been well defined. Two of them, hypertension and increased serum cholesterol, deserve special consideration. Hyperten-

---

* Registered trademark of Bristol-Myers-Squibb Company, Princeton, NJ.

sion is the most important of the known risk factors for all stroke subtypes. The risk of stroke is known to increase with increasing systolic and diastolic blood pressure, with a 3.76 relative risk increase for systolic pressures greater than 160 mm Hg and a 4.17 relative risk increase with diastolic pressures greater than 100 mm Hg.[25]

Although the link between increased cholesterol and coronary artery disease has been well described, the relation between stroke and serum cholesterol is not as well defined. Recently, the Cholesterol and Recurrent Events (CARE) trial examined the use of a 3-hydroxy-3-methylglutaryl coenzyme A reductase inhibitor (pravastatin) with stroke and TIA prevention as a defined secondary endpoint. The CARE investigators demonstrated a significant reduction (32%, $P = 0.03$) with the use of pravastatin. Similar results were reported in the Scandinavian Simvastatin Survival Study.[26]

9.5   CONCLUSIONS

Extracranial carotid artery disease accounts for a significant proportion of strokes, a leading cause of morbidity and mortality today. The two major types of pathology include carotid artery thrombosis and embolism. Patients with significant carotid artery disease can be divided into symptomatic and asymptomatic groups. Carotid endarterectomy has been demonstrated to be effective in both of these groups, and all patients should be treated with platelet inhibition and aggressive risk factor modification.

REFERENCES

1. American Heart Association, 1998 Heart and Stroke Statistical update, Dallas, Texas.
2. Schmidt, E.V., Smirnov, V.E., and Ryabova, V.S., Results of the 7-year prospective study of stroke patients, *Stroke*, 19, 942, 1988.
3. Sacco, R.L., Benjamin, E.J., Broderick, J.P., et al., Whisnant, J.P., and Wolf, P.A., Risk factors, *Stroke*, 28,1507, 1997.

4. Eaton, D., Surgery and medical management of cerebrovascular disease, in *Vascular Disease: A Multi-specialty Approach to Diagnosis and Management*, 2nd ed., Eaton, D., Ed., Landes Bioscience, Austin, 1999, 31.

5. Moore, W.S., Extracranial cerebrovascular disease: the carotid artery, in *Vascular Surgery: A Comprehensive Review*, 5th ed., Moore, W.S., Ed., W.B. Saunders, Philadelphia, 1998, 555.

6. Moneta, G.L., Edwards, J.M., and Chitwood, R.W., Correlation of North American Symptomatic Carotid Endarterectomy Trial (NASCET) angiographic definition of 70% to 99% internal carotid stenosis with duplex scanning, *J. Vasc. Surg.*, 17, 152, 1993.

7. Baker, J.D., The Vascular Laboratory: Diagnosis and Management of Cerebrovascular Disease, in *Rutherford Textbook of Vascular Surgery*, 4th ed., Rutherford, R.B., Ed., W.B. Saunders, Philadelphia, 1995, 1508.

8. Strandness, D.E., Duplex scanning in vascular disorders, in *Extracranial Arterial Disease*, 2nd ed., Strandness, D.E., Ed., Raven Press, New York, 1993, 113.

9. Modaresi, K.B., Cox, T.C.S., and Summers, P.E., Comparison of intra-arterial digital subtraction angiography, magnetic resonance angiography and duplex ultrasonography for measuring carotid artery stenosis, *Br. J. Surg.*, 86, 1422, 1999.

10. Moneta, G.L., Saxon, R.R., and Taylor, L.M., Carotid imaging before carotid endarterectomy, *Semin.Vasc. Surg.*, 8, 21, 1995.

11. NASCET Collaborators, Beneficial effects of carotid endarterectomy in symptomatic patients with high-grade stenosis, *N. Engl. J. Med.* 325, 445, 1991.

12. NASCET Collaborators, Benefit of carotid endarterectomy in patients with symptomatic moderate or severe stenosis, *N. Engl. J. Med.*, 339, 1415, 1998.

13. European Carotid Surgery Trialists' Collaborative Group, Randomised trial of endarterectomy for recently symptomatic carotid stenosis: final results of the MRC European Carotid Surgery Trial (ECST), *Lancet*, 351, 1379, 1998.

14. Mayberg, M.R., Wilson, S.E., and Yatsu, F., Carotid endarterectomy and prevention of cerebral ischemia in symptomatic carotid stenosis, *JAMA*, 266, 3289, 1991.

15. CASANOVA Study Group, Carotid surgery versus medical therapy in asymptomatic carotid stenosis, *Stroke*, 22, 1229, 1991.

16. Veterans Administration Cooperative Study, Role of carotid endarterectomy in asymptomatic carotid stenosis, *Stroke*, 17, 534, 1986.

17. Executive Committee for the Asymptomatic Carotid Atherosclerosis Study, Endarterectomy for asymptomatic carotid stenosis, *JAMA*, 273, 1421, 1995.

18. Mentzer, R.M., Jr., Finkelmeier, B.A., and Crosby, I.K., Emergency carotid endarterectomy for fluctuating neurologic deficits, *Surgery*, 89, 60, 1981.

19. Beebe, H.G., Surgery for acute stroke, *Semin. Vasc. Surg.*, 8, 55, 1995.

20. Diethrich, E.B., Ndiaye, M., and Reid, D.B., Stenting in the carotid artery: initial experience in 100 patients, *J. Endovasc. Surg.*, 3, 42, 1996.

21. Joint Council of the Society for Vascular Surgery and the International Society for Cardiovascular Surgery, North American Chapter, Statement regarding carotid angioplasty and stenting, *J. Vasc. Surg.*, 24, 900, 1996.

22. Hass, W.K., Easton, J.D., and Adams, H.P., A randomized trial comparing ticlopidine hydrochloride with aspirin for the prevention of stroke in high-risk patients, *N. Engl. J. Med.*, 321, 501, 1989.

23. CAPRIE Steering Committee, A randomized blinded trial of clopidogrel versus aspirin in patients at risk of ischemic events (CAPRIE), *Lancet*, 348, 1329, 1996.

24. Lindblad, B., Persson, N.H., and Takolander, R., Does low-dose acetylsalicylic acid prevent stroke after carotid surgery?, *Stroke*, 24, 1125, 1993.

25. Leppälä, J. M., Virtamo, J., and Fogelholm, R., Different risk factors for different stroke subtypes: association of blood pressure, cholesterol and antioxidants, *Stroke*, 30, 2535, 1999.

26. The CARE Investigators, Reduction of stroke incidence after myocardial infarction with pravastatin: the Cholesterol and Recurrent Events (CARE) Study, *Circulation*, 99, 216, 1999.

Section III

Abdominal Arterial Diseases

10 Visceral Arterial Disease

Lloyd M. Taylor, Jr., Gregory L. Moneta, Gregory Landry, and John M. Porter

CONTENTS

10.1 Introduction 192
10.2 Intestinal Artery Anatomy..192
10.3 Intestinal Artery Physiology..193
10.4 Pathophysiology of Intestinal Ischemia...............................193
10.5 Acute Intestinal Ischemia...195
    10.5.1 Superior Mesenteric Artery Thrombosis 196
    10.5.2 Superior Mesenteric Artery Embolism....................197
    10.5.3 Diagnostic Tests 197
    10.5.4 Percutaneous Interventional Treatment 198
    10.5.5 Operative Treatment..199
    10.5.6 Superior Mesenteric Artery Revascularization.........199
    10.5.7 Management of the Acutely Ischemic Intestine.......202
    10.5.8 Acute Nonocclusive Intestinal Ischemia 202
    10.5.9 Acute Colonic Ischemia ("Ischemic Colitis")..........203
    10.5.10 Colonic Ischemia after Aortic Surgery....................204
10.6 Chronic Intestinal Ischemia 206
    10.6.1 Natural History..206
    10.6.2 Diagnosis..207
    10.6.3 Percutaneous Interventional Treatment
        of Chronic Intestinal Ischemia 208
    10.6.4 Surgical Treatment of Chronic Intestinal Ischemia..208
References..216

0-8493-8413-3/01/$0.00+$1.50
© 2001 by CRC Press LLC

10.1 INTRODUCTION

Visceral arterial disease is important because it can produce intestinal infarction, a relation clearly stated in 1936 by Dunphy, who was among the first to recognize that, "The clinical importance of vascular pain in the abdomen lies in the fact that it may be the precursor of fatal mesenteric vascular occlusion."[1] A large number of diseases and conditions affecting both large and small arteries can result in intestinal ischemia or infarction (Table 10.1). Most are rare. This chapter will focus on the most frequent causes of acute and chronic visceral arterial disease, namely atherosclerosis, thromboembolism, and nonocclusive intestinal ischemia. The chapter is divided into a brief description of visceral vascular anatomy and physiology, followed by sections organized according to typical clinical presentations, including acute intestinal ischemia, chronic intestinal ischemia, and colonic ischemia.

10.2 INTESTINAL ARTERY ANATOMY

Three branches of the abdominal aorta—the celiac artery, the superior mesenteric artery, and the inferior mesenteric artery—provide the arterial supply for the intestines. In a normal situation, the majority of the

---

TABLE 10.1
Diseases and Conditions That May Result in Intestinal Ischemia

• Atherosclerosis	• Embolism
• Hypercoagulable states	• Polyarteritis nodosa
• Visceral artery dissection	• Systemic lupus erythematosis
• Fibromuscular disease	• Rheumatoid arthritis
• Ergot poisoning	• Cocaine overuse
• Radiation injury	• Neurofibromatosis
• Buerger disease	• Aortic coarctation repair
• Cogan syndrome	• Mesenteric venous thrombosis

---

celiac artery flow goes to the liver and spleen, and a minority goes to the stomach, duodenum, and pancreas. Superior mesenteric artery flow is normally distributed entirely to the small intestine and proximal colon. Inferior mesenteric artery flow normally supplies the distal colon. Many collaterals connect these three vascular distributions, notably the pancreatoduodenal arcades between the celiac and superior mesenteric vessels, the marginal artery of Drummond, and the mesenteric arc of Riolan (an ascending branch of the left colic branch of the inferior mesenteric artery), which connects the superior and inferior mesenteric circulations. The extent of these collaterals is such that extensive occlusive disease, even including occlusion of any of the three major aortic branches, is usually well tolerated.

10.3   INTESTINAL ARTERY PHYSIOLOGY

Celiac artery flow is generally constant, with a high diastolic flow component, reflecting the constant metabolic requirements of the solid organs being supplied. Fasting flow in the superior mesenteric artery exhibits high resistance characteristics, with diastolic flow reversal. Postprandially, superior mesenteric flow volume and velocity increase markedly, and there is high volume forward flow throughout diastole, reflecting the increased intestinal blood supply necessary for absorption and digestion of food.[2] Inferior mesenteric artery flow also increases postprandially.

10.4   PATHOPHYSIOLOGY OF INTESTINAL ISCHEMIA

The extensive collateral network of the three major visceral vessels is sufficient that extensive atherosclerotic occlusive disease is usually well tolerated. As an example, 27% of one series of patients undergoing aortography before peripheral vascular surgery had greater than 50% stenosis of the celiac or superior mesenteric arteries, yet none had symptoms of intestinal ischemia.[3] Indeed, chronic intestinal ischemia caused by atherosclerotic occlusive disease is one of the rarest manifestations of atherosclerosis. Even major vascular centers rarely report experience with more than 100 cases accumulated over decades. When chronic ischemic symptoms do occur, most patients have severe stenoses or occlusion of two or more of the three visceral arteries. There are occasional exceptions to this rule, and symptomatic intestinal ischemia does occur with single-vessel disease. Patients with this problem have severe occlusive disease of the superior mesenteric artery, and disruption of the normal collateral channels from the celiac and inferior mesenteric arteries. The most frequent reason for collateral interruption is previous gastric or colonic surgery. Although chronic visceral arterial occlusive disease is usually well tolerated, acute occlusion of the superior mesenteric or inferior mesenteric arteries may produce acute symptoms, including infarction. Except when normal collaterals are disrupted, both acute and chronic celiac artery occlusion are well tolerated.

With chronic intestinal ischemia, patients typically develop postprandial abdominal pain. The pain is typically attributed to intestinal hypoxia, as the increased flow requirements necessary for absorption and digestion cannot be met, a situation analogous to angina pectoris. However, the true cause of intestinal ischemic pain is unknown. Periumbilical pain typically develops 20 to 30 minutes after eating and persists for approximately 1 hour. For most patients, the pain is severe, and nearly all quickly reduce their food intake ("food fear"). Weight loss, which may become profound, is the inevitable result. There are many variations in the location and timing of the pain among individuals. Some patients have diarrhea, and some have constipation; vomiting is unusual. Most patients with chronic intestinal ischemia have sufficiently severe atherosclerosis that symptoms are present in other vascular beds (e.g., angina, stroke, claudication). Many have had previous cardiovascular surgery. Although the pain pattern may be confusing, the triad of abdominal pain, weight loss, and symptomatic vascular disease should (but frequently does not) lead to suspicion of intestinal ischemia.

The weight loss of chronic intestinal ischemia has been conclusively shown to be the result of decreased caloric intake. No studies have shown a reproducible defect in intestinal absorption as a result of ischemia.[4]

10.5   ACUTE INTESTINAL ISCHEMIA

Acute intestinal ischemia occurs when intestinal blood flow is suddenly reduced below the level required to support viability. The most frequent causes are embolism to the superior mesenteric artery and thrombosis of a chronically stenotic superior mesenteric artery. The clinical scenario resulting from these events is familiar to most surgeons. Typically, an elderly person (70% are women) is admitted to the hospital complaining of severe abdominal pain. Initially, there is a lack of accompanying physical findings (peritonitis has not yet developed, a disparity referred to as "pain out of proportion to physical findings"). This leads to an orderly and deliberate diagnostic process. Within a few hours, tachycardia, hypotension, acidosis, and marked abdominal tenderness occur (necrotic intestine produces peritoneal irritation and hemodynamic collapse), leading to laparotomy. Extensive intestinal necrosis is found, and the outcome is nearly always fatal.

There has been little improvement in this dismal scenario in the past several decades, despite general improvement in vascular diagnosis and therapy overall. As seen in Table 10.2, mortality rates for treatment of acute intestinal ischemia average 75% to 80% and are little changed from historic reports. The reason for this grim outlook is found in the time course of the clinical signs of the disease. Because the initial pain of acute intestinal ischemia is not associated with physical signs, delay in diagnosis is frequent. By the time physical signs are prominent, necrosis is nearly always present, and survival is doubtful. Even for the minority of patients who encounter an appropriately suspicious surgeon early in the course of the disease, emergency major abdominal arterial surgery and resection of significant lengths of bowel are required, a procedure poorly tolerated by elderly patients with multisystem disease.

Given these realities, mortality of acute intestinal ischemia will probably always remain high. For some patients seen early, and others

TABLE 10.2
Mortality Associated with Treatment of Acute Intestinal Ischemia from Arterial Obstructions

Study	Patients (n)	Mortality (%)
Ottinger and Austen, 1967	51	43 (84)
Slater and Elliott, 1972	4	4 (100)
Singh et al., 1975	30	24 (81)
Smith and Patterson, 1976	23	21 (91)
Kairalouma et al., 1977	44	31 (70)
Hertzer et al., 1978	10	7 (70)
Sachs et al., 1982	30	23 (77)
Levy et al., 1990	45	20(44)

From Taylor, L.M., Jr., Moneta, G.L., and Porter, J.M., Treatment of acute intestinal ischemia caused by arterial occlusions, in *Vascular Surgery*, 5th ed., Rutherford, R.B., Ed., W.B. Saunders, Philadelphia, 2000, 1512. With permission.

in whom the extent of the ischemia is limited, there is potential for salvage by prompt diagnosis and treatment. The foundation of accurate diagnosis remains a high index of suspicion. Acute abdominal pain out of proportion to physical findings occurring in an elderly person with a history of atherosclerotic cardiovascular disease should elicit recognition of the pattern of intestinal ischemia.

10.5.1 Superior Mesenteric Artery Thrombosis

An unknown number of patients with chronic severe stenosis of the superior mesenteric artery develop thrombosis with resulting acute ischemia. Most are female, and have evidence of vascular disease at other sites or a previous history of cardiovascular surgery. About one half of patients with superior mesenteric artery thrombosis have a history of chronic abdominal pain and weight loss.

10.5.2   SUPERIOR MESENTERIC ARTERY EMBOLISM

About 5% of cardiac emboli lodge in visceral vessels.[5] Obviously, embolic mesenteric artery occlusion should be strongly considered in any patient with acute abdominal pain and a history of cardiac disease that might lead to embolism, the most frequent being atrial arrhythmia and acute myocardial infarction. As the number of percutaneous intravascular diagnostic and interventional procedures continues to increase, arterioarterial embolism caused by manipulation of catheters and guidewires is an increasingly important cause of intestinal ischemia. Severe abdominal pain after cardiac catheterization or other intravascular procedures should arouse immediate consideration of acute intestinal ischemia.

10.5.3   DIAGNOSTIC TESTS

Nearly all patients with acute intestinal ischemia have profound leukocytosis (> 15,000/mL). No specific laboratory tests short of arteriography have been established as diagnostic, or even highly suggestive, of acute intestinal ischemia. Visceral artery duplex scanning, which may accurately detect visceral artery occlusions and stenoses, is not very useful in acutely symptomatic patients, who inevitably have increased intestinal gas and not infrequently have intra-abdominal fluid, both of which interfere with performance of the test. There are no specific findings on abdominal radiography or other imaging tests that are useful in diagnosis of intestinal ischemia.

Arteriography accurately detects the presence of visceral artery obstructions, whether caused by thrombosis or embolism (Figure 10.1), but at a price. Treatment of acute intestinal ischemia is a true surgical emergency, and preparing for and completing abdominal aortography typically consumes several hours, time that may be critical to patient survival. In our practice, we obtain emergency arteriograms in patients suspected of acute intestinal ischemia who have pain but an absence of other findings mandating surgery. We do not take the time for arteriography in patients with physical findings of peritonitis, in whom the need for abdominal exploration is obvious.

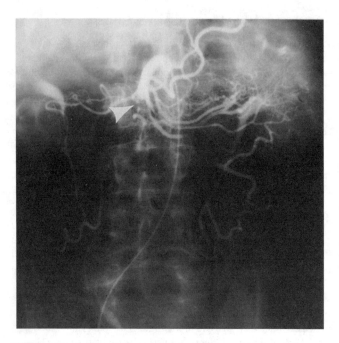

FIGURE 10.1 Acute embolic occlusion of the superior mesenteric artery (*arrowhead*) in a patient with chronic atrial fibrillation.

10.5.4 PERCUTANEOUS INTERVENTIONAL TREATMENT

The attractiveness of avoiding emergency major abdominal surgery by using percutaneous angiographic techniques to treat acute visceral artery obstructions is clear. A few case reports have described the use of balloon angioplasty or stenting to relieve acute visceral artery obstructions. Although this approach may successfully relieve the arterial obstruction, no method short of laparotomy permits assessment of the extent of bowel ischemia and resection of any necrotic segment. In a single case with survival, we have used superior mesenteric artery angioplasty and stenting to restore intestinal perfusion, followed by laparotomy and resection of necrotic bowel (unpublished case material). Whether this approach to reducing the magnitude of the emergency surgical procedure required will be more successful than conventional surgical approaches remains to be investigated. The ongoing high mortality with standard surgical treatment of acute intestinal ischemia means that investigation of innovative approaches to treatment is justified.

10.5.5 OPERATIVE TREATMENT

At laparotomy, the etiology and extent of the intestinal ischemia are determined by examination. Typically, superior mesenteric artery thrombosis results from atherosclerotic stenosis of the proximalmost part of the artery, and results in ischemia of the entire bowel, from the ligament of Treitz to the mid transverse colon. In contrast, superior mesenteric artery emboli typically lodge more distally in the artery beyond the first few large branches, so the ischemia typically spares the proximal jejunum.[6] Variation from this typical pattern is common, however, and true differentiation of thrombosis from embolism may not be possible without direct exploration of the superior mesenteric artery. With arterioarterial embolism, as occurs when intravascular manipulations dislodge atherothrombotic debris, the distribution of ischemia may be patchy and extensive.

In most patients with acute intestinal ischemia, a spectrum of ischemic changes exists with some bowel obviously necrotic, some obviously viable, and some of questionable viability. Because it is not possible to accurately predict the response of ischemic segments of intestine to restoration of arterial flow, as a general rule, revascularization should precede resection.

10.5.6 SUPERIOR MESENTERIC ARTERY REVASCULARIZATION

Embolectomy is performed by isolating the superior mesenteric artery at the base of the transverse colon mesentery, just beyond the point at which the artery emerges from beneath the inferior border of the pancreas. After arteriotomy, a balloon-tipped catheter is passed proximally into the aorta and withdrawn (Figure 10.2). Inability to pass the catheter into the aorta,

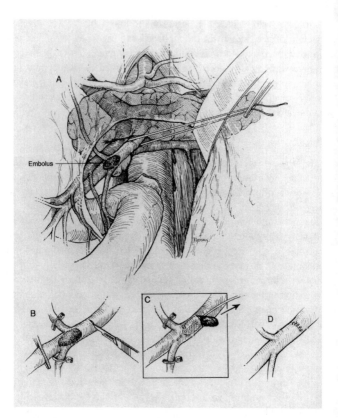

FIGURE 10.2 Superior mesenteric artery embolectomy. (A) Exposure of artery at the base of the transverse colon mesentery. (B) Transverse arteriotomy. (C) Extraction of embolus using balloon-tipped catheter. (D) Arteriotomy closure. (Reprinted from Kazmers, A., Operative management of acute mesenteric ischemia, *Ann. Vasc. Surg.*, 12, 187, 1998. With permission.)

or failure of thrombus extraction to produce copious pulsatile forward flow, makes the diagnosis of superior mesenteric artery thrombosis. In

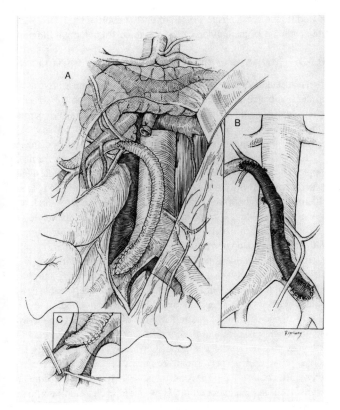

FIGURE 10.3 Bypass from aortoiliac junction for superior mesenteric artery thrombosis. (A)Prosthetic graft. (B) Autogenous vein grafting is used when intestinal resection is also required. (C) Detail of surgical closure of arteriotomy. (Reprinted from Kazmers, A., Operative management of acute mesenteric ischemia, *Ann. Vasc. Surg.*, 12, 187, 1998. With permission.)

this case, the arteriotomy serves as the anastomotic site for a bypass graft originating from the aorta or iliac artery (Figure 10.3). If adequate forward flow is reestablished, distal thromboembolectomy is performed with gentle use of the balloon catheter, and the arteriotomy is closed.

10.5.7 MANAGEMENT OF THE ACUTELY ISCHEMIC INTESTINE

After revascularization, obviously necrotic intestine must be resected and continuity reestablished. In many cases, a spectrum of ischemic changes exists, ranging from obviously viable to obviously necrotic, with varying lengths of bowel of indeterminate viability. Many techniques to assist in predicting the viability/recovery potential of damaged bowel have been evaluated, including auscultation with a sterilized Doppler ultrasonic flow detector,[6] injection of intravenous fluorescein,[7] surface oximetry,[8] infrared photoplethysmography,[9] and laser Doppler velocimetry.[10] None of these methods is completely reliable, and, perhaps most interestingly, none has been demonstrated superior to the clinical judgment of experienced surgeons.[11] We use a combination of continuous-wave Doppler insonnation and clinical judgment.

If sufficient viable intestine remains to clearly provide adequate nutrition (more than 6 feet of small intestine), all necrotic and questionably viable bowel should be resected. If the obviously viable bowel remaining is less than 6 feet in length, most surgeons choose to resect the clearly necrotic bowel and to leave the questionably viable bowel for subsequent inspection at a second-look procedure performed 18 to 36 hours after the initial operation. Obviously, it is mandatory that such an operation be performed regardless of the condition of the patient. Resection of the necrotic intestine may produce a dramatic improvement in patient condition. However, if even a small portion of the remaining questionable intestine becomes necrotic, it will result in death if not resected.

10.5.8 ACUTE NONOCCLUSIVE INTESTINAL ISCHEMIA

Intestinal ischemia occurs in the absence of visceral arterial obstruction in severely ill patients with circulatory (usually cardiogenic) shock and as a result of intoxication with cocaine or ergot. In these cases, intestinal ischemia is a result of inappropriate intestinal arterial vasospasm. Most cases have occurred when severe cardiogenic shock resulted in visceral arterial spasm, which may have been exacerbated by the use of vasopressor agents, particularly α-adrenergic agonists. Digoxin causes intestinal vasospasm in experimental animals, and many heart failure patients take this medication. Whether digoxin contributes to nonocclusive intestinal ischemia in humans has never been proven, but the association has been recognized repeatedly. In the past, nonocclusive mesenteric ischemia was the cause of as many as one half of all cases of acute mesenteric ischemia in some reported series.[13]

In modern practice, nonocclusive intestinal ischemia has become rare, most likely due to widespread use of hemodynamic monitoring and vasodilator treatment of cardiogenic shock. The condition should be suspected whenever a critically ill patient with reduced cardiac output develops abdominal pain. Initial treatment should be focused on improving the overall circulatory status and increasing cardiac output. Persistence of abdominal pain and tenderness in spite of improved cardiac output may indicate bowel that is irreversibly ischemic, and is an indication for laparotomy. Favorable response of intestinal arterial vasospasm to intra-arterial administration of vasodilators has been reported.[14] Whether improvement resulted from the local or systemic effects of the vasodilators has never been critically evaluated.

10.5.9 Acute Colonic Ischemia ("Ischemic Colitis")

Acute colonic ischemia presenting with abdominal pain and distension and bloody diarrhea may result from (1) acute occlusion of the inferior mesenteric artery; (2) atheroembolic occlusion of colonic arteries; or (3) systemic hypoperfusion producing a "watershed" colonic infarction at critical areas where overlap between the superior mesenteric and inferior mesenteric circulations is poor (e.g., "Griffith's point" near the splenic flexure). Initial management is conservative, as most patients recover with bowel rest and antibiotics. Laparotomy is reserved for persistent abdominal tenderness, leukocytosis, or signs of peritonitis or toxic megacolon.

10.5.10 Colonic Ischemia after Aortic Surgery

The inferior mesenteric artery is always interrupted during repair of infrarenal abdominal aortic aneurysms. It is also frequently interrupted during reconstruction of the infrarenal aorta for occlusive disease, thus introducing the potential for colonic ischemia. The descending and sigmoid portion of the colon is the area at risk; involvement can range from minimal mucosal ischemia that remains asymptomatic to full-thickness necrosis. In fact, colonic ischemia is a rare event (less than 1%) after elective aortic surgery but occurs not infrequently after repair of ruptured aortic aneurysms (60% in one prospective study).[15] The propensity of ruptured-aneurysm patients to develop colonic ischemia is probably related to coexisting shock and frequently extensive mesenteric hematomas that coexist with the need to interrupt the inferior mesenteric artery. This form of colonic ischemia is especially virulent, with reported mortality approaching 90% in cases with transmural involvement.[16]

Patients at highest risk for colonic ischemia after aortic surgery are those in whom coexisting superior mesenteric artery occlusive disease or vascular interruptions from previous surgery means that the normal collaterals for the inferior mesenteric artery are no longer present. The presence of a large meandering mesenteric artery (arch of Riolan) on preoperative aortography is a clue to the existence of superior mesenteric artery obstruction, which should be ruled out or confirmed by performance of lateral aortography (Figure 10.4).

Prevention of postoperative colonic ischemia involves awareness of the collateral supply of the colon and operative planning to ensure adequate colonic perfusion. Use of end-to-side aortic anastomoses when operating for occlusive disease, for example, may permit continued perfusion of the inferior mesenteric vessel when an end-to-end configuration would not. During aneurysm repair, the inferior mesenteric artery should be assessed. Patent vessels with poor back-bleeding indicate poor collateral supply. Reimplantation of the inferior mesenteric artery orifice onto the aortic graft is indicated in this situation. Intraoperative assessment of colon viability using the continuous-wave

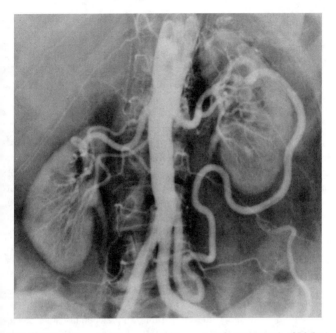

FIGURE 10.4 The very large meandering mesenteric artery (arch of Riolan) seen on this arteriogram is a collateral from the inferior mesenteric artery to the superior mesenteric branches. It indicates significant obstruction of the superior mesenteric artery. (Reprinted from Taylor, L.M., Jr. and Porter, J.M., Treatment of chronic intestinal ischemia, *Semin. Vasc. Surg.*, 3, 193, 1990. With permission.)

Doppler ultrasonic flow detector helps with the decision to reimplant the inferior mesenteric artery.

Colonic ischemia should be suspected when patients have bloody stools after aortic surgery. Given the high mortality, immediate endoscopy of the colon is indicated. Mild patchy mucosal involvement can be observed, and frequently improves spontaneously. Confluent mucosal ischemia or any extent of mucosal necrosis is an indication for laparotomy and inspection of the colon. Resection of necrotic segments might be lifesaving.

10.6 CHRONIC INTESTINAL ISCHEMIA

10.6.1 Natural History

In contrast to nearly all other clinical manifestations of atherosclerosis, chronic intestinal ischemia is rare. As mentioned previously, atherosclerotic lesions producing visceral artery obstruction are quite frequent, which leads to the inescapable conclusion that the rarity of intestinal ischemia symptoms is the result of the extensive collateral network of the three visceral arteries. Perhaps also because of the condition's rarity, the natural history of intestinal arterial obstructions is poorly documented. Only a single study by Thomas and colleagues has examined the issue of how many patients with initially asymptomatic intestinal obstructions eventually develop symptoms of intestinal ischemia.[17] These authors found 60 of 980 (6%) aortograms with significant visceral arterial obstructions of which 15 had severe involvement of all three visceral arteries. After a mean follow-up of 2.6 years, four of the 15 developed intestinal ischemia. None of the 45 patients with less than three-vessel involvement developed intestinal ischemia.

A special situation exists when intra-abdominal vascular surgery (e.g., aneurysm repair) is planned for patients with asymptomatic visceral artery lesions. As documented in a series reported by Connolly and Stemmer, intestinal infarction occasionally occurs postoperatively in such patients.[18] The best explanation is that the necessary dissection disrupted important collaterals. To prevent this complication, we usually perform reconstruction of occluded or highly stenotic superior mesenteric arteries concomitantly with abdominal aortic reconstruction in patients with no symptoms of intestinal ischemia.

The natural history of symptomatic intestinal ischemia is well documented. Patients suffer pain and progressive weight loss. Death occurs from starvation or intestinal infarction after a period of symptoms that may be quite prolonged—from many months to years.

10.6.2   DIAGNOSIS

Despite the progressive nature of intestinal ischemic symptoms, diagnosis is typically delayed. In one series, the average time from onset of symptoms to diagnosis was 18 months.[19] Perhaps this is because there are many causes of abdominal pain and weight loss (e.g., ulcer, malignancy), some of which are frequently encountered, whereas chronic intestinal ischemia remains quite rare. In our practice, patients referred with chronic intestinal ischemia have frequently had an extensive diagnostic workup lasting many months, including multiple endoscopies, imaging studies (e.g., computed tomography, magnetic resonance imaging), and malabsorption studies. Despite these difficulties, the triad of abdominal pain, weight loss, and established atherosclerotic vascular disease should lead to suspicion of intestinal ischemia.

Duplex ultrasound scanning performed in experienced laboratories can detect the intestinal arterial obstructions responsible for chronic intestinal ischemia with a high degree of accuracy. Criteria for greater than 70% stenosis or occlusion, determined from a retrospective study of 34 arteriograms and confirmed in a prospective study of 100 arteriograms in our laboratory, include fasting peak systolic velocity greater than 275 cm per second or no flow signal in the superior mesenteric artery, and fasting peak systolic velocity greater than 200 cm per second or no flow signal in the celiac artery. Accuracy of this testing, with arteriography as the "gold standard," was 85% to 90%.[20,21] Interestingly, despite the well-documented changes that occur in mesenteric arterial flow postprandially, detection of changes in this normal pattern does not substantially improve the diagnostic accuracy of duplex scanning.[22]

Mesenteric arterial duplex scanning is technically demanding, as the vessels are deep, respiratory motion interferes, and findings may be obscured by intestinal gas. Although it is possible to perform highly accurate testing in laboratories with experience, this may not be the case where testing is performed infrequently. As with any ultrasound-based test, a negative result should not prevent further investigation (arteriography) if clinical suspicion is high.

Arteriography for visceral artery lesions must include lateral aortography (Figure 10.5). This is because the lesions most frequently producing obstruction of the visceral arteries occur at the origins of the vessels from the aorta. Both the celiac and the superior mesenteric arteries overlie the aorta on routine anterior–posterior views, preventing visualization of the stenotic lesions. Selective catheterization of the visceral arteries may place the catheter tip beyond the stenoses, again failing to identify the lesions.

10.6.3   PERCUTANEOUS INTERVENTIONAL TREATMENT OF CHRONIC INTESTINAL ISCHEMIA

Surgical treatment of chronic intestinal ischemia requires major intra-abdominal arterial reconstruction most frequently in elderly patients with multiple comorbidities including profound weight loss. The attractiveness of minimally invasive percutaneous therapy as an alternative is obvious. Multiple reports have demonstrated the possibility of treating visceral artery obstructions with percutaneous transluminal balloon angioplasty. Early reports were characterized by a high recurrence rate, perhaps because the plaque producing typical origin lesions is in fact aortic in nature and somewhat resistant to dilation. For example, in the series reported by Tegtmeyer and Selby, only 48% of patients observed for 12 months after angioplasty maintained their initial successful dilation.[23] More-encouraging early results have been recently reported by Johanson and colleagues, who added intravascular stenting to the angioplasties performed.[24] Whether transluminal percutaneous techniques will improve sufficiently to achieve long-term success rates comparable to those realized with surgical treatment remains to be determined (Figure 10.6).

10.6.4   SURGICAL TREATMENT OF CHRONIC INTESTINAL ISCHEMIA

The potential to surgically correct intestinal ischemic symptoms lies in the typical distribution of the responsible atherosclerotic lesions.

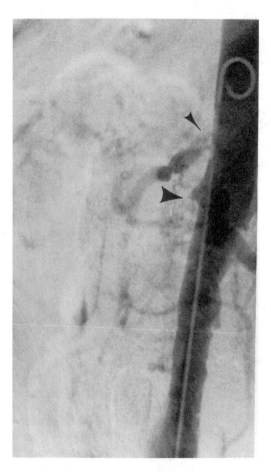

FIGURE 10.5. Lateral aortogram showing typical atherosclerotic obstruction of proximal celiac (*small arrowhead*) and superior mesenteric (*large arrowhead*) arteries.

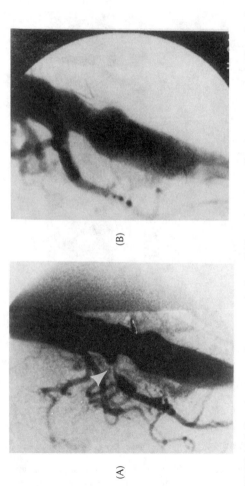

FIGURE 10.6 Superior mesenteric artery angioplasty. (A) Lateral aortogram showing severe stenosis of proximal superior mesenteric artery (*arrowhead*). (B) After angioplasty, stenosis is eliminated. This patient's symptoms were relieved by angioplasty. The symptoms and the stenosis recurred after 3 months, and she was treated by bypass grafting.

Most frequently, stenosis or occlusion involves the origin or first few centimeters of the involved vessels, with those beyond retaining a relatively normal lumen. Relief of the obstruction can be accomplished by endarterectomy[25] or by bypass grafting. The bypass grafts can be formed from autogenous vein or from prosthetic, and can originate from the proximal supraceliac aorta or from the infrarenal vessels, if unobstructed (Figure 10.7). The authors prefer to use prosthetic grafting from the infrarenal vessels for most intestinal artery reconstructions. Revascularization of the superior mesenteric artery alone is a technically simpler operation than multiple-vessel reconstructions and produces equally satisfactory results.[26] We reserve use of autogenous vein grafts for situations in which intestinal infarction has occurred, and resection will be required, at which time prosthetic grafting is contraindicated. Multiple vessel repairs are used whenever previous surgery (especially gastrectomy or colectomy) has disrupted normal collaterals between the visceral arteries. Use of the supraceliac aorta for graft origins is indicated when the infrarenal aorta is severely diseased or is otherwise difficult or dangerous to use, as when there have been multiple previous aortic operations.[27]

Multiple reports, as outlined in Table 10.3, have demonstrated the overall good results of surgical reconstruction for chronic intestinal ischemia. Long-term patency of repairs and freedom from recurrent symptoms characterize the overwhelming majority of patients who undergo this operation. Recovery from surgery is often somewhat prolonged. Many patients are severely debilitated preoperatively. The intestinal mucosa is frequently atrophic and dysfunctional because of the prolonged ischemia, and recovery of normal absorptive function may take many weeks. In addition, the pattern of voluntary food avoidance that was present preoperatively is in part a learned behavior and may require a period of time to resolve. For all these reasons, many patients treated successfully for chronic intestinal ischemia require a prolonged period of postoperative parenteral nutritional support before recovery is complete and hospital discharge is possible. It seems preferable to confirm patency of the arterial reconstruction with arteriography performed early in the postoperative period. This is

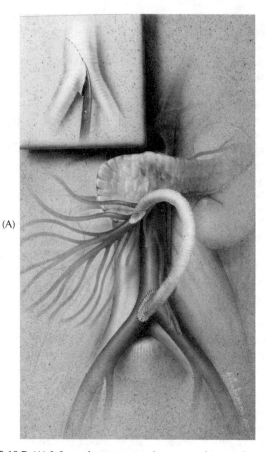

FIGURE 10.7 (A) Infrarenal aorta to superior mesenteric artery bypass. (B) Supraceliac aorta to superior mesenteric artery bypass. (Reprinted from Taylor, L.M., Jr. and Porter, J.M., Treatment of chronic intestinal ischemia, *Semin. Vasc. Surg.*, 3, 193, 1990. With permission.)

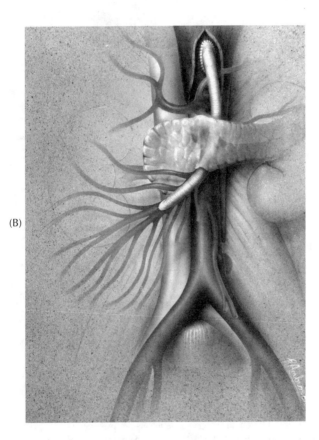

(B)

FIGURE 10.7 (B) Supraceliac aorta to superior mesenteric artery bypass. (Reprinted from Taylor, L.M., Jr. and Porter, J.M., Treatment of chronic intestinal ischemia, *Semin. Vasc. Surg.*, 3, 193, 1990. With permission.)

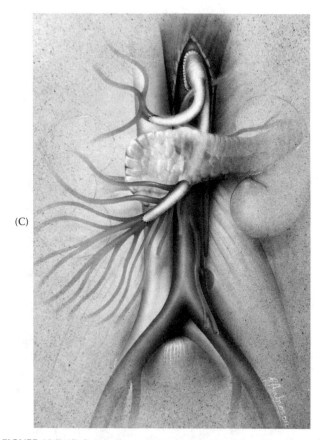

(C)

FIGURE 10.7 (C) Supraceliac aorta to superior mesenteric and hepatic artery bypass. (Reprinted from Taylor, L.M., Jr. and Porter, J.M., Treatment of chronic intestinal ischemia, *Semin. Vasc. Surg.*, 3, 193, 1990. With permission.)

because occluded repairs may be asymptomatic until adequate oral intake is resumed. If discovered early, before the development of

TABLE 10.3
Results of Surgical Treatment of Chronic Intestinal Ischemia

Study	N	Operation-Related Mortality (%)	Female (%)	Follow-up (yr)	Late Success (%)
McAfee, 1992	58	10	79	5	90
Cunningham, 1991	74	12	82	5	85
Rheudasil, 1988	41	5	51	3.5	84
Moawad, 1997	24	4	76	2.4	78
Taylor, 2000	84	11	67	11	95

Adapted from Taylor, L.M., Jr., Moneta, G.L., and Porter, J.M., Treatment of chronic visceral ischemia, in *Vascular Surgery*, 5th ed., Rutherford, R.B., Ed., W. B. Saunders, Philadelphia, 2000, 1539.

inflammatory scarring, occluded or stenotic repairs can be easily
revised. If discovery is delayed until weeks postoperatively, revision
may be technically impossible.

REFERENCES

1. Dunphy, J.E., Abdominal pain of vascular origin, *Am. J. Med.*, 192, 109, 1936.
2. Moneta, G.L., Taylor, D.C., and Helton, W.S., Duplex ultrasound measurement of postprandial intestinal blood flow: effect of meal composition, *Gastroenterology*, 95, 1294, 1988.
3. Valentine, R.J., Martin, J.D., and Myers, S.I., Asymptomatic celiac and superior mesenteric artery stenoses are more prevalent among patients with unsuspected renal artery stenoses, *J. Vasc. Surg.*, 14, 195, 1991.
4. Marston, A., Clarke, J.M.F., and Garcia, J., Intestinal function and intestinal blood supply, *Gut*, 26, 656, 1985.
5. Elliott, J.P., Jr., Hageman, J.H., and Szilagyi, E., Arterial embolization: problems of source, multiplicity, recurrence, and delayed treatment, *Surgery*, 88, 833, 1980.
6. Wright, C.B. and Hobson, R.W., Prediction of intestinal viability using Doppler ultrasound technique, *Am. J. Surg.*, 129, 642, 1975.
7. Carter, M.S., Fantini, G.A., and Sammartano, R.J., Qualitative and quantitative fluorescein fluorescence in determining intestinal viability, *Am. J. Surg.*, 147, 117, 1984.
8. Locke, R., Hauser, C.J., and Shoemaker, W.C., The use of surface oximetry to assess bowel viability, *Arch. Surg.*, 119, 1252, 1984.
9. Pearce, W.H., Jones, D.N., and Warren, G.H., The use of infrared photoplethysmography in identifying early intestinal ischemia, *Arch. Surg.*, 122, 108, 1987.
10. Oohata, Y., Mibu, R., and Hotokezaka, M., Comparison of blood flow assessment between laser Doppler velocimetry and the hydrogen gas clearance method in ischemic intestine in dogs, *Am. J. Surg.*, 160, 511, 1990.
11. Bulkley, G.B., Zuidema, G.D., and Hamilton, S.R., Intraoperative determination of small intestinal viability following ischemic injury, *Ann. Surg.*, 193, 628, 1981.

12. Bergan, J.J., Recognition and treatment of intestinal ischemia, *Surg. Clin. North Am.*, 47, 109, 1967.

13. Ottinger, L.W. and Austen, W.G., A study of 136 patients with mesenteric infarction, *Surg. Gynecol. Obstet.*, 124, 251, 1967.

14. Boley, S.J., Sprayregan, S., and Siegelman, S.S., Initial results from an aggressive roentgenological and surgical approach to acute mesenteric ischemia, *Surgery*, 82, 848, 1977.

15. Hagihara, P.F., Ernst, C.B., and Griffen, W.O., Jr., Incidence of ischemic colitis following abdominal aortic reconstruction, *Surg. Gynecol. Obstet.*, 149, 571, 1979.

16. Ernst, C.B., Colon ischemia following aortic reconstruction, in *Vascular Surgery*, 5th ed., Rutherford, R.B., Ed., W.B. Saunders, Philadelphia, 2000, 1542.

17. Thomas, J.H., Blake, K., and Pierce, G.E., The clinical course of asymptomatic mesenteric arterial stenosis, *J. Vasc. Surg.*, 27, 840, 1998.

18. Connolly, J.I. and Stemmer, E.A., Intestinal gangrene as a result of mesenteric arterial steal, *Am. J. Surg.*, 126, 197, 1973.

19. Schnieder, D.B, Schnieder, P.A., and Reilly, L.M., Reoperation for recurrent chronic visceral ischemia, *J. Vasc. Surg.*, 27, 276, 1998.

20. Moneta, G.L., Yeager, R.A., and Dalman, R., Duplex ultrasound criteria for diagnosis of splanchnic artery stenosis or occlusion, *J. Vasc. Surg.*, 14, 511, 1991.

21. Lee, R.W., Moneta, G.L., and Yeager, R.A., Mesenteric artery duplex scanning: a blinded prospective study, *J. Vasc. Surg.*, 17, 79, 1993.

22. Gentile, A.T., Moneta, G.L., and Lee, R.W., Usefulness of fasting and postprandial duplex ultrasound examinations for predicting high-grade superior mesenteric artery stenosis, *Am. J. Surg.*, 169, 476, 1995.

23. Tegtmeyer, C.J., and Selby, J.B., Balloon angioplasty of the visceral arteries, in *Endovascular Surgery*, Moore, W.S. and Ahn, S.S., Eds., W.B. Saunders, Philadelphia, 1989, 223.

24. Parikh, S. and Johansen, K. J., Balloon angioplasty and/or stenting for visceral artery stenoses, abstract presented at the Pacific Northwest Vascular Society, Vancouver, November 9, 1999.

25. Stoney, R.J., Ehrenfeld, W.K., and Wylie, E.J., Revascularization methods in chronic visceral ischemia, *Ann. Surg.*, 186, 468, 1977.

26. Gentile, A.T., Moneta, G.L., and Taylor, L.M., Jr., Isolated bypass to the superior mesenteric artery for intestinal ischemia, *Arch. Surg.*, 129, 926, 1994.

27. Beebe, H.G., MacFarlane, S., and Raker, E.J., Supraceliac aortomesenteric bypass for intestinal ischemia, *J. Vasc. Surg.*, 5, 749, 1987.

11

Etiology, Prevalence, and Natural History of Atherosclerotic Renal Artery Stenosis

Michael R. Jaff

CONTENTS

11.1 Epidemiology 219
11.2 Natural History..221
11.3 Diagnosis 223
11.4 Treatment..226
     11.4.1 Medical Therapy 226
     11.4.2 Surgical Revascularization..228
     11.4.3 Endovascular Revascularization 229
          11.4.3.1 Percutaneous Transluminal Angioplasty....229
          11.4.3.2 Endovascular Stent Placement 230
     11.4.4 Treatment of Fibromuscular Dysplasia 231
11.5 Conclusions 232
References..233

11.1 EPIDEMIOLOGY

Although generally believed to be a rare cause of hypertension, atherosclerotic renal artery stenosis (RAS) is a common finding in selected patient populations. In the general population of hypertensive patients, from 1% to 6% have some element of RAS.[1] However, there are several clinical clues that suggest a greater likelihood of RAS in certain subsets of patients, including the presence of coronary, carotid, abdominal aortic, and lower extremity arterial occlusive disease. In patients with aortoiliac occlusive disease or abdominal aortic aneurysmal disease, the prevalence of significant bilateral RAS ranges from 33% to 45%.[2,3]

Similar findings have been described in patients with significant extracranial carotid atherosclerosis. In one study of 60 patients with significant RAS, 46% had 50% to 100% stenosis of an internal carotid artery.[4] Coronary artery atherosclerosis is a similar marker for RAS. In 346 patients with aneurysmal or occlusive vascular disease prompting arteriography, 28% had significant RAS. Of the patients with RAS, 58% had clinically overt coronary artery disease. In those patients without RAS, the incidence of coronary artery stenosis was only 39%.[5] In a prospective study of 1302 patients undergoing coronary arteriography, abdominal aortography demonstrated significant RAS in 15% of patients. The number of coronary arteries involved with atherosclerosis also predicted the likelihood of RAS in this series. For example, if one coronary artery demonstrated atherosclerosis, the prevalence of significant RAS was 10.7%. If three coronary arteries demonstrated atherosclerotic involvement, the prevalence of RAS was 39.0%.[6]

The prevalence of RAS in African-American patients has been reported to be low. In a retrospective study of 819 patients referred to the Cleveland Clinic for RAS, only 40 (4.9%) were African-American. Although the location and severity of RAS were equivalent in the two groups, more African-American patients with RAS had severe or refractory hypertension and were more likely to be active tobacco users than their Caucasian counterparts. In addition, diffuse atherosclerosis (i.e., coronary, cerebrovascular, and peripheral arterial disease [PAD]) was found in 95% of African-American patients with RAS and in only 70% of Caucasian patients.[7]

Fibromuscular dysplasia (FMD) is the second most likely etiology of RAS, accounting for 40% of cases.[8] FMD is generally believed to represent a congenital arterial abnormality of the fibrous, muscular, and elastic segments. There are several types of FMD: primary intimal fibroplasia, medial fibroplasia (most common, representing 75% to 80% of cases), perimedial fibroplasia, fibromuscular hyperplasia, and periadventitial fibroplasia (extremely rare).[9]

When compared with patients with atherosclerotic RAS, patients with FMD of the renal artery are younger, more likely to be female, and have had hypertension for shorter periods of time. FMD involves the mid and distal segments of the main renal artery, as well as the branch renal arteries. These patients rarely have renal dysfunction on the basis of FMD of the renal arteries.[10]

11.2 NATURAL HISTORY

End-stage renal disease (ESRD), regardless of etiology, results in shortened life expectancy. The most frequent cause of death in patients committed to ESRD is related to cardiovascular disease, and the mortality of patients with ESRD continues to rise at alarming rates.[11] For example, elderly patients requiring dialytic support because of diabetic glomerulosclerosis have dismal survival rates. In one secondary survival analysis, no elderly patient with ESRD due to diabetes mellitus survived 5 years.[12]

The prevalence of unsuspected, significant RAS in patients with renal insufficiency is surprisingly high, up to 24 % in one series.[13] The 5-year survival of patients aged 65 to 74 years who have ESRD due to hypertension is 20%, and is only 9% in those patients aged 75 years or older. Among those patients with hypertensive ESRD, 83 of 683 dialysis patients had significant RAS.[14] The 15-year survival of patients with ESRD because of RAS was 0%, compared with 32% in patients on dialysis due to, for example, polycystic kidney disease. In a prospective angiographic trial, RAS was the cause of ESRD in 14% of new patients beginning dialysis.[15]

Once RAS is discovered, the clinical course and natural history may help predict clinical benefit from revascularization (RAR). Although there remains controversy about the true natural history of RAS, in one independent arteriographic series, 39% of patients demonstrated progression of RAS.[16] In a pooled review of five arteriographic trials, 49% of the renal arteries demonstrated progression of stenosis.[17] A total of 14% of these vessels progressed to occlusion.

In a retrospective series of 85 patients with RAS observed for a mean of 52 months, 44% demonstrated progression of RAS, 16% demonstrated progression to total occlusion, with progression occurring within the first 2 years in 46% of renal arteries.[18] In the same series, 78 initial renal arteries with less than 50% stenosis were observed. Of these renal arteries, 69% demonstrated no significant progression of stenosis. However, of 18 renal arteries with baseline stenosis of greater than 75% to 99% stenosis, 39% progressed to occlusion on sequential arteriography. Finally, deterioration in renal function as measured by increase in the serum creatinine occurred in 54% of patients with progressive stenosis of the renal artery, whereas only 25% demonstrated an increase in serum creatinine when there was no progression of disease ($P < 0.02$). Renal size decreased in 70% of patients with progressive disease, and in only 27% of patients without increasing stenosis ($P < 0.001$).

In one of only two prospective natural history studies for RAS, Dean and associates observed 41 patients with RAS whose treatment was medical, i.e., control of hypertension and correction of any coexisting renal diseases, if possible.[19] Progression of RAS occurred when blood pressure was well controlled; 40% of patients developed an increase in serum creatinine, and 37% of patients demonstrated a decrease in renal mass. The second prospective study involved the use of renal artery duplex ultrasonography (RADUS). In this study, 84 patients with at least one abnormal renal artery whose therapy did not involve RAR were included. Of 139 renal arteries over the course of a mean follow-up of almost 13 months, progression of RAS as documented by RADUS was 42% at 2 years. The occlusion rate at 2 years was 11%. The overall progression rate was 20%.[20]

Until recently, the correlation between progressive RAS and deterioration in renal function had not been demonstrated. This is the critical issue, as many patients presently undergo RAS in an effort to preserve renal function. Caps et al[21] have demonstrated that untreated

RAS leads to renal atrophy. Of 204 kidneys with varying degrees of RAS in 122 patients observed for a mean of 33 months, the 2-year incidence of renal atrophy (> 1 cm) was 20.8% in patients with severe baseline RAS ($P = 0.009$ compared with normal or mild baseline RAS). Baseline systolic blood pressure > 180 mm Hg and duplex ultrasound findings suggestive of significant RAS also predicted a higher likelihood of progressive renal atrophy. Of greatest importance, these data revealed that patients who demonstrated bilateral renal atrophy also experienced a greater rise in serum creatinine than those patients who were found to have no renal atrophy ($P = 0.03$).

This natural history suggests progression of moderate RAS to a more severe form, and progression of severe baseline RAS to occlusion, with a gradual deterioration in serum creatinine and renal mass. In patients requiring hemodialysis whose renal parenchyma is being supplied by stenotic renal arteries,[22,23] or in patients with recurrent flash pulmonary edema or angina pectoris with RAS,[24–26] early RAR seems appropriate. The "wait and see" approach[27] may lead to dialysis dependence with a worse outcome.

11.3 DIAGNOSIS

Figure 11.1 presents an algorithm for the diagnosis of renal artery disease. Although a number of noninvasive methods of diagnosis in RAS have been proposed, none have obviated the role of the "gold standard"—renal arteriography. Each screening test has significant limitations that prevent widespread acceptance. Plasma renin activity was commonly measured several years ago, but has inadequate sensitivity and specificity to be used as the sole diagnostic test for RAS, even with stimulation with an angiotensin-converting enzyme (ACE) inhibitor. Captopril-stimulated nuclear renal flow scanning is an accurate screening test for the diagnosis of unilateral RAS in a patient with normal renal function. However, in cases of bilateral RAS, and in patients with impaired renal function, the accuracy of this test decreases, and cannot be used in screening. Renal vein renin ratios can be helpful; however, this is an invasive diagnostic test that also

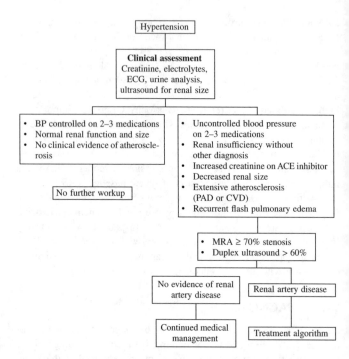

FIGURE 11.1 Diagnosis algorithm for renal artery disease. ACE = angiotensin-converting enzyme; BP = blood pressure; CVD = cardiovascular disease (including coronary and carotid artery disease); ECG = electrocardiogram; MRA = magnetic resonance angiography; PAD = peripheral arterial disease.

requires that most, if not all, antihypertensive agents be withdrawn before sampling. Given that many of these patients have poorly controlled hypertension, hospitalization and use of parenteral antihypertensive agents would be required to adequately perform this test.

Several investigators have demonstrated the validity of duplex ultrasonography to diagnose RAS. In one prospective series, 29 patients (58 renal arteries) underwent duplex ultrasonography and contrast arteriography. The sensitivity of RADUS was 84%, specificity 97%, and positive predictive value 94% for a detection of greater than 60% stenosis.[28] Using criteria of peak systolic velocity (PSV) (> 180 cm/s) within the renal artery, duplex scanning was able to discern between normal and diseased renal arteries with a sensitivity of 95% and specificity of 90%.[29] The ratio of PSV in the area of RAS compared with the PSV within the aorta (renal–aortic ratio > 3.5) predicts the presence of greater than 60% RAS. Using this criterion, RADUS demonstrated a sensitivity of 92%.

In a large prospective series of 102 consecutive patients who underwent both duplex ultrasonography and contrast arteriography within 1 month, 62 of 63 arteries with less than 60% stenosis, 31 of 32 arteries with 60% to 79% stenosis, and 67 of 69 arteries with 80% to 99% stenosis were correctly identified by duplex ultrasonography. Occluded renal arteries were correctly identified by ultrasonography in 22 of 23 cases. The overall sensitivity of duplex ultrasonography was 98%, specificity 99%, positive predictive value 99%, and negative predictive value 97%.[30]

Limitations of direct visualization of the renal arteries include body habitus and overlying bowel gas obscuring identification of the renal arteries. Some authors have suggested that renal hilar scanning is easier and as accurate as complete interrogation of the renal arteries. However, direct comparison of both techniques has revealed limitations of hilar scanning, including low sensitivity, inability to discriminate between stenosis and occlusion, and inadequate determination of accessory renal arteries.[31] The sensitivity was 67% for hilar scanning, with a specificity of 89% to 99%.[32] Given that many patients have both main RAS and intraparenchymal disease, the addition of resistive indices within the parenchyma may help predict which patients will benefit from RAR.[33]

Magnetic resonance angiography (MRA) has the potential to become the ideal diagnostic test for RAS. Minimally invasive, requiring only a peripheral intravenous cannula and use of non-nephrotoxic contrast, the results of renal MRA are very impressive. However, approximately 10% of patients cannot undergo MRA owing to implanted metal (i.e., permanent pacemakers) or claustrophobia. Finally, in patients who have undergone RAR with metallic endoluminal stents, MRA cannot be used to determine patency of the stent because of signal dropout from the metal.

Duplex ultrasonography is the ideal method of determining the adequacy of RAR.[34] Given the proliferation of endovascular therapy (percutaneous angioplasty with stent deployment),[35] duplex ultrasonography is helpful in detecting important areas of restenosis.

11.4   TREATMENT

Once a stenosis of the renal artery due to atherosclerosis has been identified, the optimal method of treatment must be chosen. Figure 11.2 shows an algorithm for treatment of renal artery disease. Three alternatives presently exist: medical therapy alone (control of hypertension and risk factor modification), surgical bypass or endarterectomy, or percutaneous transluminal angioplasty (PTA) and/ or endovascular stent deployment. To make the appropriate choice, a basic understanding of the complication rates and clinical outcomes for each option is necessary.

11.4.1   MEDICAL THERAPY

In the 1970s, 32% of patients with severe hypertension were found to have RAS.[36] However, antihypertensive therapy for atherosclerotic RAS was quite ineffective in the 1970s, offering adequate control in fewer than 50% of patients.[37] With the advent of ACE inhibitors and calcium channel blockers, over 80% of patients in several series have demonstrated excellent blood pressure control.[38] In fact, bilateral nephrectomy as urgent therapy for uncontrollable hypertension, formerly considered a viable therapeutic option, is now rarely, if ever, performed. Therefore, RAR for "cure" of true renovascular hypertension has been an uncommon scenario since the 1990s.

However, progressive renal insufficiency may still occur in the face of controlled hypertension and RAS. Although the use of ACE

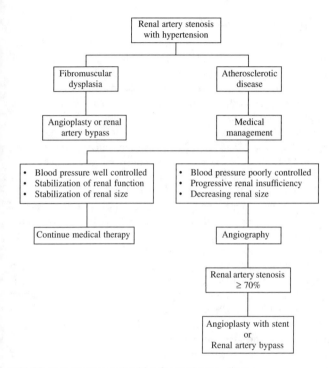

FIGURE 11.2 Treatment algorithm for renal artery disease.

inhibitors is relatively contraindicated in patients with bilateral RAS, in one series azotemia occurred in only 38% in this scenario and never occurred in patients with unilateral RAS.[39] Therefore, progressive renal insufficiency likely represents a decrease in renal blood flow below the level of "critical perfusion pressure." Identification of deteriorating renal function or decrease in renal size over time, even in the face of well-controlled hypertension, may suggest the need for more-aggressive treatment of atherosclerotic RAS.

11.4.2 SURGICAL REVASCULARIZATION

Several centers have demonstrated proficiency with surgical RAR. Surgical techniques differ based on the individual surgeon's experience, and the presence of aortic atherosclerosis, bilateral disease, and branch renal artery lesions. Techniques available to the surgeon include aortorenal bypass with saphenous vein or hypogastric artery as the bypass conduit, synthetic material when autogenous conduits are unavailable, endarterectomy, or "extra-anatomic bypass" using the splenic (left renal artery) or hepatic (right renal artery) arteries as the inflow. More recently, the thoracic aorta or supraceliac aorta has been used when there is significant atherosclerosis of the abdominal aorta. Extracorporeal RAR for branch RAS can also be performed.

Experienced centers performing large numbers of these surgical procedures demonstrate technical and clinical success. In one series of 323 surgical RAR procedures over 15 years, the overall mortality rate from the procedure was 5.6%.[40] In those surgical cases that avoided the aorta, the mortality rate was 4.1% versus 8.1% with grafts arising from the aorta. Major postoperative complications occurred in 5.9% of patients with aortorenal bypass alone and in 21.4% of patients with combined aortic replacement and aortorenal bypass. Early (less than 30-day) graft failure occurred in 2.1% of combined procedures and 17.6% of aortorenal bypass cases.

Hallett and others from the Mayo Clinic reported their experience with surgical RAR in 304 patients, demonstrating a 30-day operative mortality rate of 10.2%.[41] In this series, combined aortic replacement and RAR resulted in a 30-day mortality rate of 11.8% as compared with a 3.6% 30-day mortality rate with RAR alone.

Novick et al. reviewed their experience with 254 surgical RAR procedures, demonstrating a mortality rate of only 2.1%.[42] The overall incidence of graft thrombosis or stenosis was 4.3%. Hansen et al. reported an operative mortality rate of 2.5% in 291 procedures, with a 1.4% primary failure rate within 30 days of the procedure.[43]

The clinical impact of surgical RAR has also been extensively reported. In Hansen's series of 291 RAR procedures, cure of hypertension was seen in 21%, and improvement in control of hypertension occurred in 70% of survivors.[43] Effects of surgical RAR on renal function revealed improved renal function in 49%, caused no change in 36%, and resulted in deterioration in 15% of patients. This beneficial impact on hypertension control and renal function has also been shown in patients with diabetes and RAS. Of 54 patients undergoing surgical RAR, cure or improvement in hypertension was seen in 72%, and 40% of patients demonstrated improved renal function.[44]

Even in patients with solitary kidneys and RAS, surgical RAR appears to have a positive impact. In one series of 35 patients with RAS to a solitary functioning kidney, the 30-day mortality rate was 6%, with major postoperative complications occurring in 43% of patients.[45] However, postoperative renal function improved in 21% of patients, and remained stable in 70%. Hypertension was cured in 14% and improved in 71% of patients.

11.4.3 ENDOVASCULAR REVASCULARIZATION

11.4.3.1 Percutaneous Transluminal Angioplasty

Interest in nonsurgical methods of RAR began after Sos et al. published their initial series of 89 patients with RAS who underwent PTA.[46] The procedure was technically successful in 57% of patients with unilateral RAS and in only 10% of patients with bilateral RAS. Antihypertensive response was impressive, with cure or improvement in hypertension in 84% of patients with atherosclerotic disease. Sos and others noted the lack of benefit of PTA on ostial atherosclerotic lesions by stating that the ostial lesions "… are, more precisely, lesions of the thickened aortic wall that encroach on the renal-artery ostium, rather than lesions in the renal artery itself." Although an initial relief of the pressure gradient occurs after PTA of an ostial atherosclerotic lesion, "… most of them probably return to their pre-angioplasty state within hours or days."

Canzanello et al. reported the effect of PTA on blood pressure and renal function in 100 consecutive patients with 125 renal artery stenoses.[47] Technical success ranged from 67.7% (solitary kidneys) to

76.2% (unilateral RAR). Over a mean follow-up of 29 months, 59% of patients demonstrated improvement or cure of hypertension. Patients with ostial RAS demonstrated the poorest benefit in blood pressure control (32.5%). Complications resulting from PTA occurred in 14% of patients, with two deaths as a result of the procedure. Acute renal insufficiency occurred in 26% of patients after PTA.

In a retrospective series of 320 patients who underwent RAR using PTA, technical success was seen in 82% of patients with atherosclerotic RAS.[48] Cure of hypertension was noted in only 8.4% of patients; however, 70% demonstrated improvement in blood pressure control. The 30-day overall mortality rate was 2.2%. Dissection of the renal artery occurred in 5.6% of cases, with 1.6% suffering guidewire perforation of the renal artery. Thrombotic occlusion of the renal artery occurred in only 0.9% of cases. Contrast-induced acute renal failure was seen in 5.6% of patients, with only one patient requiring dialysis.

RADUS has been used to determine the anatomic impact of PTA. In a recent series of 41 patients who underwent 52 RAR procedures with PTA, the initial post-PTA duplex demonstrated normal renal arteries in 23 patients, less than 60% stenosis in 19, and 60% or greater stenosis in 10.[49] The restenosis rate from a normal renal artery to less than 60% was 13% and 19% after 1 and 2 years, respectively. If the immediate post-PTA renal artery was classified as less than 60%, the restenosis rate to 60% or more was 44% and 55% after 1 and 2 years, respectively.

11.4.3.2   Endovascular Stent Placement

Because of the limitations of PTA in effectively treating ostial atherosclerotic RAS, endovascular stent placement has emerged as an RAR procedure that may prevent recoil and offer a more durable result. This procedure is technically sound, with one series demonstrating technical success in 100% of 92 renal arteries undergoing stent deployment.[50] Henry et al. also demonstrated 100% technical success in 64 procedures, with a 6-month restenosis rate of 1.6% and a primary 1-year patency rate of 92%.[51] Cure or improvement in hypertension was found in 76% of patients.

Complications of endovascular stent deployment can occur. Iannone et al. performed RAR with stent deployment in 83 lesions among 63 patients, with 99% technical success.[52] Ten patients required transfusion after the procedure, three suffered renal artery perforation, and eight patients had acute renal failure. Two died as a result of the procedure.

In a series of 100 patients with 133 renal arteries, renal artery stent deployment was technically successful in 99% of cases.[53] Cure or improvement in blood pressure control was seen in 76% of patients 6 months after the procedure. Restenosis occurred in 19% of cases at a mean follow-up of 8.7 months. No patients died as a result of the procedure, and only one stent thrombosis occurred. Two patients experienced contrast-induced acute renal failure, but neither required dialysis. In this series, 76% of patients demonstrated normalization of the blood pressure on the same or fewer antihypertensive agents. No significant adverse effects on renal function were noted.

In a prospective series of 74 consecutive renal artery stenoses that were revascularized with stent deployment, technical success was 100%, with a restenosis rate of 11% after 60 months.[54] No major complications occurred, and no patients required emergency surgery after the procedure.

Recent data in 163 patients who underwent renal artery stent placement and were observed for 4 years revealed some important information. This study demonstrated a marked benefit in overall survival and reduction in progressive renal insufficiency if the baseline serum creatinine before stent RAR was less than 1.5 mg/dL, as compared with those patients whose present serum creatinine was greater than 2.0 mg/dL.[55]

11.4.4 TREATMENT OF FIBROMUSCULAR DYSPLASIA

Treatment of renal artery FMD is indicated for patients with true renovascular hypertension. The ideal method of treatment for main renal artery FMD is PTA. Technical success is high (85.7% in one series of 120 vessels[46]), clinical blood pressure response is consistent with atherosclerotic RAS (22% cure, 63% clinical benefit[3]). However, in patients with branch RAS, surgical RAR with "bench" procedures is often required and can be quite effective.[56]

11.5   CONCLUSIONS

Choosing the appropriate method for treatment of atherosclerotic RAS requires a basic understanding of the natural history of the disorder, as well as benefits and risks of the therapy. Medical therapy is appropriate if the patient's blood pressure can be easily controlled, if the renal function remains stable, and if there is no objective evidence of renal atrophy. However, if renal RAR is required, the method of RAR depends on the local level of expertise. Certainly, if a skilled and experienced surgeon is available, and there is no physician with the ability to perform endovascular therapy, surgery would likely be the preferred method of RAR. However, if both modalities are available, a choice must be made.

In a prospective randomized trial of PTA versus surgical RAR in 58 nondiabetic patients with atherosclerotic RAS, procedural success was seen in 83% of patients treated with PTA and 97% treated with surgery.[57] Major complications occurred in 17% of patients undergoing PTA and 31% of patients receiving surgical RAR. This suggests that PTA should be the initial treatment for atherosclerotic RAS. However, none of these patients received a stent as part of their endovascular therapy. An economic analysis has suggested cost benefit in favor of PTA, as surgical RAR resulted in a 12% higher cost than PTA.[58]

There have been no prospective comparative trials of medical therapy, surgery, and endovascular therapy. However, the emerging data on the technical success, low complication rates, durability, and clinical benefit of stent RAR suggest that a comparison is warranted. In skilled hands, renal artery stent deployment rivals the technical and clinical results of surgical RAR, even in ostial atherosclerotic RAS, and should be considered a primary treatment option.

REFERENCES

1. Simon, N., Franklin, S.S., Bleifer, K.H., et al., Clinical characteristics of renovascular hypertension, *JAMA*, 220, 1209, 1972.
2. Olin, J.W., Melia, M., and Young, J.R., Prevalence of atherosclerotic renal artery stenosis in patients with atherosclerosis elsewhere, *Am. J. Med.*, 88, 46N, 1990.
3. Missouris, C.G., Buckenham, T., Cappucio, F.P., et al., Renal artery stenosis: a common and important problem in patients with peripheral vascular disease, *Am. J. Med.*, 96, 10, 1994.
4. Louie, J., Isaacson, J.A., and Zierler, R.E., Prevalence of carotid and lower extremity arterial disease in patients with renal artery stenosis, *Am. J. Hypertens.*, 7, 436, 1994.
5. Valentine, R.J., Clagett, G.P., and Miller, G.L., The coronary risk of unsuspected renal artery stenosis, *J. Vasc. Surg.* 18, 433, 1993.
6. Harding, M.B., Smith, L.R., and Himmelstein, S.I., Renal artery stenosis: prevalence and associated risk factors in patients undergoing routine cardiac catheterization, *J. Am. Soc. Nephrol.*, 2, 1608, 1992.
7. Novick, A. C., Zaki, S., Goldfarb, D., et al., Epidemiologic and clinical comparison of renal artery stenosis in black patients and white patients, *J. Vasc. Surg.*, 20, 1, 1994.
8. Olin, J.W. and Novick, A.C., Renovascular disease, in *Peripheral Vascular Diseases*, 2nd ed., Young, J.R., Olin, J.W., and Bartholomew, J.R., Eds., Mosby, St. Louis, 1996, 321.
9. Harrison, H.G. and McCormack, L.J., Pathologic classification of renal artery disease in renovascular hypertension, *Mayo Clin. Proc.*, 46,161, 1971.
10. Luscher, T.F., Lie, J.T., and Stanson, A.W., Arterial fibromuscular dysplasia, *Mayo Clin. Proc.*, 62, 931, 1987.
11. Huting, J., Cardiovascular survival of patients undergoing long-term dialysis, *Prim. Cardiol.*, 20, 21, 1994.
12. Byrne, C., Vernon, P., and Cohen, J. J., Effect of age and diagnosis on survival of older patients beginning chronic dialysis, *JAMA*, 271, 34, 1994.
13. O'Neil, E.A., Hansen, K.J., and Canzanello, V.J., Prevalence of ischemic nephropathy in patients with renal insufficiency, *Am. Surg.*, 58, 485, 1992.

14. Mailloux, L.U., Napolitano, B., and Bellucci, A. G., Renal vascular disease causing end-stage renal disease, incidence, clinical correlates, and outcomes: a 20-year clinical experience, *Am. J. Kidney Dis.*, 24, 622, 1994.

15. Scoble, J.E., Maher, E.R., and Hamilton, G., Atherosclerotic renovascular disease causing renal impairment—a case for treatment, *Clin. Nephrol.*, 31, 119, 1989.

16. Meaney, T.F., Dustan, H.P., and McCormack, L.J., Natural history of renal arterial disease, *Radiology*, 9, 877, 1968.

17. Greco, B. A. and Breyer, J.A., The natural history of renal artery stenosis: who should be evaluated for suspected ischemic nephropathy?, *Semin. Nephrol.*, 16, 2, 1996.

18. Schreiber, M.J., Pohl, M.A., and Novick, A.C., The natural history of atherosclerotic and fibrous renal artery disease, *Urol. Clin. North Am.*, 11, 383, 1984.

19. Dean, R.H., Kieffer, R.W., and Smith, B.M., Renovascular hypertension: anatomic and renal function changes during therapy, *Arch. Surg.*, 116, 1408, 1981.

20. Zierler, R.E., Bergelin, R.O., and Isaacson, J.A., Natural history of atherosclerotic renal artery stenosis: a prospective study with duplex ultrasonography, *J. Vasc. Surg.*, 19, 250, 1994.

21. Caps, M.T., Zierler, R.E., and Polissar, N.L., Risk of atrophy in kidneys with atherosclerotic renal artery stenosis, *Kidney Int.*, 53, 735, 1998.

22. Novick, A.C., Pohl, M.A., and Schreiber, M., Revascularization for preservation of renal function in patients with atherosclerotic renovascular disease, *J. Urol.*, 129, 907, 1983.

23. Kaylor, W.M., Novick, A.C., Ziegelbaum, M., vReversal of end stage renal failure with surgical revascularization in patients with atherosclerotic renal artery occlusion, *J. Urol.*, 141, 486, 1989.

24. Pickering, T.G., Devereux, R.B., and James, G.D., Recurrent pulmonary edema in hypertension due to bilateral renal artery stenosis: treatment by angioplasty or surgical revascularisation. *Lancet*, 2, 551, 1988.

25. Messina, L.M., Zelenock, G.B., Yao, K.A., et al., Renal revascularization for recurrent pulmonary edema in patients with poorly controlled hypertension and renal insufficiency: a distinct subgroup of patients with arteriosclerotic disease, *J. Vasc. Surg.*, 15, 73, 1992.

26. Tami, L.F., McElderry, M.W., and Al-Adli, A., Renal artery stenosis presenting as crescendo angina pectoris, *Cath. Cardiovasc. Diagn.*, 35, 252, 1995.

27. Scoble, J.E., Is the "wait-and-see" approach justified in atherosclerotic renal artery stenosis?, *Nephrol. Dial. Trans.*, 4,588, 1995.

28. Taylor, D.C., Kettler, M.D., and Moneta, G.L., Duplex ultrasound scanning in the diagnosis of renal artery stenosis: a prospective evaluation, *J. Vasc. Surg.*, 7, 363, 1988.

29. Strandness, D.E., Duplex imaging for the detection of renal artery stenosis, *Am. J. Kidney Dis.*, 24, 674, 1994.

30. Olin, J.W., Piedmonte, M.R., and Young, J.R., The utility of duplex ultrasound scanning of the renal arteries for diagnosing significant renal artery stenosis, *Ann. Intern. Med.*, 122, 833, 1995.

31. Munier, M.N.S., Hoballah, J.J., and Miller, E.V., Renal hilar doppler analysis is of value in the management of patients with renovascular disease, *Am. J. Surg.*, 174, 164, 1997.

32. Isaacson, J.A., Zierler, R.E., Spittell, PC., et al., Noninvasive screening for renal artery stenosis: comparison of renal artery and renal hilar duplex scanning, *J. Vasc. Technol.*, 19, 105, 1995.

33. Cohn, E.J., Benjamin, M.E., and Sandager, G.P., Can intrarenal duplex waveform analysis predict successful renal artery revascularization?, *J. Vasc. Surg.*, 28, 471, 1998.

34. Eidt, J.F., Fry, R.E., and Clagett, G.P., Postoperative follow-up of renal artery reconstruction with duplex ultrasound, *J. Vasc. Surg.*, 8, 667, 1988.

35. Dorros, G., Jaff, M., and Mathiak, L., Four-year follow-up of Palmaz-Schatz stent revascularization as treatment for atherosclerotic renal artery stenosis, *Circulation*, 98, 642, 1998.

36. Davis, B.A., Crooke, J.E., Vestal, R.E., et al., Prevalence of renovascular hypertension in patients with grade III or IV hypertensive retinopathy, *N. Engl. J. Med.*, 301, 1273, 1979.

37. Hollenberg, N.K., Medical therapy for renovascular hypertension: a review, *Am. J. Hypertens.*, 1, 338, 1988.

38. Textor, S.C., ACE inhibitors in renovascular hypertension, *Cardiovasc. Drugs Ther.*, 4, 229, 1990.

39. Jackson, B., Matthews, P.G., McGrath, B.P., et al., Angiotensin converting enzyme inhibition in renovascular hypertension: frequency of reversible renal failure, *Lancet*, 1, 225, 1984.

40. Cambria, R.P., Brewster, D.C., and L'Italien, G.J., The durability of different reconstructive techniques for atherosclerotic renal artery disease, *J. Vasc. Surg.*, 20, 76, 1994.

41. Hallett, J.W., Textor, S.C., and Kos, P.B., Advanced renovascular hypertension and renal insufficiency: trends in medical comorbidity and surgical approach from 1970 to 1993, *J. Vasc. Surg.*, 21, 750, 1995.

42. Novick, A.C., Ziegelbaum, M., and Vidt, D.G., Trends in surgical revascularization for renal artery disease, ten years' experience, *JAMA*, 257, 498, 1987.

43. Hansen, K.J., Starr, S.M., and Sands, R.E., Contemporary surgical management of renovascular disease, *J. Vasc. Surg.*, 16, 319, 1992.

44. Hansen, K.J., Lindberg, A.H., and Benjamin, M.E., Is renal revascularization in diabetic patients worthwhile?, *J. Vasc. Surg.*, 24, 383, 1996.

45. Reilly, J.M., Rubin, B.G., and Thompson, R.W., Revascularization of the solitary kidney: a challenging problem in a high-risk population, *Surgery*, 120, 732, 1996.

46. Sos, T.A., Pickering, T.G., and Sniderman, K., Percutaneous transluminal renal angioplasty in renovascular hypertension due to ahteroma or fibromuscular dysplasia, *N. Engl. J. Med.*, 309, 274, 1983.

47. Canzanello, V.J., Millan, V.G., and Spiegel, J.E., Percutaneous transluminal renal angioplasty in management of atherosclerotic renovascular hypertension: results in 100 patients, *Hypertension*, 13, 163, 1989.

48. Bonelli, F.S., McKusick, M.A., and Textor, S.C., Renal artery angioplasty: technical results and clinical outcome in 320 patients, *Mayo Clin. Proc.*, 70, 1041, 1995.

49. Tullis, M.J., Zierler, R.E., and Glickerman, D.J., Results of percutaneous transluminal angioplasty for atherosclerotic renal artery stenosis: a follow-up study with duplex ultrasonongraphy, *J. Vasc. Surg.*, 25, 46, 1997.

50. Dorros, G., Jaff, M., and Jain, A., Follow-up of primary Palmaz-Schatz stent placement for atherosclerotic renal artery stenosis, *Am. J. Cardiol.*, 75, 1051, 1995.

51. Henry, M., Amor, M., and Henry, I., Stent placement in the renal artery: 3-year experience with the Palmaz stent, *J. Vasc. Interv. Radiol.*, 7, 343, 1996.

52. Iannone, L.A., Underwood, P.L., and Nath, A., Effect of primary balloon expandable renal artery stents on long-term patency, renal function, and blood pressure in hypertensive and renal insufficient patients with renal artery stenosis, *Cath. Cardiovasc. Diagn.*, 37, 243, 1996.

53. White, C.J., Ramee, S.R., and Collins, T.J., Renal artery stent placement: utility in lesions difficult to treat with balloon angioplasty, *J. Am. Coll. Cardiol.*, 30, 1445, 1997.

54. Blum, U., Krumme, B., and Flugel, P., Treatment of ostial renal artery stenoses with vascular endoprostheses after unsuccessful balloon angioplasty, *N. Engl. J. Med.*, 336, 459, 1997.

55. Dorros, G., Jaf, M., and Mathiak, L., Four-year follow-up of Palmaz-Schatz stent revascularization as treatment for atherosclerotic renal artery stenosis, *Circulation*, 98, 642, 1998.

56. Anderson, C.A., Hansen, K.J., and Benjamin, M.E., Renal artery fibromuscular dysplasia: results of current surgical therapy, *J. Vasc. Surg.*, 22, 207, 1995.

57. Weibull, H., Bergqvist, D., and Sven-Erik, B., Percutaneous transluminal renal angioplasty versus surgical reconstruction of atherosclerotic renal artery stenosis: a prospective randomized study, *J. Vasc. Surg.*, 18, 841, 1993.

58. Weibull, H., Bergqvist, D., and Jendteg, S., Clinical outcome and health care cost in renal revascularization: percutaneous transluminal renal angioplasty versus reconstructive surgery, *Br. J. Surg.*, 78, 620, 1991.

Section IV

Diseases of the Aorta

12 Abdominal Aortic Aneurysms

William C. Krupski

CONTENTS

12.1 Introduction 241
12.2 Definition and Classification..243
12.3 Epidemiology 244
12.4 Natural History..249
12.5 Pathogenesis 253
12.6 Diagnosis and Evaluation..255
     12.6.1 Screening for Abdominal Aortic Aneurysms 258
     12.6.2 Economic Analysis..261
12.7 Treatment...262
12.8 Conclusions 271
References..271

12.1 INTRODUCTION

One of the first credible manuscripts, the Ebers Papyrus (2000 BC), describes aneurysms of the peripheral arteries.[1] Galen (131–200), the Roman historian, defined an aneurysm as a localized pulsatile swelling that disappeared on pressure[2] and Antyllus first reported operative treatment of an aneurysm, which consisted of ligation of the artery above and below the aneurysm, incision of the sac, and evacuation of its contents.[3] Few other operative procedures have stood the test of time so well, because, for the next 15 centuries, Antyllus's recommendations for aneurysm repair remained the basis for arterial operations.

During the Middle Ages, traumatic aneurysms of the brachial artery frequently occurred after attempted puncture of the median cubital vein for bloodletting. Ambrose Paré (1510–1590) vividly described the death of a patient after application of a caustic solution to such an aneurysm (against Paré's advice) produced massive fatal hemorrhage.[4] Paré's contemporary, the 16th-century Flemish anatomist Andreas Vesalius (1514–1564) wrote one of the first treatises on abdominal aortic aneurysms (AAAs).[5]

The distinguished English anatomist John Hunter (1728–1793) ligated a popliteal artery aneurysm in a coachman. The aneurysm was possibly caused by repetitive trauma against the seat while the patient was driving on cobblestone streets. Another renowned British surgeon, and Hunter's adversary, Percival Pott (1714–1788), recommended above-knee amputations for popliteal aneurysms.[6] Although Hunter is most frequency remembered for descriptions of female breast anatomy and inguinal hernia repair, in 1817 his most renowned student, Sir Astley Cooper (1768–1841), ligated the abdominal aorta in a patient who had a leaking iliac artery aneurysm.[7] The operation was initially successful, but the patient died suddenly after 40 hours, presumably from delayed aneurysmal rupture. In addition, Cooper was the first to document spontaneous aortoenteric fistulae due to aneurysmal disease and reported that patients with one aneurysm often have others elsewhere.[7] Mistakes of the past have been repeated in contemporary times. For example, arterial ligation accompanied by extra-anatomic bypass was reintroduced for treatment of AAAs in high-risk patients in the 1970s by the Albany, NY group; outcomes were similar to those in Cooper's patient.[8]

In the early 19th century, several ingenious (albeit unsuccessful) treatments for arterial aneurysms were introduced. Monteggia (1762–1815) attempted to obliterate an aneurysm by injecting it with a sclerosant—a scheme that predictably failed because of rapid blood flow. Conducting an electric current between needles stuck into the vessel in an effort to thrombose it was first attempted in 1832, a technique still used in the 1930s. In London, in 1864, Charles Moore (1821–1870) described the generally unsuccessful obliteration of aneurysms by insertion of steel wires, once inserting 26 yards of metal![9] We have reported rupture of a large iliac artery aneurysm treated by embolization with stainless steel coils as recently as 1998.[10]

Modern treatment of arterial aneurysms was introduced by the legendary New Orleans surgeon Rudolph Matas (1860–1957). Matas performed the first successful proximal ligation of an aortic aneurysm in 1923, some 106 years after Astley Cooper's pioneering operation.[11] He later developed endoaneurysmorrhaphy, which entailed aortic clamping above and below the aneurysm, opening it, ligating branches from within, and buttressing the wall with imbricating sutures. Endoaneurysmorrhaphy paved the way for the current technique of intrasaccular interposition grafting devised by Creech and DeBakey.[12] Using lessons learned from his countryman Jacques Oudot, who in 1950 reconstructed an occluded abdominal aorta using freeze-dried homograft,[13] Charles Dubost reportedly performed the first successful interposition graft for AAA repair using a freeze-dried homograft.[14] In fact, Schaffer and Hardin actually preceded Dubost in a case subsequently recounted.[15] When Voorhees et al. replaced the unreliable homograft with durable Vinyon "N" cloth, the modern era of aneurysm repair had decidedly begun.[16] In 1953, Bahnson described the first successful repair of a ruptured aortic aneurysm.[17] During the late 1950s and early 1960s, AAA repair became a safe and common surgical procedure.

12.2 DEFINITION AND CLASSIFICATION

It is ironic that no universally accepted definition of aneurysm exists, because arterial aneurysms are among the most common and important arterial disorders. An aneurysm is most frequently defined as a permanent localized dilation of an artery, but the amount of enlargement required for an artery to be categorized as aneurysmal is controversial. Johnston et al.[18] have defined aneurysms as focal dilations of arteries with an increase in diameter of at least 50% compared with the expected normal diameter. However, determination of expected normal diameter is confounded by differences in sex, total body surface area, and other factors. The dimensions of the abdominal aorta have been analyzed in large numbers of individuals using computed tomography (CT) measurements,[19] but there is no universal agreement about what size constitutes an aneurysm. Moreover, diffusely enlarged arteries are often present in patients with aneurysms, a condition known as arteriomegaly, arteriectasis, or dolichomegaly. Thus, a more generally applicable definition of an aneurysm is dilatation more than twice the size of the more proximal artery. For abdominal aortas, which measure about 2.0 cm in the general population, the controversy is illustrated by variable definitions of aneurysmal dilatation from 3.0 cm (50% increase in size) to 4.0 cm (twice the size of the more proximal artery).

Numerous classification systems for aneurysms have been proposed (Table 12.1). The classification systems have been designed to help establish the correct diagnosis and plan treatment. In general, classifications based on shape, location, and structure are less useful than those based on etiology. A classification system of aneurysms should include categories whose features are unique and sufficiently distinctive to warrant individual consideration. Obviously, no single strategy satisfies every clinical application.

12.3   EPIDEMIOLOGY

Many famous individuals have had AAAs. In 1868, Kit Carson, the 19th-century American frontiersman, died of a ruptured AAA in rural Colorado.[20] Albert Einstein also died of a ruptured AAA.[21] He had been treated for his AAA by Nissen, who wrapped the aneurysm in cellophane, a technique popularized by Rea in 1948.[22] French general and president Charles DeGaulle and cowboy-actor Roy Rogers also had AAAs. More recently, baseball pitcher Johnny VanDemeer, country singer Conway Twitty, and actor George C. Scott died of ruptured AAAs.

Aneurysms occur most commonly in the infrarenal abdominal aorta. In an epidemiologic study in the United States from 1951 to 1981, Lilienfeld et al. reported that the ratio of abdominal:thoracic aneurysms was 7:1 in men and 3:1 in women.[23] The incidence (number

TABLE 12.1
Classification of Arterial Aneurysms

- Shape
- Fusiform
- Saccular
- Location
- Central
- Peripheral
- Visceral
- Cerebral
- Etiology

- Size
- Macroaneurysms
- Microaneurysms
- Structure
- True
- False

Degenerative
- Nonspecific (atherosclerotic)
- Fibrodysplasia
- Graft

Inflammatory

Dissecting

Aneurysms Associated With Pregnancy

Congenital

- Idiopathic
- Tuberous sclerosis
- Turner syndrome
- Berry (cerebral)

Inherited Abnormality of Connective Tissue
- Marfan syndrome
- Ehlers-Danlos syndrome
- Cystic medial necrosis

Infection
- Bacterial
- Syphilitic
- Infection of false aneurysm
- Fungal

Mechanical
- Post-Stenotic
- Traumatic
- Anastomotic
- Prosthetic

(continued)

TABLE 12.1 (CONTINUED)
Classification of Arterial Aneurysms

Aneurysms Associated With Arteritis
- Systemic lupus erythematosis
- Takayasu disease
- Giant cell arteritis
- Polyarteritis nodosa
- Beçhet disease

of new cases) of AAAs in the homogeneous population of Rochester, MN, during 1976 to 1980 was about seven times higher than the incidence of thoracic aneurysms.[24] Repair of arterial aneurysms constitutes about 13% of the vascular experience of general surgical residents, and probably accounts for an even higher proportion of operations performed by vascular surgeons in practice.[25]

In an autopsy study from the Massachusetts General Hospital, AAAs were found in 2% of 24,000 consecutive postmortem examinations.[26] Studies in unselected populations using autopsies, ultrasound examinations, and CT scans have reported a similar prevalence (number of existing cases) of about 2% to 3%.[27–29] AAAs are mostly a disease of elderly white men. Johnson et al. found more aneurysms in Caucasian men (4.2%) than in Caucasian women, African-American men, and African-American women (all about 1.5%).[28] In general, AAAs increase steadily in frequency after age 50, are about five times more common in men than women, and 3.5 times more common in Caucasian than African-American men.[30] The likelihood of developing an AAA varies from 3 to 117 per 100,000 person-years.[31]

Prevalence of AAAs in a given population depends on risk factors associated with this disorder, including, age, male sex, white race, positive family history, smoking, hypertension, hypercholesterolemia, peripheral arterial disease, and coronary artery disease (CAD).[32] In a recent report from a Department of Veterans Affairs cooperative study (Aneurysm Detection and Management [ADAM]), in more than 73,000 individuals aged 50 to 79, the prevalence of abdominal aortas 3.0 cm or greater was 4.6%; 1.4% had AAAs greater than 4.0 cm.[33] This study and others have shown that age, sex, and smoking have the largest impact on AAA prevalence.[30,31,33] Curiously, diabetes mellitus is associated with a negative relative risk for AAAs.

The coexistence of other vascular disorders in the study population substantially increases the prevalence of aortic aneurysms. Statistics show that 5% of individuals with symptomatic CAD have aneurysms, and 10% of patients with peripheral or cerebrovascular disease have AAAs.[34–36] Patients with peripheral arterial aneurysms (especially those involving the popliteal artery) have a prevalence of aortic aneurysms approaching 50%..[37] Hypertensive patients may also be more likely to develop AAAs, but reports are conflicting. One European study indicated a 7% prevalence of AAAs in hypertensive men over age 50,[38] whereas an investigation in Sweden found only one of 245 hypertensive patients had an aneurysm (0.4%).[39]

Numerous studies have documented familial clustering of AAAs. In 1977, Clifton reported increased likelihood of developing AAAs in first-order relatives, describing a family in which all three male siblings had undergone operations for ruptured aneurysms.[40] Subsequent studies confirmed the observation that AAAs can be familial; a positive family history is present in 15% to 25% of patients undergoing AAA repair.[27,41–45] Genes responsible for synthesis and degradation of collagen and elastin are fundamental focal points in AAA research. Investigators have suggested that autosomal-dominant, autosomal-recessive, and sex-linked inheritance modes of transmission are possible.[46] About 18% of patients with AAAs have a first-degree relative (FDR) also affected. In Marfan syndrome, which is associated with arterial dilations and dissections of the entire aorta, mutations in the fibrillin-1 gene (FBN1) on chromosome 15 have been identified.[47] In patients with Ehlers-Danlos syndrome, who are at risk for sudden death from rupture of large arteries, defects in the type III collagen gene (COL3A1) have been described.[48]

The incidence of AAAs is increasing. Two separate studies from the Mayo Clinic examining the period 1951 to 1980 showed a threefold increase in prevalence from 12.2 per 100,000 to 36.2 per 100,000.[24,49] Some of this increase in frequency may be related to improved detection owing to technological advances, but the magnitude of the difference suggests a genuine increase.[50] The aging of the population also plays a role in the increasing incidence. This was emphasized in a European autopsy study in which aneurysms occurred with a steadily increasing frequency in men after age 55, peaking at 5.9% in those aged 90.[51] Women developed an increased incidence of aneurysms after age 70, peaking at 4.5% at 90 years of age.

Mortality rates from ruptured AAAs also reflect a genuine increase in the prevalence of AAAs. In the past 5 decades, the number of deaths due to ruptured aneurysms in individuals under age 65 has remained low but rates have risen in older age groups. Compared with 30 years earlier, a 1984 study in England and Wales revealed a 20-fold and 11-fold increase in deaths from ruptured aortic aneurysms for men and women, respectively. [52] The ratio of male:female death rates decreases from 11:1 in younger age groups to 3:1 in octogenarians. Wilmink et al., also from Great Britain, recently reported a 2.4% per year increase in the age-adjusted incidence of death from AAA rupture between 1952 and 1998. [31] In another English population-based study, Chosky et al. reported an incidence of ruptured AAAs of 76 per 100,000 person-years for men and 11 per 100,000 person-years for women over 50 years of age, for a male:female ratio of 4.8:1.[53] A 1995 analysis of hospital deaths in the United States indicates that AAA rupture rates stabilized at about four deaths per 100,000 Caucasian males from 1979 to 1990.[54] Curiously, deaths from ruptured AAAs, like those from CAD, most commonly occur in the winter months.[55] It is intriguing that deaths from aneurysms are increasingly common, whereas deaths from coronary heart disease, which shares many of the same risk factors, have decreased by 20% in the past decade.[56]

12.4   NATURAL HISTORY

Rupture and death are the most important and frequent complications of AAAs. Unfortunately, estimates of rupture risk are imprecise and are largely based on old, retrospective reviews conducted before widespread application of surgical repair. No prospective randomized series are currently available. Available data are handicapped by inaccurate measurement methods (often physical examination or plain abdominal radiograms). In addition, many of these AAAs were not only large but also symptomatic.[57,58] Contemporary studies have analyzed natural history of small aneurysms, because larger ones are nearly always repaired when detected.[59]

Risk of rupture increases directly with AAA diameter. Although aneurysms are not ideal cylinders, they appear to follow the law of Laplace: $T = pr$, where T is wall tension, p is intraluminal pressure, and r is radius. Thus, larger AAAs in patients with hypertension are most likely to rupture. Decreasing wall strength (or thickness) should theoretically increase rupture risk, though this is difficult to measure.[59]

Szilagyi et al. are credited with the sentinel 1966 report correlating AAA size and risk of rupture.[60] Patients with large (greater than 6 cm) or small (less than 6 cm) AAAs were managed either operatively or nonoperatively, even though more than half were considered fit for surgery in that era. During follow-up, 43% of the patients with large AAAs suffered rupture compared with only 20% of those with small AAAs, although the exact size at the time of rupture was unknown. Because of this difference in rupture rates, patients with large AAAs had a 5-year survival of only 6% compared with 48% for those with small AAAs. In 1969, Foster et al. confirmed these findings, reporting a rupture rate of 51% for AAAs greater than 6 cm compared with 16% for AAAs smaller than 6 cm managed expectantly.[61] It is likely that the diameter of AAAs in these studies was overestimated by physical examination and radiography, such that what was called a 6-cm aneurysm would be closer to 5 cm by current standards. Nevertheless, the influence of size on AAA rupture rates was firmly established by these studies, which also showed improved survival with operative intervention.[60,61]

Correlation of AAA diameter and likelihood of rupture has also been shown in autopsy studies. In 1977, Darling et al. analyzed 473 consecutive patients who had an AAA at autopsy; 25% had ruptured.[62] Postmortem aneurysm diameter varied directly with rupture rates; rates were 10%, 25%, 46%, and 61% for AAA diameters less than 4 cm, 4 cm to 7 cm, 7 cm to 10 cm, and greater than 10 cm, respectively. More recently, Sterpetti et al. reported an autopsy study of 297 patients with AAAs; rupture rates were 5%, 39%, and 65% for AAAs measuring less than 5 cm, 5 to 7 cm, and greater than 7 cm, respectively.[63] However, autopsy studies probably overestimate true rupture risk, because they are biased toward patients with larger AAAs that rupture, which more often lead to postmortem examinations than those with smaller asymptomatic AAAs who die of other causes. In addition, after rupture, AAA diameter tends to be underestimated because the AAA is not distended by blood pressure, i.e., what is judged to be a 4-cm AAA may have been much larger *in vivo*.

Because of the inherent flaws in the aforementioned studies, it is impossible to determine precise rupture rates for AAAs of various diameters. It is well established that larger aneurysms rupture more frequently than smaller ones, and the transition point is generally considered to be between 5 cm and 6 cm. A recent survey of vascular surgeons documented wide variation in estimates of rupture risk; median estimates for annual rupture risk were 20% per year for a 6.5-cm AAA and 30% per year for a 7.5-cm AAA.[64] Over 90% of the vascular surgeons estimated that the annual rupture risk of a 6-cm or larger AAA is at least 10% per year. Thus, operative repair is recommended for nearly all patients with large AAAs, and a precise determination of rupture risk for large AAAs is relevant only for patients with high operative risk or reduced life expectancy.

Based on the above discussion, interest has focused on patients with small, asymptomatic aneurysms. Many studies have examined selective management of these patients, whose AAAs are followed periodically until they reach a threshold size or produce symptoms.[65–68] Design of and results from these investigations were remarkably similar. In general, elective repair was recommended at a threshold diameter of 5 cm for low-risk patients and 6 cm for higher-risk patients, or for expansion greater than 1 cm per year, or for development of symptoms. After an average follow-up of about 2.5 years, 38% of patients met these criteria and had elective AAA repair and 6% required emergent operation for rupture or acute expansion; 27% were alive with intact AAAs at final follow-up and 29% died of other causes.[69]

It is difficult to calculate estimates of rupture risk for small aneurysms, because most studies used selective management in which 30% to 40% of patients with small AAAs had elective repair during follow-up, thus eliminating the possibility of rupture. Because of differences in management and populations studied, disparate results have been reported with respect to small AAA rupture rates. Cronenwett et al. described a 3% per year rupture rate in AAAs that remained less than 5 cm in diameter; only 3% of 167 patients observed with 4 to 6 cm AAAs underwent elective repair at 3-year follow-up.[70] In a homogeneous, mostly Caucasian, stable population in a single county in Minnesota, Nevitt et al. observed that 176 patients with AAAs over 5 years had no ruptures in AAAs less than 5 cm but a 5% annual rupture rate for AAAs larger than 5 cm at initial presentation.[71] A higher risk was described by Limet et al. in a referral-based study.[72] A total of 114 patients with small AAAs selected for expectant management were observed for 2 years; 12% suffered ruptured AAAs, despite elective repair in 38% because of rapid expansion. These authors estimated annual rupture risks of 0%, 5.4%, and 16% for AAAs less than 5 cm, 4 cm to 5 cm, and greater than 5 cm in diameter, respectively.

Cronenwett et al. and Sterpetti et al. used multivariate analyses to examine clinical variables that might predict rupture risk.[66,73] The Cronenwett study found that larger initial AAA diameter, hypertension and chronic obstructive pulmonary disease (COPD) were independent predictors of AAA rupture.[66] Similarly, by comparing ruptured and nonruptured AAA in postmortem examinations, the Sterpetti study concluded that larger initial diameter, hypertension, and bronchiectasis were independent predictors of rupture.[73] In a review of 75 patients managed expectantly, Foster et al. corroborated the importance of hypertension in AAA rupture; death from rupture occurred in 72% of patients with diastolic hypertension, but in only 30% of the entire group.[61] Similarly, in a review of patients thought to be "unfit" for surgery, Szilagyi et al. found that hypertension occurred in 67% patients who suffered AAA rupture compared with only 23% of those without rupture.[74] The association of hypertension with AAA rupture fits easily into Laplace's law, whereas the causative role of pulmonary disease is less apparent. Speculation has focused on a "systemic emphysema" of sorts, perhaps related to an imbalance in proteinase activity affecting connective tissue in the lungs and aorta.[69]

Cigarette smoking has also been associated with AAA rupture. In the ADAM Study, smoking was the best predictor for the presence of AAAs in veteran patients.[33] In a large population study of English civil employees, the relative risk from AAA rupture increased 4.6-fold for cigarette smokers, 2.4% for cigar smokers, and 14.6-fold for smokers of hand-rolled cigarettes.[75] (Incidentally, no study has addressed the possible association of marijuana smoking and AAAs.) It has not been possible, however, to separate the effects of smoking and COPD either in these large epidemiologic studies or the smaller reports previously discussed.[70,73]

In addition to contributing to the occurrence of AAAs, positive family history also appears to increase the risk of rupture. The presence of AAAs in FDRs increases risk of rupture significantly. Darling et al. described ruptured AAAs in 15% of patients with two FDRs, 29% with three FDRs, and 36% with more than four FDRs.[76] Women with familial AAAs were more likely to suffer rupture (30%) than men with familial AAAs (17%). Verloes et al. reported a 32% rupture rate in patients with familial aneurysms compared with 9% in those with sporadic aneurysms, whereas familial aneurysms ruptured 10 years sooner than the sporadic variety (65 versus 75 years of age).[42] It is unclear, however, whether family history is an independent risk factor for AAA rupture, because studies did not account for other confounding variables such as AAA size, which might have been different in the familial group.

It is generally accepted that rapid AAA expansion increases AAA rupture risk, but it is difficult to differentiate this from the influence of absolute diameter that independently increases risk. On average, AAAs expand at about 4 mm per year.[77] In addition to aforementioned variables, aneurysm architectural characteristics may play a role in this rate; for example, the authors and others have shown that increased thrombus content within AAAs is associated with more rapid expansion.[78,79] Several studies have suggested that more rapidly expanding AAAs are more likely to rupture, but most of the ruptured AAAs were large.[80,81]

In summary, it has been well established that the rupture risk of AAAs correlates directly with diameter. Surprisingly, the estimated risk of rupture for a given aneurysm diameter is based on old, imperfect data, and precise figures are unavailable. Most authorities estimate that a 5- to 6-cm AAA carries a rupture risk between 2% to 15% per year, or about 45% over 5 years. Hypertension and COPD are independent risk factors for rupture. Smoking is also a risk factor, although interactions between smoking and COPD require clarification. Rapid expansion and family history are probably risk factors for rupture, whereas the influence of patient gender, AAA shape, and thrombus content, and the ratio of AAA diameter to proximal "normal" aortic diameter are more equivocal risk factors.

12.5 PATHOGENESIS

AAAs are more accurately designated degenerative or nonspecific in etiology rather than the traditional term atherosclerotic. Indeed, the characteristics of atherosclerosis are present within AAAs (e.g., macrophages, cholesterol, foam cells, etc. within atherosclerotic plaques), but these changes coexist with aneurysms, which are most likely related to different pathogenesis despite some shared risk factors. A wealth of research is being conducted to better elucidate the etiology of AAAs, and several reviews of this subject have been published.[82,83]

Aortic aneurysms affect the infrarenal aorta far more commonly than the suprarenal. The aortic wall consists of an organized structure of layers of smooth muscle cells with the matrix proteins, such as collagen, alternating with layers of elastin. The number of medial elastin layers is greater in the proximal thoracic aorta (60 to 80 layers) than in the infrarenal aorta (28 to 32 layers), accompanied by medial thinning and intimal thickening in the more distal aorta.[84] In addition, collagen and elastin content is reduced in the more distal aorta.[82] Elastin is the principal load-bearing element in the aorta that resists aneurysm formation, whereas collagen serves as a strong "safety net" to prevent rupture after an aneurysm occurs.[30] Hemodynamic factors, such as reflected waves from the aortic bifurcation and increased pulsatility (e.g., after lower-extremity amputations), have been associated with AAAs. Minimal vasa vasora in the infrarenal aorta may reduce nutrient blood supply and potentiate degeneration.[85] Tilson et al. found more immunoreactive proteins in the abdominal than in the thoracic aorta, and have implicated an autoimmune mechanism for aneurysm formation.[30]

Matrix metalloproteinases (MMPs) are proteolytic enzymes that are increased in both expression and activity in the walls of aortic aneurysms.[82,85,86] The most important elastolytic enzyme, MMP-9, is three times higher in larger (5 to 7 cm) than smaller (less than 5 cm) AAAs, consonant with increased expansion rates in larger AAAs. Other MMPs, including serine proteases such as plasmin and neutrophil elastase, are increased in AAAs compared with normal aortic tissue, whereas their inhibitors are unchanged; thus, there is a net increase in matrix degradation in AAAs.[82] In animal experiments, elastase infusion results in an inflammatory aneurysm-producing response, which is blocked by inhibiting inflammatory cell recruitment or MMP activity with such agents as doxycycline.[87]

In addition to decreased elastin content and fragmentation of elastin fibers, AAAs, in contrast with occlusive arterial disease, have transmural inflammatory infiltrates rather than mostly inflammatory changes in the intima. Although it is incompletely understood, this transmural inflammatory response appears central to AAA development. Infection with *Chlamydia pneumoniae* has been implicated as a possible stimulus for the inflammatory response, because this common organism has been found in AAA walls.[88] Conversely, the characteristics of the transmural infiltrate (B-lymphocytes, plasma cells, immunoglobulins) suggest an autoimmune reaction.[89] Tilson and others have summarized the highly complex nature of the biochemical, molecular, and genetic factors related to AAA formation. [82,83,89–91]

12.6 DIAGNOSIS AND EVALUATION

AAAs are difficult to detect because they are usually asymptomatic. Although low-back pain occurs frequently in patients, rarely is it caused by an AAA. Whereas rupture or acute expansion produces severe and dramatic abdominal, back, and flank pain, these symptoms are unassociated with intact AAAs. Mild to moderate chronic back pain may be caused by large AAAs that erode posteriorly into adjacent vertebrae. Even without bony involvement, AAAs can cause chronic back or abdominal pain that is vague and ill defined. Occasionally, large AAAs produce compressive symptoms, including hydronephrosis, early satiety, nausea, or vomiting from duodenal involvement, or swelling due to venous compromise. Rarely, acute arterial ischemia can occur from embolization of thrombotic intraluminal debris or, less frequently, from AAA thrombosis; ischemia from embolism or thrombosis has been estimated to occur in fewer than 2% to 5% of patients.[92] In most cases, any symptoms definitely related to AAAs warrant repair, although it is unusual for AAAs smaller than 4 cm to produce symptoms.

Most patients who develop symptoms related to AAAs do so because of rupture or acute expansion. Classically, patients with ruptured AAAs present with the triad of severe abdominal or back pain, hypotension, and a pulsatile abdominal mass. However, all three findings are discovered in only 26% of patients with proven AAA rupture.[93] Thus, a high index of suspicion is required, especially in patients with unexplained pain and loss of consciousness, which occur together in as many as 50% of patients; loss of consciousness alone is the only initial symptom in 17% of patients with AAA rupture.[94] Ruptures occur anteriorly into the peritoneal cavity in about 20% of cases and then are almost uniformly fatal.[62] Fortunately, 80% of ruptures occur posteriorly into the retroperitoneum; because they are initially contained, survival is possible. Usually, even patients with contained AAA ruptures have a period of hypotension that eventually results in shock over a period of hours. In rare patients, chronic contained ruptures develop, causing symptoms that mimic inflammatory conditions.

When a ruptured aneurysm is strongly suspected clinically, additional diagnostic studies are often unwarranted. It is preferable to perform a "negative celiotomy" than to have a patient suffer shock and hypotension while in the CT scanner. Older patients with risk factors for AAAs who are clearly ill (i.e., severe abdominal and back pain with moderately unstable vital signs, even without a palpable AAA) usually benefit from exploratory laparotomy because other surgical pathology is discovered (e.g., perforated ulcer, pancreatic tumor, diverticulitis, colonic tumor). On the other hand, if the patient is completely stable and an aneurysm cannot be palpated, an abdominal imaging study is helpful. Ultrasound can confirm the presence of an AAA but not rupture. In contrast, CT scanning can document an AAA, diagnose or exclude rupture, and provide information concerning alternate diagnoses. CT scans have more than 90% accuracy for demonstrating rupture; Kvilekval et al. reported a sensitivity of 94% and a specificity of 95% for CT scanning in 65 hemodynamically stable but symptomatic patients with AAAs who were considered for a diagnosis of ruptured AAA.[95] In this series, AAA rupture was found in 30%, a nonruptured AAA in 50%, and other pathology to explain the symptoms in 20%.[95]

Occasionally, patients themselves describe or palpate a pulsatile mass, but AAAs are often difficult to detect by palpation, even by experienced physicians. In a review of 243 patients who underwent elective AAA repairs, vascular surgeons from the University of Texas Southwestern found that only 38% were initially discovered by physical examination, whereas 62% were detected by incidental radiologic studies.[96] Notably, 23% of these clinically significant AAAs were not palpable even when the diagnosis was established, and in obese patients, two thirds of AAAs were not palpable.

Such findings underscore the importance of imaging studies for diagnosing AAAs. Abdominal B-mode ultrasound is the least expensive, safest, and most commonly used modality for both confirmation and follow-up of AAAs. Limitations of ultrasound include interobserver variability in measurements, inability to measure the suprarenal aorta and iliac arteries reliably, inaccuracy in obese patients or those with a large amount of bowel gas, and inability to diagnose ruptured AAAs.[97,98] Although CT scanning involves radiation, may require intravenous contrast, and is more expensive than ultrasound, it more accurately determines AAA size, with over 90% of studies associated with less than 5 mm interobserver variability.[99] Moreover, CT scans provide important additional details about aneurysm architecture, including proximal extent of the AAA, iliac artery involvement, severity of calcification, the presence of an inflammatory AAA, amount and extent of intraluminal thrombus, and venous anomalies such as retroaortic or circumaortic left renal vein, and left-sided or duplicated inferior vena cava. Knowledge of these features helps develop a prudent operative plan. Associated disorders such as ureteral obstruction, coexistent malignancy (most commonly colon and pancreas), renal anomalies (e.g., horseshoe or pelvic kidneys), and biliary disease may also be elucidated by CT scans. CT scans are particularly useful for excluding a ruptured AAA in a symptomatic but stable patient. Spiral CT scans are a new, rapid, and accurate method for AAA assessment. Thin slices permit good visualization of visceral vessels and three-dimensional reconstructions provide satisfactory images for planning endovascular AAA repairs. However, both CT and ultrasound can overestimate AAA size if an oblique rather than perpendicular section is obtained in a tortuous aneurysm; ultrasound and CT measurements of maximum AAA diameter can differ by over 1 cm.[100]

Magnetic resonance imaging (MRI) for AAAs provides information similar to CT scanning. Although it avoids radiation exposure, it is less widely available, more expensive, and less well tolerated by claustrophobic patients than CT scanning. MRI is especially useful when intravenous contrast is contraindicated in patients with renal dysfunction. Likewise, magnetic resonance angiography can demonstrate coexistent occlusive disease in patients with AAAs and renal disease precluding contrast administration. Arteriography may help define arterial anatomy (e.g., status of the mesenteric and renal arteries) in selected patients, but is notoriously inaccurate in confirming the diagnosis of an AAA or determining diameter because mural thrombus may produce what erroneously appears to be a normal lumen.

12.6.1 SCREENING FOR ABDOMINAL AORTIC ANEURYSMS

Because asymptomatic AAAs often are not discovered until they rupture, there has been great interest in potential benefits of ultrasound screening programs. Numerous studies have been reported concerning ultrasound screening for AAAs. Among 9777 subjects screened by ultrasound in 15 combined studies, relatively few aneurysms 6 cm or greater in diameter were discovered in unselected populations.[36,101–114] In contrast, screening selected populations detects significant numbers of AAAs. The coexistence of peripheral vascular disease markedly increases the likelihood of a positive scan. Galland et al. in Great Britain performed abdominal ultrasound examinations in 242 patients with peripheral vascular disease.[110] AAAs were found in 34 (14%); half of these aneurysms were over 4 cm in diameter. The presence of aortoiliac disease increased the likelihood of AAA. In another study from the United Kingdom, 104 patients with claudication or rest pain were surveyed for AAA.[108] Eight (7.7%) aneurysms, ranging from 2.8 cm to 6.9 cm in diameter, were discovered. Allardice et al., also in the United Kingdom, screened 100 consecutive patients with claudication compared with a control group.[36] In the control group, the incidence of AAA was 2%. In the study group, 20% of the men and 12% of the women had aortic aneurysms or ectasia. Of note, of the abnormal aortas identified by ultrasound, only 31% were palpable. Bengtsson et al. in Malmo, Sweden, screened 372 patients with claudication for AAAs, mostly using abdominal ultrasound. The overall frequency of AAAs was 13.7%. More recently, Carty et al. found that hemodynamically significant carotid artery disease was a definite marker for an increased incidence of AAA in a prospective study of 131 patients.[114]

In addition, screening relatives of patients with AAAs discloses more aneurysms than screening unselected populations. In a Swedish study, 87 siblings from 32 different families of AAA patients underwent ultrasound screening.[105] Their median age was 63 years (range, 39 to 82 years). Aortic dilatation (greater than 29 mm) was found in 10 brothers (29%) and three sisters (6%).

These results were confirmed by Adamson et al. in the United Kingdom, who screened 28 families (25 brothers and 28 sisters) of patients with known AAAs.[113] Remarkably similar findings were reported by Webster et al. in Pittsburgh.[112] These investigators screened 103 FDRs of patients with AAAs. Of siblings aged 55 years or older, five of 20 men (25%) and two of 29 women (6.9%) were found to have a previously undiagnosed AAA. Thus, consideration should be given to screening those with a family history of aneurysm, patients between ages 55 and 80 with peripheral vascular disease, and those with known extremity artery aneurysms, such as popliteal and femoral.

Three large-scale screening programs (combined with trials to investigate the prognosis and optimal management of small asymptomatic AAAs) were introduced in the 1990s in the United Kingdom, Canada, and the United States. These three studies are remarkably similar in design. The Canadian Small Aneurysm Trial has been discontinued because of inadequate patient accrual. The United Kingdom Small Aneurysm Trial has enrolled 1000 patients aged 60 to 76 years old with AAAs of 4.0 cm to 5.4 cm. Results of the United Kingdom trial have recently been published.[115] Curiously, the meaning of the United Kingdom screening program was not addressed in this important report, but the main conclusion from results in 1090 patients, who were randomly assigned to early surgery versus serial ultrasound examinations, was that early surgery does not provide a long-term survival advantage. However, the study has been criticized for a high elective operative mortality rate (5.8%) and low autopsy rate (29%).[116] Of note, a recent screening study from Cambridge and Huntington, United Kingdom, found that screening for asymptomatic AAAs can reduce the incidence of ruptured AAAs by 49%.[117]

The small-aneurysm study conducted in the United States is designated by the acronym ADAM; details of the study design have recently been reported.[118] This prospective randomized clinical trial is being carried out by the Department of Veterans Affairs (VA) Cooperative Studies Program in 15 VA Medical Centers. Aneurysms discovered by ultrasound screening are categorized by size. Patients with AAAs 3.0 cm to 3.9 cm are observed using serial abdominal ultrasonography. Patients with aneurysms measuring 4.0 cm to 5.4 cm in diameter (as confirmed by CT scan) were carefully evaluated with respect to operative risk. If they were good candidates for operative repair, these patients were randomized to expeditious elective surgery or serial ultrasonography/CT scans. Patients in this latter group, designated "selective surgery," were offered operative repair of AAAs if they expanded rapidly, enlarged to 5.5 cm, or became symptomatic. Aneurysms of 5.5 cm were electively repaired unless the patients were not surgical candidates because of comorbid conditions. The primary outcome measure was all-cause mortality, and secondary outcome measures were AAA-related death, morbidity, and general health status. In all, 73,451 veterans aged 50 to 79 with no history of AAAs have been screened. An AAA of 4.0 or larger was detected in 1031 participants (1.4%). Smoking was the risk factor most strongly associated with AAAs (odds ratio, 5.57); smoking accounted for 78% of all AAAs that were 4.0 cm or larger in the study sample.[119]

The discrepancy in prevalence of AAAs in screening programs can be attributed to differences in the definitions of aneurysms and, most importantly, variance in the populations studied. Owing to economic considerations, it is unlikely that mass population screening will ever be implemented. However, based on available data, the individual physician should carefully consider recommending ultrasound screening for AAAs in FDRs of patients with aneurysms (over age 50), and patients over 50 with hypertension, CAD, and peripheral vascular disease, particularly if body habitus makes aortic palpation difficult.

12.6.2 Economic Analysis

The economic cost of ruptured aneurysms is staggering. In 1984, Pasch et al. estimated that $50 million and 2000 lives could have been saved if aneurysms had been repaired before they ruptured.[120] In 1991, Breckwoldt et al. reviewed financial data of 102 patients undergoing elective and emergent AAA repair between 1986 and 1989.[121] Postoperative length of stay, net revenue, total standard cost, and net profit–loss margin were the principal variables analyzed. A net loss of $409,459 was noted for the entire series. Although emergent operations (mostly for ruptured AAAs) accounted for only 12% of the procedures, they accounted for 73% of the losses, with an average loss of $24,655 per patient. Moreover, the average loss among survivors of emergent AAA repair was $36,672 per patient. Predictably, length of stay correlated closely with overall costs.

Because of the high costs of ruptured aneurysms, it would seem economically reasonable to screen individuals for AAAs and repair them electively. However, because of the variable incidence of aneurysms, determination of cost effectiveness is complicated. In a cost–benefit analysis of AAA screening, Quill et al. noted that, in 1985, there were 28,536,000 persons over age 65 in the United States.[122] During that year, 12,499 deaths in the same age group were caused by ruptured AAAs (a "soft" value considering the declining rate of autopsies in recent decades). Using an average cost of $150 for an abdominal ultrasound examination, these investigators calculated that it would cost about $4.3 billion to scan all persons at risk. This amounts to a cost of $360,000 per life saved, provided that all patients found to have an AAA undergo operation and there are no operative deaths (another unlikely assumption). Frame et al. recently concluded that screening for AAAs in men aged 60 to 80 years is "cost-effective but of small benefit."[123] However, the accuracy of this conclusion is questionable because the report is based on references identified from bibliographies of pertinent articles and computerized literature searches; a computer spreadsheet model was constructed to simulate the costs and effectiveness of various protocols.

However, if the population screened consists of patients with increased risk of AAAs, the cost–benefit ratio improves. For example, if patients with concomitant peripheral vascular disease are screened (with a prevalence of AAA approaching 10%), Quill et al. calculated that ultrasound screening would save 1500 lives at a cost of $78,000 per life saved.[122] The National Academy of Sciences has estimated that the average cost of death is $200,000,[124] thereby suggesting that ultrasound screening for AAA is cost-effective in carefully selected groups.

Figure 12.1 presents a diagnostic algorithm for AAA.

12.7 TREATMENT

Patients with ruptured AAAs nearly always warrant surgical repair because the death rate associated with untreated rupture approaches 100%. Occasionally, patients with ruptured AAAs deemed excessive operative risks before the rupture or patients with virtually no chance of survival or reasonable quality of life are best treated with analgesia and comfort measures (see Figure 12.2). According to most authorities, almost half of patients with ruptured AAAs do not make it to the hospital alive. Of those admitted with ruptured AAAs, mortality varies greatly and is a function of efficiency of emergency medical service (EMS) systems, patient stability on admission to the emergency department, and patient-related variables (age, hemodynamic status, comorbidities such as CAD, heart failure, renal insufficiency, and COPD). Operative mortality rates for ruptured AAAs vary enormously, ranging from less than 30% to over 90%. For example, Cohen et al. reported mortality of only 42% for ruptured AAA repair in patients under age 60 compared with 81% for those aged 60 to 69.[125] In a recognized center of excellence, led by a surgeon of experience and superb technical abilities, Johansen et al. reported a disappointing overall mortality rate of 70% in 186 patients with ruptured AAAs treated at Harborview Hospital in Seattle.[126] Although this report engendered criticism by others, it likely represents reality in a community with one of the best and fastest EMS systems in the country.

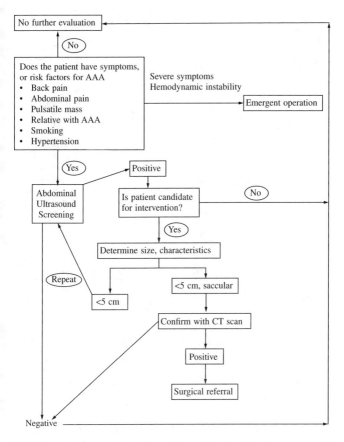

FIGURE 12.1 Diagnostic algorithm. AAA = abdominal aortic aneurysm; CT = computed tomography.

Patients with symptomatic aneurysms (e.g., embolization, thrombosis, severe abdominal or back pain) have a high likelihood of limb loss or death and should be treated by urgent operation. For

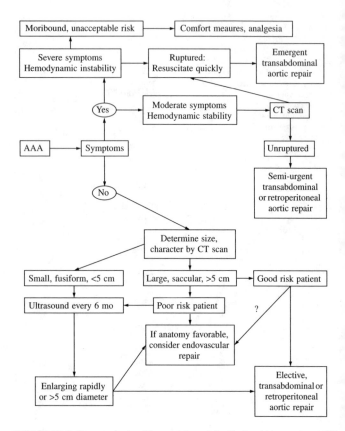

FIGURE 12.2 Treatment algorithm. AAA = abdominal aortic aneurysm; CT = computed tomography.

patients with asymptomatic AAAs, however, surgical decision-making is often difficult. Because AAA repairs are basically prophylactic operations designed to avoid rupture and prolong life, appropriate decision-making requires an accurate estimate of AAA rupture risk versus elective operative risk. These factors must be considered in the context of an individual patient's life expectancy. In the United States, a 60-year-old man can expect to live 18 years, whereas an 85-year-old man's life expectancy decreases to 5 years.[69] Coexistent medical problems and family history of longevity clearly must also be considered. Moreover, after successful AAA repair, long-term survival is reduced in patients with CAD, renal insufficiency, hypertension, and peripheral atherosclerosis.

Decision analysis models have been constructed to aid in the process of determining the best course of action for patients with AAAs of various sizes and coexistent conditions.[127–129] These models take into consideration the three most important variables in determining the prudence of recommending operative repair of AAAs: (1) risk of rupture, (2) life expectancy, and (3) operative risk. For example, in a 70-year-old man with average life expectancy and average operative mortality (about 5%), AAA repair will improve life expectancy if annual AAA rupture risk exceeds 1.5% per year.[128] For younger patients, the threshold AAA diameter that justifies elective repair is lower than for older patients. Of the three key factors above, the operative risk is most accurately determined, followed by life expectancy and rupture risk, which is most difficult to assess for individual AAAs. Thus, decision analyses are most relevant for policy-making for large populations than for individual patients.

With respect to operative risk, center-specific mortality is a crucial consideration. Differences in results between centers and individual surgeons vary independently of patient-specific risk factors. Volume and experience are important; low-volume hospitals and surgeons have demonstrably worse outcomes for AAA repair than higher-volume centers. For example, in New York State in 1985 to 1987, age- and severity-adjusted operative mortality was 9% for elective AAA repair among surgeons who performed fewer than five procedures per year compared with only 4% for those who performed more than 26 procedures per year.[130] Mortality rates for elective AAA repairs were 12% versus 5% in hospitals with fewer than five versus more than 38 procedures per year, respectively. Of note, the average number of AAA repairs per surgeon was only 3.6 annually; per hospital, it was 10.2 annually. In Norway, the operative mortality after elective AAA repair was 2.7-fold higher in hospitals performing fewer than 10 cases per year, and 2.6-fold lower in hospitals in which more than 100 major vascular operations were performed annually.[131] Similar observations have been made in other large series.[132,133]

Conventional surgical repair of AAAs has improved steadily. There has been a steady decline in operative mortality associated with open repair of AAAs over the last 4 decades. This is in part attributed to advances in anesthetic and intraoperative monitoring, improved patient selection, better preoperative patient preparation, refinements in surgical technique, and major improvements in postoperative care. Modern series from vascular centers of excellence describe operative mortality rates less than 5% for elective AAA repair.[30,133,134] Two recent publications reviewing the results of surgery for infrarenal AAAs reported operative mortality of 2.1% and 3.5%, respectively.[135] Sedwitz reported no operative deaths in 109 consecutive elective aortic operations performed by residents in a veterans hospital—a most impressive accomplishment considering the average health status of the veteran population.[136] Table 12.2 summarizes the results of elective AAA repair in individual institutions in the l990s. Even geographically based multi-institutional, multisurgeon studies document acceptable operative mortality rates (Table 12.3). Graft-related complications (i.e., durability of repair) occur in fewer than 10% of patients even with 30-year follow-up.[137]

The technical details of AAA repair, complications, and specific anatomic considerations (e.g., thoracoabdominal aneurysms, peri- or juxtarenal AAAs, inflammatory AAAs, aortocaval fistulas, associated developmental abnormalities such as retro- or circumaortic renal veins or duplicated vena cavas, aortoenteric fistula-infected aneurysms, coexistent occlusive disease, preservation of bowel perfusion) are beyond the scope of this text. For example, there is great debate over the relative merits of transabdominal versus retroperitoneal repair of AAAs; each has its relative merits. Randomized trials have reached different conclusions about the potential advantages of retroperitoneal

TABLE 12.2
Abdominal Aortic Aneurysm Repair in the Modern Era: Individual Series with More Than 100 Patients

Study	N	Mortality (%)
Sedwitz, 1990	109	0.0
Golden, 1990	500	1.6
Shah, 1991	280	4.0
Bunt, 1992	156	2.0
Seeger, 1994	146	3.5
Baron, 1994	457	4.4
Lord, 1994	329	3.5
Sicard, 1995	145	1.4
Schueppert, 1996	144	3.5
D'Angelo, 1997	113	2.7
Allen, 1998	637	2.1

TABLE 12.3
Abdominal Aortic Aneurysm Repair in the Modern Era: Multi–Institutional Series

Study (Location)	N	Mortality (%)
Hertzer, 1984 (Cleveland)	840	6.5
Johnston, 1988 (Canada)	666	4.8
Richardson, 1991 (Kentucky)	136	6.0
Katz, 1994 (Michigan)	8,185	7.5[a]

[a] Mortality decreased from 13.6% in 1980 to 5.6% in 1990.

over transabdominal incisions. Cambria et al. found no difference in morbidity or postoperative complications, except slightly prolonged return to oral intake after the transperitoneal approach.[138] In contrast,

Sicard et al. reported more prolonged ileus, small bowel obstruction, and overall complications after transabdominal compared with retroperitoneal aortic surgery, although pulmonary complications were similar.[139] The most recent prospective comparison of these two approaches found no difference in operating time, cross-clamp time, blood loss, fluid requirement, analgesia requirement, gastrointestinal function, intensive-care-unit stay, or length of hospital stay between these methods.[140] The author's personal preference is a retroperitoneal approach for most cases because it facilitates exposure of the perirenal aorta and, after a brief learning curve, it is easier on both the patient and the surgeon. Retroperitoneal exposure is particularly useful in the case of a "hostile abdomen" due to multiple previous transperitoneal operations, an abdominal wall stoma, a horseshoe kidney, an inflammatory aneurysm, or need for suprarenal aortic control. A transperitoneal approach is superior for ruptured AAAs, coexistent abdominal pathology, and requirement for extensive exposure of the right iliac artery (e.g., for aneurysm repair) or the right renal artery (e.g., for renal artery revascularization).

Although routine preoperative arteriography before AAA repair is controversial, it is widely accepted that preoperative CT scanning to define the anatomy precisely is essential (Figure 12.3). Similarly, it is well known that patients with aortic aneurysmal disease frequently have coexistent CAD, but the appropriateness of cardiac screening remains contentious. In general, the incidence of the most serious adverse cardiac outcomes—myocardial infarction (MI) and cardiac death—is relatively low. However, up to half of postoperative MIs are fatal.[141,142] The uncommon but dangerous occurrence of postoperative MI has given rise to four major approaches to preoperative risk assessment: (1) an aggressive interventional strategy such as that evaluated by Hertzer and others in Cleveland,[143,144] (2) a rigid protocol requiring extensive preoperative testing proposed by Bunt in Loma Linda,[142] (3) a selective evaluation recommended by several groups in Boston,[145-147] and (4) a minimalist policy championed by Taylor et al. in Oregon.[148] Numerous variations of these approaches have also been

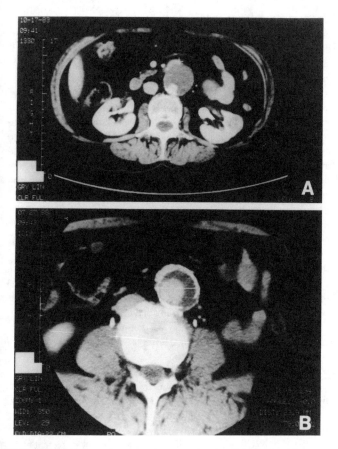

FIGURE 12.3 Computed tomography scans showing abdominal aortic aneurysms (with intravenous contrast). In panel A there is a large amount of intraluminal thrombus and little calcification in the aortic wall. In panel B there is less intraluminal thrombus but a large amount of calcium in the wall.

recommended by other authorities. We recently reported that extensive cardiac evaluation before vascular operations can result in morbidity, delays, and refusal to undergo vascular surgery. The underlying indication for vascular operations and the local iatrogenic cardiac complication rates must be considered before ordering special studies.[149]

The minimally invasive nature of the endoluminal method of abdominal aneurysm repair has gained increasing popularity. Endovascular repair was first reported by Parodi et al. in 1991.[150] Development of grafts has flourished during the past decade, and currently two commercially available grafts have been approved by the U.S. Food and Drug Administration (Guidant™* and AneuRx™**). A thorough description of endovascular aneurysm repair has been provided by May and White.[151] The durability of endoluminal AAA repair remains in question. Nassim et al. reported their experience in placing endoluminal grafts in 29 patients.[152] Overall, 24 procedures (83%) were completely successfully placed. Complications included two deaths due to microembolization, five early conversions, two chest infections, three patients with buttock claudication, and three patients with trash foot. Perigraft leaks were detected in four patients (three proximal and one distal). Continued AAA expansion was observed in three of the patients. One of the leaks was discovered at 1-year follow-up. In this patient, the aneurysmal process was not retarded by endoluminal repair. These findings are dismal in comparison with the excellent results using conventional methods.

In one of the few concurrent comparisons of endoluminal versus open repair in the treatment of AAAs, May et al. studied 303 patients by life table analysis.[153] They found no significant difference in the perioperative mortality rate for open repair (11 deaths, or 5.6%, in 195 patients) and endovascular repair (six deaths, or 5.6%, in 108 patients). Three of the six deaths in the latter group occurred in patients with successful endovascular repair, and three occurred among 18 patients who were converted to open repair. Similarly, there was no difference

---

* Registered trademark of Guidant Corporation, Indianapolis, IN.
** Registered trademark of Medtronic, Inc., Minneapolis, MN.

in survival rate between endoluminal and open-repair groups when analyzed by the log-rank test ($P = 0.14$). The rate of graft failure, however, was significantly higher in the endovascular group than the open-repair group ($P < 0.001$). However, the endoluminal method results in shorter length of hospital stay, shorter length of intensive-care-unit stay, and less blood loss than the open method. Despite these savings, the high cost of endoluminal grafts and need for lifelong CT scan follow-up negate most potential cost savings.

12.8   CONCLUSIONS

Conventional repair remains the "gold standard" for AAA treatment. Endoleak rates average 10% to 20%, and cost considerations become less important when one considers the costs of endoluminal grafts and follow-up. Conventional AAA repairs by transabdominal or retroperitoneal approaches are safe, effective, and durable.

REFERENCES

1. Osler, W., Aneurysm of the abdominal aorta, *Lancet*, ii,1089, 1905.
2. Erichsen, J. E., *Observations on Aneurism*, C. and J. Allard Co., London, 1844.
3. Osler, W., Remarks on arterio-venous aneurysm, *Lancet*, ii, 949, 1915.
4. Johnson, T., *The Works of That Famous Surgeon Ambrose Paré*, Coates and Dugard Co., London, 1649.
5. Leonardo, R., *History of Surgery*, Froben, New York, 1943.
6. Pott, P., *Remarks of the Necessity and Propriety of the Operation of Amputation in Certain Cases*, J. Johnson, London, 1779.
7 Cooper, A.P., *Lectures on the Principles and Practice, Surgery*, 2nd ed., F. C. Westley, London, 1830.
8. Cho, S.I., Johnson, W.C., Bush, H.L., et al., Lethal complications associated with nonresective treatment of abdominal aortic aneurysms, *Arch. Surg.*, 117, 1214, 1982.
9. Haeger, K. *The Illustrated History of Surgery*, Bell, New York, 1988.
10. Krupski, W.C., Selzman, C.H., and Floridia, R., Contemporary management of isolated iliac artery aneurysms, *J. Vasc. Surg.*, 28, 1, 1998.

11. Matas, R., Ligation of the abdominal aorta: report of the ultimate result, 1 year, 5 months and 9 days after the ligation of the abdominal aorta for aneurysm of the bifurcation, *Ann. Surg.*, 81, 457, 1925.

12. Creech, O., Jr., Endoaneurysmorrhaphy and treatment of aortic aneurysm, *Ann. Surg.*, 164, 935, 1966.

13. Oudot, J., La greffe vasculaire dans les thromboses du carrefour aortique, *Press. Med.*, 59, 234, 1951.

14. DuBost, C., Allary, M., and Deconomos, N., Resection of an aneurysm of the abdominal aorta: reestablishment of the continuity by a preserved human arterial graft with a result after 5 months, *Arch. Surg.*, 64, 405, 1952.

15. Schaffer, P.W. and Hardin, C.W., The use of temporary and polyethylene shunts to permit occlusion, resection and frozen homologous artery graft replacement of vital vessel segments, *Surgery*, 31, 186, 1952.

16. Voorhees, A., Jaretzki, A., and Blakemore, A.H., The use of tubes constructed from Vinyon "N" cloth in bridging arterial defects, *Am. Surg.*, 135, 332, 1952.

17. Bahnson, H.T., Considerations in the excision of aortic aneurysms, *Am. Surg.*, 97, 257, 1953.

18. Johnston, K.W., Rutherford, R.B., Tilson, M.D., et al., Suggested standards for reporting on arterial aneurysms, *J. Vasc. Surg.*, 13, 452, 1991.

19. Ouriel, K., Green, J.R.M., Donayre, C., et al., An evaluation of new methods of expressing aortic aneurysm size; relationship to rupture, *J. Vasc. Surg.*, 15, 12, 1992.

20. Abernathy, C.M., Baumgartner, R., and Butler, H.G., The management of ruptured abdominal aortic aneurysms in rural Colorado: with a historical note on Kit Carson's death, *JAMA*, 256, 597, 1986.

21. Cohen, J.R. and Graver, L.M., The ruptured abdominal aortic aneurysm of Albert Einstein, *Surg. Gynecol. Obstet.*, 170, 455, 1990.

22. Rea, C.E., The surgical treatment of aneurysm of the abdominal aorta, *Minn. Med.*, 31, 153, 1948.

23. Lilienfield, C.E., Gunderson, P.D., Sprafka, J.M., et al., Epidemiology of aortic aneurysms: 1, mortality trends in the United States, 1951–1981, *Arteriosclerosis*, 7, 637, 1987.

24. Melton, L.J., Bickerstaff, L.K., and Hollier, L.H., Changing incidence of abdominal aortic aneurysms: a population-based study, *Am. J. Epidemiol.*, 120, 379, 1984.

25. Wheeler, H.B., Myth and reality in general surgery, *Bull. Am. Coll. Surg.*, 78, 21, 1993.

26. Darling, R.C., Messina, C.R., and Brewster, D.C., Autopsy study of unoperated abdominal aortic aneurysms, the case for early resection, *Circulation*, 56, II-161, 1977.

27. Johansen, K. and Koepsell, T., Familial tendency for abdominal aortic aneurysms, *JAMA*, 256, 1934, 1986.

28. Johnson, G., Jr., Avery, A., and Mcdougal, G., Aneurysms of the abdominal aorta: incidence in blacks and whites in North Carolina, *Arch. Surg.*, 120, 1138, 1985.

29. Leopold, G.R., Goldberger, L.E., and Bernstein, E.F., Ultrasonic detection and evaluation of abdominal aortic aneurysms, *Surgery*, 939: 939, 1972.

30 Cronenwett, J.L., Krupski, W.C., and Rutherford, R.B., Abdominal aortic and iliac aneurysms, in *Vascular Surgery*, 5th ed., Rutherford, R.B., Ed., W.B. Saunders Co., Philadelphia, 2000, 1246.

31. Wilmink, A.B.M., Hubbard, C.S., and Quick, C.R.G., The influence of screening for asymptomatic abdominal aortic aneurysms in the Huntington district, *Br. J. Surg.*, 84, S11, 1997.

32. Alcorn, H.G., Wolfson, S.K., Jr., and Sutton-Tyrell, K., Risk factors for abdominal aortic aneurysms in older adults enrolled in the cardiovascular health study, *Art. Thromb. Vasc. Biol.*, 16, 963, 1996.

33. Lederle, F.A., Johnson, G.R., and Wilson, S.E., Prevalence and associations of abdominal aortic aneurysm detected through screening. Aneurysm Detection and Management (ADAM) Veterans Affairs Study Group, *Ann. Intern. Med.*, 126, 441, 1997.

34. Cabellon, S., Jr., Moncrief, C.L., and Pierre, D.R., Incidence of abdominal aortic aneurysms in patients with atheromatous arterial disease, *Am. J. Surg.*, 146, 575, 1983.

35. Graham, M. and Chan, A., Ultrasound screening for clinically occult abdominal aortic aneurysm, *Can. Med. Assoc. J.*, 138, 627, 1988.

36. Allardice, J.T., Allwright, G.J., Wafula, J.M.C., et al., High prevalence of abdominal aortic aneurysm in men with peripheral vascular disease: screening by ultrasonography, *Br. J. Surg.*, 75, 240, 1988.

37. Anton, G.E., Hertzer, N.R., and Beven, K.G., Surgical management of popliteal aneurysms: trends in presentation, treatment, and results from 1952 to 1984, *J. Vasc. Surg.*, 3, 125, 1986.

38. Twomey, A., Twomey, E., and Wilkins, R.A., Unrecognized aneurysmal disease in male hypertensive patients, *Int. Angiol.*, 5, 269, 1986.

39. Lindholm, L., Ejlertsson, G., and Forsberg, L., Low prevalence of abdominal aortic aneurysm in hypertensive patients: a population-based study, *Acta. Med. Scand.*, 218, 305, 1985.

40. Clifton, M.A., Familial abdominal aortic aneurysms, *Br. J. Surg.*, 64, 765, 1977.

41. Webster, M.W., Ferrell, R.E., and St. Jean, P.I., Ultrasound screening of first-degree relatives of patients with an abdominal aortic aneurysm, *J. Vasc. Surg.*, 13, 9, 1991.

42. Verloes, A., Sakalihasan, N., and Koulischer, L., Aneurysms of the abdominal aorta: familial and genetic aspects in three hundred thirteen pedigrees, *J. Vasc. Surg.*, 21, 646, 1995.

43. Tilson, M.D., Seashore. Fifty families with abdominal aortic aneurysms in two or more first-order relatives, *Am. J. Surg.*, 147, 551, 1984.

44. Norrgard, O., Angquist, K.A., and Rais, O., Familial occurrence of abdominal aortic aneurysms, *Surgery*, 95, 650, 1984.

45. Webster, M.W., St. Jean, P.I., and Steed, D.L., Abdominal aortic aneurysm: results of a family study, *J. Vasc. Surg.*, 13, 366, 1991.

46. Tilson, M.D., Ozsvath, K.J., and Hirose, H., A genetic basis for autoimmune manifestations in the abdominal aortic aneurysm resides in the MHC class II locus DR-beta–1, *Ann. N.Y. Acad. Sci.*, 800, 208, 1996.

47. Lee, B., Godfrey, M., and Vitale, E., Linkage of Marfan syndrome and a phenotypically related disorder to two different fibrillin genes, *Nature*, 352, 330, 1991.

48. Kuivaniemi, H., Tromp, G., and Prockop, D.J., Mutations in collagen genes; causes of rare and some common diseases in humans, *FASEB J*, 5, 2025, 1991.

49. Bickerstaff, L.K., Hollier, L.H., Van Peenen, H.J., et al., Abdominal aortic aneurysms: the changing natural history, *J. Vasc. Surg.*, 1, 6, 1984.

50. Ernst, C.B., Abdominal aortic aneurysm, *N. Engl. J. Med.*, 328, 1167, 1993.

51. Bengtsson, H., Bergqvist, D., and Sternby, N.H., Increasing prevalence of abdominal aortic aneurysm: a necropsy study, *Eur. J. Surg.*, 158, 19, 1992.

52. Fowkes, F.G.R., Macintyre, C.C.A., and Ruckley, C.V., Increasing incidence of aortic aneurysms in England and Wales, *BMJ*, 298, 33, 1989.

53. Chosky, S.A., Wilmink, A.B.M., and Quick, C.R.G., Ruptured abdominal aortic aneurysm in the Huntington District: a 10-year experience, *Br. J. Surg.*, 84, 44, 1997.

54 Gillum, R.F., Epidemiology of aortic aneurysm in the United States, *J. Clin. Epidemiol.*, 48, 1289, 1995.

55. Castleden, W.M. and Mercer, J.C., Abdominal aortic aneurysms in Western Australia: descriptive epidemiology and patterns of rupture, *Br. J. Surg.*, 72, 109, 1985.

56. Stern, M.P., The recent decline in ischemic heart disease mortality, *Ann. Intern. Med.*, 91, 630, 1979.

57. Estes, W., Abdominal aortic aneurysm: a study of one hundred and two cases, *Circulation*, 2, 258, 1950.

58. Schatz, I.J., Fairbairn, J.F., and Jugens, J.L., Abdominal aortic aneurysms: a reappraisal, *Circulation*, 26, 200, 1962.

59 Krupski, W.C., Bass, A., and Thurston, D.W., Utility of computed tomography for surveillance of small abdominal aortic aneurysms, *Arch. Surg.*, 125, 1345, 1990.

60. Szilagyi, D.E., Smith, R.F., and DeRusso, F.J., Contribution of abdominal aortic aneurysmectomy to prolongation of life, *Ann. Surg.*, 164, 678, 1966.

61. Foster, J.H., Bolasny, B.L., and Gobbel, W.G., Comparative study of elective resection and expectant treatment of abdominal aortic aneurysm, *Surg. Gynecol. Obstet.*, 129, 1, 1969.

62. Darling, P.C., Messina, C.R., and Brewster, D.C., Autopsy study of unoperated abdominal aortic aneurysms: the case for early resection, *Circulation*, 56, II-161, 1977.

63. Sterpetti, A.V., Cavallaro, A., and Cavallari, N., Factors influencing the rupture of abdominal aortic aneurysm, *Surg. Obstet. Gynecol.*, 173, 175, 1991.

64 Lederle, F.A., Risk of rupture of large abdominal aortic aneurysms, Disagreement among vascular surgeons, *Arch. Intern. Med.*, 156, 1007, 1996.

65. Bernstein, E.F. and Chan, E.F., Abdominal aortic aneurysms in high risk patients: outcome of selective management based on size and expansion rate, *Ann. Surg.*, 200, 255, 1984.

66. Cronenwett, J.L., Sargent, S.K., and Wall, M.H., Variables that affect the expansion rate and outcome of small abdominal aortic aneurysms, *J. Vasc. Surg.*, 11, 260, 1990.

67. Littooy, F.N., Steffan, G., and Greisler, H.P., Use of sequential B-mode ultrasonography to manage abdominal aortic aneurysms, *Arch. Surg.*, 124, 419, 1989.

68. Sterpetti, A.V., Schultz, R.D., and Feldhaus, R.J., Factors influencing enlargement rate of small abdominal aortic aneurysms, *J. Surg. Res.*, 43, 211, 1987.

69. Cronenwett, J.L. and Katz, D.A., When should infrarenal abdominal aortic aneurysms be repaired: what are the critical risk factors and dimensions?, in *Current Critical Problems in Vascular Surgery*, Veith, F.J., Ed., Quality Medical Publishing, St. Louis, 1996, 256.

70. Cronenwett, J.L., Murphy, T.F., and Zelenock, G.B., Actuarial analysis of variables associated with rupture of small abdominal aortic aneurysms, *Surgery*, 98, 256, 1985.

71. Nevitt, M.P., Ballard, D.J., and Hallett, J.W., Jr., Prognosis of abdominal aortic aneurysms: a population based study, *N. Engl. J. Med.*, 321, 1009, 1989.

72. Limet, R., Sakalihassan, N., and Albert, A., Determination of the expansion rate and incidence of rupture of abdominal aortic aneurysms, *J. Vasc. Surg.*, 14, 540, 1991.

73 Sterpetti, A.V., Cavallaro, A., and Cavallari, N., Factors influencing the rupture of abdominal aortic aneurysm, *Surg. Obstet. Gynecol.*, 173, 175, 1991.

74. Szilagyi, D.E., Elliott, J.P., and Smith, R.F., Clinical fate of the patient with asymptomatic aortic aneurysm and unfit for surgical treatment, *Arch. Surg.*, 115, 299, 1984.

75. Strachan, D.P., Predictors of death from aortic aneurysm among middle-aged men; the Whitehall Study, *Br. J. Surg.*, 78, 401, 1991.

76. Darling, R.C., Brewster, D.C., and Darling, R.C., Jr., Are familial abdominal aortic aneurysms different?, *J. Vasc. Surg.*, 10, 39, 1989.

77. Bernstein, E.F., and Chan, E.L., Abdominal aortic aneurysms in high risk patients; outcome of selective management based on size and expansion rate, *Ann. Surg.*, 200, 255, 1984.

78. Krupski, W.C., Bass, A., and Thurston, D.W., Utility of computed tomography for surveillance of small abdominal aortic aneurysms, *Arch. Surg.*, 125, 1345, 1990.

79. Wolf, Y.G., Thomas, W.S., and Brennan, F.J., Computed tomography scanning findings associated with rapid expansion of abdominal aortic aneurysms, *J. Vasc. Surg.*, 20, 529, 1994.

80 Limet, R., Sakalihassan, N., and Albert, A., Determination of the expansion rate and incidence of rupture of abdominal aortic aneurysms, *J. Vasc. Surg.,* 14, 540, 1991.

81. Schewe, C.K., Schwokart, H.P., and Hammel, G., Influence of selective management on the prognosis and the risk of rupture of abdominal aortic aneurysms, *Clin. Invest.,* 72, 585, 1994.

82. Grange, J.J., Davis, V., and Baxter, B.T., Pathogenesis of abdominal aortic aneurysm; an update and look to the future, *Cardiovasc. Surg.,* 5, 256, 1997.

83. Van der Vliet, J.A., and Boll, A.P., Abdominal aortic aneurysm, *Lancet,* 349, 864, 1997.

84. Halloran, B.G., Davis, V.A., and McManus, B.M., Localization of aortic disease is associated with intrinsic differences in aortic structure, *J. Surg. Res.,* 59, 17, 1995.

85. Patel, M.I., Hardman, D.T., and Fischer, C.M., Current views on the pathogenesis of abdominal aortic aneurysms, *J. Am. Coll. Surg.,* 181, 371, 1995.

86. McMillan, W.D., Tamarina, N.A., and Cipollone, M., Size matters: the relationship between MMP-9 expression and aortic diameter, *Circulation,* 96, 2228, 1997.

87. Boyle, J.R., McDermott, E., and Crowther, M., Doxycycline inhibits elastin degradation and reduces metalloproteinase activity in a model of aneurysmal disease, *J. Vasc. Surg.,* 27, 354, 1998.

88. Petersen, E., Boman, J., and Persson, K., *Chlamydia pneumoniae* in human abdominal aortic aneurysms, *Eur. J. Vasc. Endovasc. Surg.,* 15, 138, 1998.

89. Tilson, M.D., Ozsvath, K.J., and Hirose, H., A genetic basis for autoimmune manifestations in the abdominal aortic aneurysm resides in the MHC class II locus DR-beta-l, *Ann. N. Y. Acad. Sci.,* 800, 208, 1996.

90. Gregory, A.K., Yin, N.X., and Capella, J., Features of autoimmunity in the abdominal aortic aneurysm, *Arch. Surg.,* 131, 85, 1996.

91. Ozsvath, K.J., Hirose, H., and Xia, S., Molecular mimicry in human aortic aneurysmal diseases, *Ann. N. Y. Acad. Sci.,* 800, 288, 1996.

92. Baxter, B.T., McGee, G.S., and Flinn, W.R., Distal embolization as a presenting symptom of aortic aneurysms, *Am. J. Surg.,* 160, 197, 1990.

93. Marston, W.A., Ahliquist, R., and Johnson, G., Misdiagnosis of ruptured abdominal aortic aneurysm, *J. Vasc. Surg.,* 16, 17, 1992.

94. Bengstsson, H. and Bergqvist, D., Ruptured abdominal aortic aneurysm: a population-based study, *J. Vasc. Surg.,* 18, 74, 1993.

95. Kvilekval, K.V.H., Best, I.M., and Mason, R.A., The value of computed tomography in the management of symptomatic abdominal aortic aneurysms, *J. Vasc. Surg.*, 12, 28, 1990.

96. Chervu, A., Clagett, G.P., and Valentine, R.J., Role of physical examination in detection of abdominal aortic aneurysms, *Surgery*, 117, 454, 1995.

97. Jaakkola, P., Hippelainen, M., and Farin, P., Interobserver variability in measuring the dimensions of the abdominal aorta: comparison of ultrasound and computed tomography, *Eur. J. Vasc. Endovasc. Surg.,* 12, 230, 1996.

98. Shuman, W.P., Hastrup, W.J., and Hohler, T.R., Suspected leaking abdominal aortic aneurysm: use of sonography in the emergency room, *Radiology*, 168, 117, 1988.

99. Jaakkola, P., Hippelainen, M., and Farrin, P., Interobserver variability in measuring the dimensions of the abdominal aorta: comparison of ultrasound and computed tomography, *Eur. J. Vasc. Endovasc. Surg.,* 12, 230, 1996.

100. Lederle, F.A., Wilson, S.E., and Johnson, G.R., Variability in measurement of abdominal aortic aneurysms, *J. Vasc. Surg.*, 21, 945, 1995.

101 Thurmond, A.S. and Semler, H.J., Abdominal aortic aneurysm: incidence in a population at risk, *J. Cardiovasc. Surg.*, 27, 457, 1986.

102. Collin, J., Araujo, L., Walton, J., et al., Oxford screening program for abdominal aortic aneurysm in men aged 65–74 years, *Lancet*, ii, 613, 1988.

103. Lederle, F.A., Walker, J.M., and Reinke, D.B., Selective screening for abdominal aortic aneurysms with physical examination and ultrasound, *Arch. Intern. Med.*, 148, 1753, 1988.

104. Scott, R.A.P., Ashton, H.A., and Kay, D.N., Routine ultrasound screening in management of abdominal aortic aneurysm, *BMJ*, 296, 1709, 1988.

105. Bengtsson, H., Norrgard, O., Angquist, K.A., et al., Ultrasonic screening of the abdominal aorta among siblings of patients with abdominal aortic aneurysms, *Br. J. Surg.*, 76, 589, 1989.

106. O'Kelly, T.J. and Heather, B.P., General practice-based population screening for abdominal aortic aneurysms: a pilot study, *Br. J. Surg.*, 76, 479, 1989.

107. Bengtsson, H., Ekberg, O., Aspelin, P., et al., Ultrasound screening of the abdominal aorta in patients with intermittent claudication, *Eur. J. Vasc. Surg.*, 3, 497, 1989.

108. Berridge, D.C., Griffith, C.D.M, Amar, S.S., et al., Screening for clinically unsuspected abdominal aortic aneurysms in patients with peripheral vascular disease, *Eur. J. Vasc. Surg.*, 3, 421, 1989.

109. Akkersdijk, G.J.M., Puylaert, J.B.C.M., and deVries, A.C., Abdominal aortic aneurysm as an incidental finding in abdominal ultrasonography, *Br. J. Sur.*, 78, 1261, 1991.

110. Galland, R.B., Simmons, M.J., and Tonie, E.P.H., Prevalence of abdominal aortic aneurysm in patients with occlusive peripheral vascular disease, *Br. J. Surg.*, 78, 1259, 1991.

111. Scott, R.A.P., Ashton, H.A., and Kay, D.N., Abdominal aortic aneurysm in 4237 screened patients: prevalence, development and management over 6 years, *Br. J. Surg.*, 78, 1122, 1991.

112. Webster, M.W., Ferrell, R.E., St. Jean, P.L., et al., Ultrasound screening of first-degree relatives of patients with an abdominal aortic aneurysm, *J. Vasc. Surg.*, 13, 9, 1991.

113. Adamson, J., Powell, J.T., and Greenhalgh, R.M., Selection for screening for familial aortic aneurysms, *Br. J. Surg.*, 79, 897, 1992.

114. Carty, G.A., Nachtigal, T., Magyar, R., et al., Abdominal duplex ultrasound screening for occult aortic aneurysm during carotid arterial evaluation, *J. Vasc. Surg.*, 17, 696, 1993.

115. The UK Small Aneurysm Trial Participants, Mortality results for randomised controlled trial of early elective surgery or ultrasonographic surveillance for small abdominal aortic aneurysms, *Lancet*, 352, 1649, 1998.

116. Cronenwett, J.L. and Johnston, K.W., The United Kingdom small aneurysm trial: implications for surgical treatment of abdominal aortic aneurysms, *J. Vasc. Surg.*, 29, 191, 1999.

117. Wilmink, T.B.M., Quick, C.R.G., Hubbard, C.S., and Day, N.E., The influence of screening on the incidence of ruptured abdominal aortic aneurysms, *J. Vasc. Surg.*, 30, 203, 1999.

118. Lederle, F.A., Wilson, S.E., and Johnson, G.R., Design of the abdominal aortic Aneurysm Detection and Management Study, *J. Vasc. Surg.*, 20, 296, 1994.

119. Lederle, F.A., Johnson, G.R., and Wilson, S.E., Prevalence and associations of abdominal aortic aneurysm detected through screening, *Ann. Intern. Med.*, 126, 441, 1997.

120. Pasch, A.R., Ricotta, J.J., May, A.G., et al., Abdominal aortic aneurysm: the case for elective resection, *Circulation*, 70, I-1, 1984.

121. Breckwoldt, W.L., Mackey, W.C., and O'Donnell, T.F., Jr., The economic implications of high-risk abdominal aortic aneurysms, *J. Vasc. Surg.*, 13, 798, 1991.

122. Quill, D.S., Colgan, M.P., and Sumner, D.S., Ultrasonic screening for the detection of abdominal aortic aneurysms, *Surg. Clin. North Am.*, 69, 713, 1989.

123. Frame, P.S., Fryback, D.G., and Patterson, C., Screening for abdominal aortic aneurysm in men ages 60 to 80 years: a cost-effective analysis, *Ann. Intern. Med.*, 119, 411, 1993.

124. Richardson, E.L., *The Creative Balance*, Holt, Rinehart and Winston, New York, 1977, 138.

125. Cohen, J.R., Birnbaum, E., Kassan, M., et al., Experience in managing 70 patients with ruptured abdominal aneurysms, *N. Y. State J. Med.*, 91, 97, 1991.

126. Johansen, K., Kohler, T.R., and Nicholls, S.C., Ruptured abdominal aortic aneurysm: the Harborview experience, *J. Vasc. Surg.*, 13, 240, 1991.

127. Katz, D.A. and Cronenwett, J.L., The cost-effectiveness of early surgery versus watchful waiting in the management of small abdominal aortic aneurysms, *J. Vasc. Surg.*, 19, 980, 1994.

128. Katz, D.A., Littenberg, B., and Cronenwett, J. L., Management of small abdominal aortic aneurysms: early surgery vs. watchful waiting, *JAMA*, 268, 2678, 1992.

129. Michaels, J.A., The management of small abdominal aortic aneurysms: a computer simulation using Monte Carlo methods, *Eur. J. Vasc. Surg.*, 6, 551, 1992.

130. Veith, F.J., Goldsmith, J., and Leather, R.P., The need for quality assurance in vascular surgery, *J. Vasc. Surg.*, 14, 523, 1991.

131. Amundsen, S., Skjaerven, R., and Trippestad, A., Abdominal aortic aneurysms: is there an association between surgical volume, surgical experience, hospital type and operative mortality?, *Acta. Chir. Scand.*, 156, 323, 1990.

132. Katz, D.A., Stanley, J.C., and Zelenock, G.B., Operative mortality rates for intact and ruptured abdominal aortic aneurysms in Michigan: an eleven-year statewide experience, *J. Vasc. Surg.*, 19, 804, 1994.

133. Kazmers, A., Abdominal aortic aneurysm repair in Veterans Affairs medical centers, *J. Vasc. Surg.*, 23, 191, 1996.

134. Johnson, K.W., and Scobie, T.K., Multicenter prospective study of nonruptured abdominal aortic aneurysms. Population and operative management. *J. Vasc. Surg.*, 7,69, 1988.

135. Allen, B.T., Hovsepien, D.M., and Reilly, J.M., Endovascular stent grafts for aneurysmal and occlusive vascular disease; an initial institutional experience, *Am. J. Surg.*, 45, 437, 1998.

136. Sedwitz, M.M., Hye, R.J., Freischlag, J.A., et al., Zero operative mortality in 109 consecutive elective aortic operations by residents, *Surg. Gynecol. Obstet.*, 170, 385, 1990.

137. Hallett, J.W., Jr., Marshall, J., and Peterson, T.M., Graft-related complication after abdominal aortic aneurysm repair: reassurance from a 36-year population-based experience, *J. Vasc. Surg.*, 25, 277, 1997.

138. Cambria, R.P., Brewster, D.C., and Abbott, W.M., Transperitoneal versus retroperitoneal approach for aortic reconstruction: a randomized prospective study, *J. Vasc. Surg.*, 11, 314, 1990.

139. Sicard, G.A., Transabdominal versus retroperitoneal incision for abdominal aortic surgery: report of a prospective randomized trial, *J. Vasc. Surg.*, 21,174, 1995.

140. Sieunarine, K. and Lawrence-Brown, M.M., Comparison of transperitoneal and retroperitoneal approaches for infrarenal aortic surgery: early and late results, *Cardiovasc. Surg.*, 5, 71, 1997.

141. Mangano, D.T., London, M.J., and Hollenberg, M., Perioperative myocardial ischemia in patients undergoing noncardiac surgery-I: incidence and severity during the four-day perioperative period, *J. Am. Coll. Cardiol.*, 17, 843, 1991.

142. Bunt, T.J., The role of a defined protocol for cardiac risk assessment in decreasing perioperative myocardial infarction in vascular surgery, *J. Vasc. Surg.*, 15,626, 1992.

143. Hertzer, N.R., Beven, K.G., and Young, J.R., Coronary artery disease in peripheral vascular patients: a classification of 1000 coronary angiograms and results of surgical management, *Ann. Surg.*, 199, 223, 1984.

144. Hertzer, N.R., Basic data concerning associated coronary disease in peripheral vascular patients, *Ann. Vasc. Surg.*, 1, 616, 1987.

145. Boucher, C.A., Brewster, D.C., Darling, R.C., et al., Determination of cardiac risk by dipyridamole-thallium imaging before peripheral vascular surgery, *N. Engl. J. Med.*, 312, 389, 1985.

146. Eagle, K.A., Coley, D.M., and Newell, J.B., Combining clinical and thallium data optimizes preoperative assessment of cardiac risk before major vascular surgery, *Ann. Intern. Med.*, 110, 859, 1989.

147. Golden, M.A., Whittemore, A.D., Donaldson, M.C., et al., Selective evaluation and management of coronary artery disease in patients undergoing repair of abdominal aortic aneurysms, *Ann. Surg.*, 212, 415, 1990.

148. Taylor, L.M., Yeager, R.A., Moneta, G.L., et al., The incidence of perioperative myocardial infarction in general vascular surgery, *J. Vasc. Surg.*, 15, 52, 1991.

149. Krupski, W.C., Nehler, M.R., Whitehill, T.A., et al., Negative impact of cardiac evaluation before vascular surgery, *Vasc. Med.*, 5, 3, 2000.

150. Parodi, J., Palmaz, J., and Barone, H., Transfemoral intraluminal graft implantation for abdominal aortic aneurysm, *Vasc. Surg.*, 5, 491, 1991.

151. May, J. and White, G.H., Endovascular treatment of aortic aneurysms, in *Vascular Surgery,* 5th ed., Rutherford, R.B., Ed., W. B. Saunders, Philadelphia, 2000, 1281.

152. Nassim, A., Thompson, M.W., and Sayers, R.D., Results of endovascular grafting for abdominal aortic aneurysms, *Ann. Vasc. Surg.*, 12, 222, 1997.

153. May, J., White, G.H., and Yu, W., Concurrent comparison of endoluminal versus open repair in the treatment of abdominal aortic aneurysms: analysis of 303 patients by life table method, *J. Vasc. Surg.*, 27, 213, 1998.

13 Aortic Dissection

Mark R. Nehler and Alden Harken

CONTENTS

13.1 Epidemiology 283
13.2 Pathophysiology 283
13.3 Natural History...289
13.4 Diagnosis and Evaluation...291
13.5 Treatment..292
13.6 Conclusions 295
References...296

13.1 EPIDEMIOLOGY

Acute dissection is one of the most common lethal conditions of the aorta, with a mortality rate (1.2 to 1.5/100,000 males) slightly less than that reported for ruptured aortic aneurysms.[1] This figure likely under-appreciates the disease, as many patients who die acutely from dissection are presumed to have a fatal myocardial infarction (MI) or arrhythmia. Males have a two- to threefold increased risk compared with females.[2] Dissection is rarely seen before age 50 (except in Marfan disease). Uncontrolled hypertension and structural weakness in the aortic wall are considered to be primary risk factors for aortic dissection.[3]

13.2 PATHOPHYSIOLOGY

The initial abnormality in aortic dissection is a tear in the wall of the aorta allowing blood to dissect into the media, separating the intimal layer and the adventitial layer of the vessel (Figure 13.1). In general, 60% of aortic

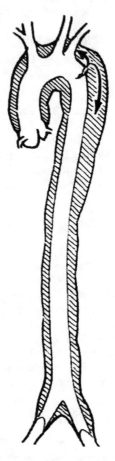

FIGURE 13.1 Illustration demonstrating intimal tear in the descending aorta that has dissected both distally and proximally to involve both the descending and ascending aorta with false lumen of blood. (From Pretre, R. and Segesser, L.K., Aortic dissection, *Lancet,* 349, 1461, 1997. With permission.)

dissections originate in the convex ascending aorta 2 cm above the coronary sinus, 10% in the aortic arch, and 30% in the descending aorta just distal to the left subclavian artery.[4] The two important permissive factors are an inherent structural weakness in the arterial wall and an initiating event (dilation of the aorta and hypertension). The proximal ascending aorta is vulnerable to stress because it expands most during systole, and its convexity is repeatedly exposed to the greatest shear stress. The origin of the descending aorta is a point of relative fixation of the mobile arch, and is therefore also predisposed to mechanical stress.

A minority of all patients with hypertension will suffer aortic dilation. Additional structural aortic weakness is also necessary. Table 13.1 outlines the majority of recognized predisposing factors. A small subset of aortic dissections (fewer than 10%) originate from the external layer of the aorta due to hemorrhage in the vasa vasorum, leading to an intra-aortic hematoma that then spreads via the media to disrupt the intima and initiate the false channel.

TABLE 13.1
Predisposing Factors for Aortic Dissection

- Hypertension
  - Descending (type B)

- Congenital structural
  - Bicuspid aortic valve, aortic coarctation

- Pregnancy
  - 50% of all dissections in women <40 yr occur during during pregnancy (third trimester). Only 50% of these pregnant women have connective tissue disease

- Connective tissue
  - Marfan syndrome, Ehlers-Danlos syndrome

- Iatrogenic
  - (Aortic cross clamp, balloon pump)

- Other
  - Turner syndrome, Noonan syndrome, polycystic kidney disease, giant cell aortitis, systemic lupus erythematosus, relapsing polychondritis

---

Aortic dissections generally propagate distally, but can also extend retrograde. There are frequently multiple sites of reentry into the aortic lumen via secondary tears distally. The extent of dissection can be limited by atherosclerotic plaque, existent infrarenal aneurysmal disease, or coarctation. Not surprisingly, therefore, in young patients, the dissection often extends the length of the entire thoracic and abdominal aorta. The primary causes of morbidity and mortality are related to complications from progression of the dissection channel, including branch vessel occlusion with end-organ ischemia, and external rupture with hemorrhage.

Major changes in clinical decision-making have occurred based on the site of aortic involvement, and, therefore, classification systems have been adopted to describe the pertinent issues. Any dissection involving the ascending aorta is considered a surgical emergency due to the high risk of extension proximally with aortic rupture into the pericardium and cardiac tamponade, acute aortic valve incompetence, or coronary artery occlusion. Two classification systems have been used to describe the degree of aortic involvement, the DeBakey and the Stanford. DeBakey types I and II both involve the ascending aorta, with type I also involving the descending aorta. DeBakey type III involves only the descending aorta. The Stanford system is simpler to remember and has essentially replaced the DeBakey classification. Any aortic dissection involving the ascending aorta is type A, and any not involving the ascending aorta is type B. Figure 13.2 illustrates the Stanford classification system.

As stated, most of the morbidity and mortality is related to complications from dissection progression. The most immediately lethal problem is external rupture with overwhelming hemorrhage. The two sites most common for this are the pericardial sac and the left chest. This is almost always fatal and accounts for the majority of early (within hours of onset) mortality. The second potentially lethal problem involves end-organ ischemia due to branch vessel occlusion from the false channel (Figure 13.3).[5] These occlusions can affect the arch vessels with stroke, the intercostal arteries with spinal cord ischemia, the renal arteries with acute renal failure, the mesenteric circulation

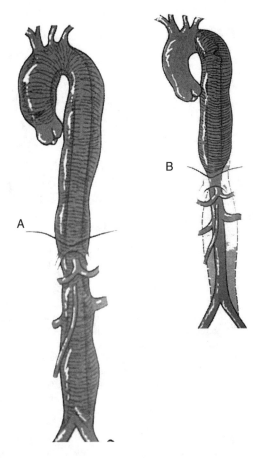

FIGURE 13.2 Anatomic classifications of aortic dissection types A and B used in the Stanford classification system. Stanford type A is any dissection involving the ascending aorta. Stanford type B is any dissection not involving the ascending aorta.

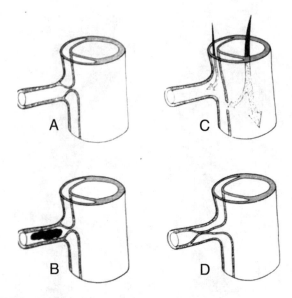

FIGURE 13.3 Mechanisms of branch artery obstruction in acute aortic dissection. (A) Bulging of the false lumen compresses flow in the true lumen. (B) Subsequent thrombosis distal to the area compressed, further potentiating ischemia. (C) Intimal detachment resulting in the majority of the perfusion occurring through the false channel (D) Dissection proceeds into the branch, causing the point of obstruction to occur beyond the branch point. (From Cambria, R.P., Brewster, D.C., Gertler, J., Moncure, A.C., Gusberg, R., Tilson, M.D., Darling, R.C., Hammond, G., Mergerman, J., and Abbott, W.M., Vascular complications associated with spontaneous aortic dissection, *J. Vasc. Surg.*, 7, 199, 1988. With permission.[5])

with visceral ischemia, and the iliac–femoral arteries with leg ischemia. Because of abundant collateral circulation, limb-threatening upper extremity ischemia is rare. It is important to understand that the dissecting false lumen is often spiral in orientation, with frequent reentry points via second intimal tears distally. Therefore, organs can be supplied by either true or false lumens and interpretation of arteriograms can be difficult.

13.3 NATURAL HISTORY

It is important to make an early diagnosis of aortic dissection, because, left untreated (including failure to control hypertension), the mortality rate climbs rapidly for type A dissections (8% in 6 hours, 20% in 24 hours, 50% in 48 hours, and 75% in the first 2 weeks; Figure 13.4).[6-8] As stated previously, the risk of early death due to rupture is much greater for dissections involving the ascending aorta. Other factors predisposing to rupture include poorly controlled hypertension, absent or small-sized reentry sites, high flow within the false channel, and increased aortic diameter. Although the left chest is the most common site of rupture in dissections involving the descending aorta, other sites (mediastinum, right chest, retroperitoneum, peritoneal cavity, and, rarely, esophagus or bronchus) can occur. In general, dissections are classified as acute (symptoms for 14 days or less) and chronic (more

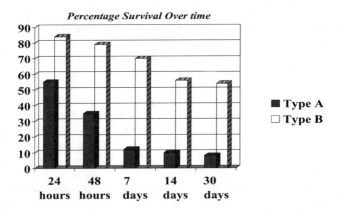

FIGURE 13.4 Projected mortality rates over time for untreated type A and B aortic dissections.

than 14 days of symptoms) due to the much higher likelihood of rupture during the acute phase.

Ischemic complications can involve any branch of the ascending or descending aorta, with various mechanisms involved. The majority of ischemic complications are caused by obstruction of the true lumen by the false lumen. Aortic obstruction via this process is most often located at the thoracoabdominal junction. This leads to acute renovascular hypertension with simultaneous mesenteric, spinal, renal, and lower-extremity ischemia. Blockage of branches of the thoracic and abdominal aorta is most common due to compression of the true lumen by the false lumen at the origin of the arterial branch from the aorta; however, other pathology can occur. The dissection can extend into the branch artery with lumen reduction, or can disrupt the aortic intima with an occlusion from the intimal flap. Regardless of the mechanism, the occluded artery may thrombose distal to the site of obstruction, further exaggerating organ ischemia. The incidence of aortic branch vessel occlusion is between 30% and 50%, depending on the type of diagnostic technique (aortography versus computed tomography [CT] or transesophageal echocardiography).[5,9,10]

Clinical symptoms relate to the degree of ischemia and organs involved. In general, due to collateral blood flow, many branch vessel obstructions can be relatively asymptomatic. Stroke occurs in 3% to 7% of cases, with a wide range of symptoms from focal deficits to coma and death. Spinal symptoms (2% to 6%) can include paraplegia, paraparesis, or other partial neurologic deficits. Lower-extremity ischemia usually involves loss of one or both femoral pulses with associated threatened limbs. This occurs in 25% of patients and resolves spontaneously in up to one third due to reentry of the false lumen into the true lumen. Renal (5% to 25%) and mesenteric (3% to 5%) involvement can be asymptomatic (contralateral kidney uninvolved or single mesenteric artery involved), or can lead to acute renal failure or acute abdomen. The interpretation of creatinine changes and hypertension can be difficult, as preexisting kidney disease (most often from long-standing hypertension) and administered antihypertensive agents can markedly influence these parameters.

In up to 85% of patients who survive acute descending aortic dissection, the false lumen initially remains patent.[11] Of patients who survive acute descending aortic dissection, 35% will develop an aneurysm.[12] Aneurysm formation usually is limited to the upper portion of the descending thoracic aorta or the infrarenal abdominal aorta. Aneurysm rupture is related to increased size or rapid expansion rate. Thrombosis of the false lumen does not protect against potential rupture. Aneurysm rupture is a major cause of late mortality.

13.4   DIAGNOSIS AND EVALUATION

The majority of patients with acute aortic dissection experience sudden onset of intense interscapular pain. The pain is presumably caused by intimal tearing in well-innervated large vessels. The pain frequently migrates to the lower back and abdomen. Any unexplained chest pain, especially if radiating to the back or abdomen in an older hypertensive man, should include acute aortic dissection as part of the diagnostic differential in addition to MI and ischemia. Painless dissection with presentation related to end-organ ischemia from aortic branch occlusion is limited to neuropathic or diabetic patients on corticosteroids typically leading to significant diagnostic delay. Acute aortic dissection should be considered any time a patient who presents with an acute unexplained illness involving apparently unrelated organ systems develops acute arterial occlusion(s). One potential confounding situation to avoid is emergently taking a patient to the operating room for a presumed acute lower-extremity embolus when he or she has an acute type A dissection and iliac occlusion. Another is admitting a patient with acute type A dissection and renal insufficiency to the coronary care unit for presumed cardiogenic shock and making the correct diagnosis postmortem—after death from pericardial rupture and tamponade.

Most patients with acute aortic disease are hypertensive. If hypotensive, then aortic rupture should be suspected. Physical examination may reveal unequal arm blood pressures or absent peripheral pulses. Patients may demonstrate signs of acute cardiac failure related to tamponade or aortic valve insufficiency. Acute neurologic deficits related to cerebral or spinal cord ischemia may be present. Acute renal failure with anuria or oliguria may be present. Acute abdomen due to visceral ischemia may be present. Acute limb ischemia with pain, pallor, pulselessness, paresthesias, or paralysis may be found.

Chest radiography is usually not helpful but may demonstrate widening of the mediastinum. CT with intravenous contrast of the chest and abdomen (particularly spiral) can determine the type and extent of the dissection. To provide adequate visualization of the aorta, intravenous contrast is needed, but this can be problematic in patients with compromised renal function. Nevertheless, CT is available in most centers, and is clearly the first study usually obtained. Magnetic resonance imaging (MRI) is excellent for the delineation of aortic anatomy and does not require intravenous contrast. However, it is difficult to perform MRI in unstable patients. The historic "gold standard" has been arteriography. It is time-consuming, and false negatives can occur due to difficulties interpreting the false lumen (thrombosed, faint opacification, or simultaneous opacification). The primary screening modality that is gaining enthusiasts is transesophageal echocardiography (TEE). It does not require contrast and can determine ascending aortic involvement. It can also determine aortic insufficiency, pericardial rupture, and tamponade. However, it is not universally available, and is not the first diagnostic study to be obtained (Figure 13.5).

The study chosen should optimally delineate (1) whether a dissection is present and (2) whether it involves the ascending or descending aorta (the extent of the false lumen, not the site of the intimal tear). If the ascending aorta is involved, then the status of the aortic valve (regurgitation) and the status of the coronary arteries (significant concomitant coronary disease) are useful data points.

13.5 TREATMENT

As stated earlier, the type and urgency of therapy depend on whether the ascending aorta is involved. The therapy of choice for ascending (type A) aortic dissections is emergency ascending aorta replacement grafting.

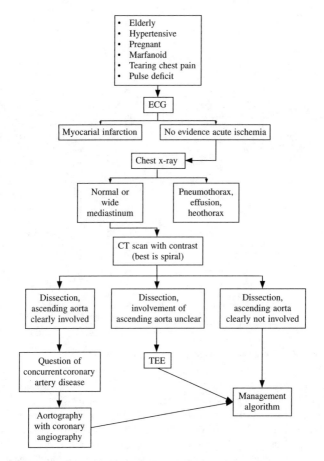

FIGURE 13.5 Evaluation algorithm for aortic dissection. CT = computed tomography; ECG = electrocardiogram; TEE = transesophageal echocardiography.

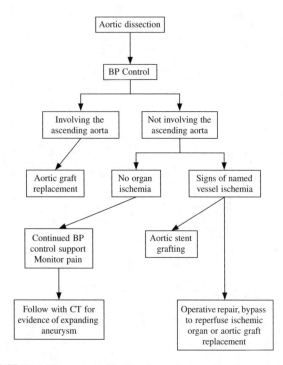

FIGURE 13.6 Management algorithm for aortic dissection. BP = blood pressure; CT = computed tomography.

If acute aortic regurgitation is present, salvage of the aortic valve is attempted unless the patient has Marfan syndrome or severe annuloaortic ectasia that requires aortic valve conduit replacement. Operative mortality for acute ascending (type A) dissection ranges from 5% to 27%.

Descending (type B) aortic dissection management is rapidly evolving. Traditionally, patients with descending (type B) aortic dissection were managed medically with blood pressure control (intravenous β-blockers and vasodilators) in the intensive care unit to try to limit the extension of the dissection channel. Surgical intervention was reserved for patients with persistent pain (presumably continued dissection despite medical therapy), unstable (enlarging) dissection, or end-organ ischemia from branch occlusion (particularly visceral). Operative mortality ranges from 6% to 50% but can be as high as 85% if visceral ischemia is involved.[8,13] Both surgically and interventionally created fenestrations (defect created between the true and false lumen) have been performed in select centers to provide circulation for branch vessel occlusions and renal or visceral ischemia. Extra-anatomic bypass (femoral to femoral or axillobifemoral) has been a potential surgical approach to provide circulation to the lower extremities when the dissection occludes flow in the iliac or femoral arteries and direct operation on the aorta is avoidable. Select centers have advocated direct aortic replacement in the setting of branch artery organ ischemia. The argument is that direct replacement of the descending aorta sutures the false and true lumens together at the distal anastomosis and decompresses the false lumen, frequently resolving organ ischemia. However, operative mortality can be substantial (see above).

Most recently, two reports with a combined 31 patients have demonstrated excellent results using aortic stent grafts to treat dissections originating in the descending aorta.[14,15] In all, three patients (10%) died at 30 days. All patients in each study underwent sophisticated aortic imaging (spiral CT and three-dimensional magnetic resonance angiography) to provide maximal anatomic detail for both patient selection and correct graft placement. A total of 75% of patients experienced relief of end-organ ischemia from branch vessel occlusion due to the false lumen after endograft treatment. Importantly, the majority of patients (> 80%) demonstrated thrombosis of the false lumen on follow-up imaging. Mean follow-up for these patients was only 12 to 13 months, but these preliminary reports are very encouraging.

13.6   CONCLUSIONS

Aortic dissection is a life-threatening problem. Even in the best of reports with aortic stent grafting, mortality is 10%. The majority of clinical series report much higher mortality rates. Clearly, failure to make an expedient diagnosis will lead to early death. Cardiothoracic and or vascular surgical consultation must be obtained early, as a great number of early management decisions will center around the need to perform operative or interventional therapy based on anatomic and clinical variables. For type B dissections, blood pressure control and organ support are globally important.

REFERENCES

1. Wheat, M.W., Jr. and Palmer, R.F., Dissecting aneurysms of the aorta, *Curr. Probl. Surg.*, July 1, 1971.
2. Lilienfeld, D.E., Gunderson, P.D., Sprafka, J.M., et al., Epidemiology of aortic aneurysms: I, Mortality trends in the United States, 1951 to 1981, *Arteriosclerosis*, 7, 637, 1987.
3. Melchior, T., Hallam, D., and Johansen, B.E., Aortic dissection in the thrombolytic era: early recognition and optimal management is a prerequisite for increased survival, *Int. J. Cardiol.*, 42, 1, 1993.
4. Hirst, A.E., Dissecting aneurysm of the aorta: a review of 505 cases, *Medicine*, 37, 217, 1958.
5. Cambria, R.P., Brewster, D.C., Gertler, J., et al., Vascular complications associated with spontaneous aortic dissection, *J. Vasc. Surg.*, 7, 199, 1988.
6. Bickerstaff, L.K., Pairolero, P.C., Hollier, L.H., et al., Thoracic aortic aneurysms: a population-based study, *Surgery*, 92, 1103, 1982.
7. Roberts, W.C., Aortic dissection: anatomy, consequences, and causes, *Am. Heart J.*, 101, 195, 1981.
8. Fann, J.I., Smith, J.A., Miller, D.C., et al., Surgical management of aortic dissection during a 30-year period, *Circulation*, 92, II–113, 1995.
9. Fann, J.I., Sarris, G.E., Mitchell, R.S., et al., Treatment of patients with aortic dissection presenting with peripheral vascular complications, *Ann. Surg.*, 212, 705, 1990.
10. Fann, J.I., Sarris, G.E., Miller, D.C., et al., Surgical management of acute aortic dissection complicated by stroke, *Circulation*, 80, I-257, 1989.

11. Yamaguchi, T., Naito, H., Ohta, M., et al., False lumens in type III aortic dissections: progress CT study, *Radiology*, 156, 757, 1985.

12. Kato, M., Bai, H., Sato, K., et al., Determining surgical indications for acute type B dissection based on enlargement of aortic diameter during the chronic phase, *Circulation*, 92, II-107, 1995.

13. Fann, J.I. and Miller, D.C., Aortic dissection, *Ann. Vasc. Surg.*, 9, 311, 1995.

14. Nienaber, C.A., Fattori, R., Lund, G., et al., Nonsurgical reconstruction of thoracic aortic dissection by stent-graft placement [see comments], *N. Engl. J. Med.*, 340,1539, 1999.

15. Dake, M.D., Kato, N., Mitchell, R.S., et al., Endovascular stent-graft placement for the treatment of acute aortic dissection [see comments], *N. Engl. J. Med.*, 340, 1546, 1999.

14 Aortic Disease: Atheroembolism and Thromboembolism

Paul A. Tunick

CONTENTS

14.1 Introduction 299
14.2 Epidemiology 301
14.3 Natural History..301
    14.3.1 Atheroembolism...301
    14.3.2 Thromboembolism..302
14.4 Pathophysiology 306
14.5 Diagnosis and Evaluation..309
    14.5.1 Atheroembolism...309
    14.5.2 Thromboembolism..311
14.6 Treatment...311
    14.6.1 Atheroembolism...312
    14.6.2 Thromboembolism..314
        14.6.2.1 Medical Therapy......................................314
        14.6.2.2 Surgical Therapy 315
References...317

14.1 INTRODUCTION

Severe atherosclerosis of the aorta and its branches may result in spontaneous or iatrogenic embolic phenomena ranging from asymptomatic findings on tissue biopsy to organ infarction and fatal multi-

0-8493-8413-3/01/$0.00+$1.50
© 2001 by CRC Press LLC

system failure. Atherosclerotic disease of the abdominal aorta has long been recognized as an embolic source.[1] Over the last decade, imaging of thoracic aortic atherosclerosis (especially with transesophageal echocardiography [TEE]) has rekindled interest in the embolic potential of this more proximal part of the vascular tree.[2] Although emboli from the aorta were once thought to be rare, suitable only for inclusion in clinical pathologic conferences, they are now commonly recognized as an important cause of disability and death.

There are two embolic syndromes resulting from aortic atherosclerosis. The first is the "classic" atheroemboli syndrome[3] (most commonly found with "blue toes" [Figure 14.1] and renal failure), also known as cholesterol crystal embolization. The second is the syndrome of embolic arterial occlusion caused by thrombus emanating from aortic atherosclerotic plaque.[4] This can result in stroke, acute limb ischemia (ALI), and infarction of various organs. This chapter

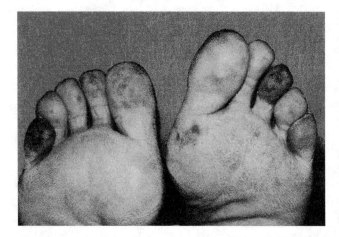

FIGURE 14.1 Blue toes due to atheroemboli (cholesterol crystal embolization). (From Pai, R.G. and Heywood, J.T., Atheroembolism, *N. Engl. J. Med.*, 33, 852, 1995. With permission.)

discusses both of these sometimes coexistent problems, with delineation of their epidemiology, presenting symptoms, natural history, diagnosis, and treatment.

14.2 EPIDEMIOLOGY

Aortic atherosclerosis is typically associated with traditional risk factors for cardiovascular disease[5] such as age, male sex, hypertension, diabetes, smoking, elevated low-density lipoprotein (LDL) cholesterol and triglyceride levels, low high-density lipoprotein cholesterol levels, and family history of atherosclerosis.

The average age of patients with thromboemboli from thoracic aortic atherosclerosis is approximately 70 years. Hypertension, diabetes, smoking, and hypercholesterolemia have been reported in approximately 50%, 30%, 25%, and 40% of patients, respectively.[6] The atheroemboli syndrome is rare, and usually occurs in elderly men.[7]

More recently, elevated levels of homocysteine[8] and fibrinogen[9] have also been implicated. Surprisingly, in a study of 73,451 patients screened for the presence of abdominal aortic aneurysm (detected in 1.4%), diabetes was a negative risk factor for aneurysm formation (perhaps due to earlier calcification) as were female sex and African American race.[10]

14.3 NATURAL HISTORY

14.3.1 ATHEROEMBOLISM

The presenting symptoms are most often related to skin embolization, which is found in approximately one third of patients.[11] This may result in blue toes or livedo reticularis (a diffuse, mottled discoloration of the skin), usually involving the lower extremities, as well as petechiae, ulcers, and gangrene. A series of 62 cases from one institution[12] has pointed out other important presenting problems: renal insufficiency (29%) (often with hypertension) and intestinal infarction (6%). In addition, patients may have lower gastrointestinal (GI) bleeding (with ischemic colitis or polyp formation) and amaurosis fugax (with cholesterol crystals (Hollenhorst plaques), seen in the retinal arteries on fundoscopy). More rarely, atheroemboli may result in a wide variety of syndromes, including pancreatitis, cholecystitis, nephrotic syndrome, myocardial infarction (MI), myositis, peripheral neuropathy, and infarction of the spleen or prostate. When a combination of signs and symptoms is present, the diagnostic picture may at first suggest a multisystem disorder such as vasculitis or sepsis with disseminated intravascular coagulation. It is therefore important to maintain a high index of suspicion of atheroemboli, especially in patients with multiple other manifestations of, or risk factors for, atherosclerosis. This is especially critical in patients who have had recent vascular instrumentation or trauma (see discussion of pathophysiology, below).

Although the manifestations of atheroembolism may be transient and self-limited, they can also progress to permanent organ damage and death. The natural history of patients with atheroemboli is manifested by a relatively high recurrence rate and mortality (15% and 17%, respectively, in only 2 years in one series of 41 patients).[13] Renal failure can occur in several patterns[3]: stabilization after the initial insult, steady deterioration after one episode, or repetitive insults ultimately leading to dialysis. In addition, some patients may have some recovery of function after requiring dialysis, although permanent loss of function is more common.

14.3.2 Thromboembolism

Using TEE to document large atherosclerotic plaques in the thoracic aorta of patients with embolic phenomena (Figure 14.2), it has been shown that these plaques often have superimposed mobile components that move freely with the blood flow (Figure 14.3).[14] These mobile thrombi are seen in 25% to 40% of patients with significant aortic plaques. Surgical exploration of the femoral arteries of patients with such plaques who had ALI documented that they were indeed embolizing thrombus in amounts large enough to occlude medium- and large-size arteries (Figure 14.4).[15] The most common thromboembolic

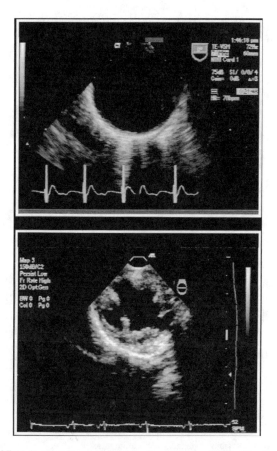

FIGURE 14.2. (Top) Transesophageal echocardiogram (TEE) of the descending thoracic aorta, in a patient being evaluated for prosthetic valve malfunction. Note the normal, smooth intimal surface. (Bottom) TEE of the descending thoracic aorta, in a patient being evaluated for embolic phenomena. Note the multiple large, protruding, and ulcerated atheromas impinging on the lumen.

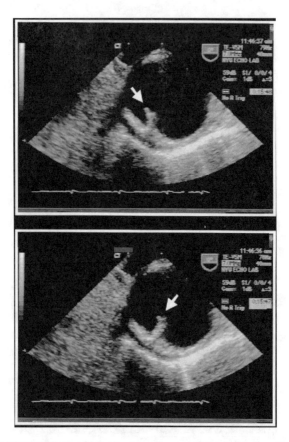

FIGURE 14.3 Transesophageal echocardiogram of the descending thoracic aorta in a patient being evaluated for embolic phenomena. The top and bottom images are taken less than 0.5 seconds apart. Note the mobile thrombus (*arrows*) attached to the atherosclerotic plaque, which can be seen in different positions in the top and bottom images as it moves back and forth with the blood flow.

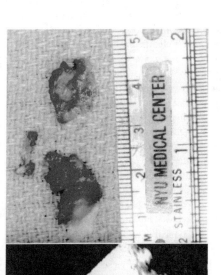

FIGURE 14.4 (Left) Transesophageal echocardiogram of the descending thoracic aorta in a patient with emboli to both legs and the left arm. Note the two large thrombi (*arrows*) that moved freely with the blood flow. (Right) Surgical pathology of the two thrombi seen on transesophageal echocardiography in the image on the left. (From Tunick, P.A., Lackner, H., Katz, E.S., Culliford, A.T., and Kronzon, I. Multiple emboli from a large aortic arch thrombus in a patient with thrombotic diathesis, *Am. Heart J.*, 124, 239, 1992. With permission.[15])

phenomenon in patients with thoracic aortic plaque is stroke, but such thromboemboli can also result in ischemia or infarction of the limbs, intestine, kidneys, and other abdominal organs. The risk of recurrent stroke in 1 year in patients with significant thoracic aortic plaque is high, and was remarkably consistent in three separate prospective studies: 12%.[16–18] An additional 21% of patients had peripheral thromboembolism over the same short period.[14] This high risk of recurrent embolism illustrates the unstable nature of these plaques, and mobile thrombi may be seen to appear in new locations when the same patients have repeat TEE over time.[19] The natural history of these patients is also characterized by a high mortality rate: in one study of the ascending aorta, the death rate over 7 years was 15.4% for patients with a normal ascending aorta, and much higher, 43.4%, in those with severe ascending aortic atherosclerosis.[20]

Although patients who have thromboembolism emanating from thoracic aortic plaque may also have cholesterol crystals demonstrated on muscle or skin biopsy, the typical atheroemboli syndrome is quite uncommon in follow-up (and occurred in only 0.7% in the Stroke Prevention in Atrial Fibrillation study).[16,21]

14.4   PATHOPHYSIOLOGY

Both atheroembolism and thromboembolism originating from the aorta may occur spontaneously. However, both are more likely to occur after instrumentation of the aorta.[3,22] The risk of catheter- or balloon pump-induced embolization is actually surprisingly low, considering the protruding lesions that may be present and the size of the mobile thrombi seen in some patients. In one large series, the stroke rate after cardiac catheterization was only 0.5%.[23] However, instrumentation does significantly increase the incidence of embolization, which was six times more likely to be found on autopsy in patients who had recently undergone arteriography.[24] In one study of 1000 patients undergoing coronary artery interventions, atherosclerotic debris was retrieved from 50% of the guiding catheters used.[25] Figure 14.5 shows a transesophageal echocardiogram of the descending aorta in a patient

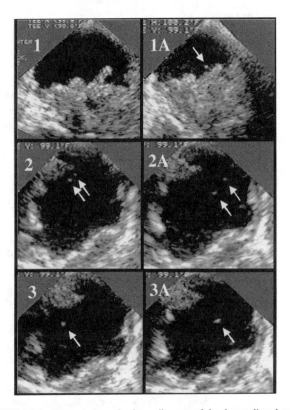

FIGURE 14.5. Transesophageal echocardiogram of the descending thoracic aorta in a patient who died of multisystem failure due to atheroembolism following cardiac catheterization. Images in the right column were taken a very short time (one to two video frames) after the corresponding figures on the left. Note the multiple pieces of small particulate matter (*arrows*) that can be seen to move (left vs. right images) across the aorta adjacent to the very large atheroma. (From Freedberg, R.S., Tunick, P.A., and Kronzon, I., Emboli in transit: the missing link, *J. Am. Soc. Echocardiogr.,* 11, 826, 1998. With permission.)

who died of multisystem failure due to atheroembolism after cardiac catheterization. Multiple pieces of small particulate matter can be seen to be moving across the field adjacent to the voluminous atheroma.

Other precipitating causes of embolization are trauma, aortic surgery, and cardiac surgery using cardiopulmonary bypass. Stroke is a devastating complication of cardiac surgery, with a general incidence of about 2%. However, if a significant aortic arch plaque is seen on TEE, the stroke risk is six times greater (12%).[26] Most of these strokes appear to occur because of cannulation of the aorta for the initiation of cardiopulmonary bypass, which results in the dislodging of thrombus and plaque.

Controversy surrounds the ability of anticoagulants and thrombolytic agents to precipitate the atheroembolism syndrome.[27] Starting in the 1960s, reports began to appear implicating anticoagulants in the genesis or worsening of this syndrome. In theory, these drugs could increase plaque hemorrhage and instability. However the incidence of this complication appears to be low: there was only one case of atheroembolism (0.7%) in patients with aortic plaque treated with warfarin in the Stroke Prevention in Atrial Fibrillation III study.[18] Although it may be prudent to discontinue heparin or warfarin if atheroemboli occur, it may not be necessary to do so if there is an overriding indication for anticoagulation.[3] Patients who have had atheroembolism after thrombolytic therapy have also been reported. However, skin and muscle biopsies were done prospectively in 60 patients undergoing bypass surgery after MI.[28] This study showed no significant association of thrombolytic therapy with atheroembolism (which was seen on biopsy in four of 29 patients after thrombolysis and in three of 31 who had not had thrombolysis).

The pathophysiologic factors that lead to plaque instability in the aorta are not fully understood. It is possible that plaques that are more lipid-laden are less stable and more likely to undergo thrombosis. This theory is supported by a pathologic study that evaluated the size of the lipid pool in human aortic plaques that were intact as compared with those that had superimposed thrombi.[29] These authors found that the presence of superimposed thrombus is characteristic of aortic plaques with a high proportion of their volume occupied by extracellular lipid. The plaques that had thrombosed also had a preponderance of mono-cytes/macrophages (as opposed to smooth muscle cells) in the cap. The role of these cells in inflammation that may lead to plaque instability is unknown. Markers of inflammation such as C-reactive protein have been noted in patients with atherosclerosis involving the coronary arteries, and *Chlamydia pneumoniae* antigens have been identified in aortic ath-erosclerotic lesions using immunocytochemical staining.[30] There has also been recent interest in free radicals and the oxidation of LDL cholesterol in the pathogenesis of atherosclerotic plaque. One study looked at antioxidant enzyme activity in the aorta of patients with aortic occlusive disease and aneurysms, and found evidence of high levels of lipid peroxide fluorochromes and decreased antioxidant activity.[31]

14.5   DIAGNOSIS AND EVALUATION

14.5.1   ATHEROEMBOLISM

As mentioned above, the diagnosis of the atheroembolism syndrome can be elusive, as patients may present with multisystem findings. They may be thought to have necrotizing vasculitis, meningococcemia or gonococcemia, endocarditis, or other sepsis with disseminated intra-vascular coagulation. However, in patients with diffuse atherosclerosis (coronary disease, carotid disease, peripheral arterial disease, or aortic aneurysm) a high index of suspicion will lead to the correct diagnosis. The diagnosis should be especially entertained if there has been recent aortic instrumentation for angiography, cardiac catheterization, or intra-aortic balloon pump placement. The high risk of aortic cannula-tion for heart surgery involving cardiopulmonary bypass should also be kept in mind.

In the typical patient with diffuse atherosclerosis who acutely develops livedo reticularis or blue toes and renal insufficiency after aortic instrumentation, there is usually no diagnostic dilemma. How-ever, the findings may be more subtle and may not be noticed by the physician or the patient (who is now routinely discharged on the same day as angiography or catheterization, and thus escapes observation). In such a patient, an elevation in serum creatinine first noted on the follow-up visit 1 or 2 weeks after angiography may be the first tip-off. Laboratory evaluation[32] may reveal an elevated sedimentation rate and eosinophilia, with leukocytosis and occasionally thrombocytopenia. Hypocomplementemia has also been reported. Although none of these findings is specific, eosinophilia is very common in patients with atheroemboli (reported in 71%[7]) and it is associated with fewer other conditions, making it a cost-effective measure. It may be the most common laboratory abnormality along with an elevated blood urea nitrogen and creatinine.

On physical examination, in addition to a careful evaluation for the typical skin findings and evidence of atherosclerosis (bruits, pulsatile abdominal mass), the retinae should always be inspected for intra-arterial cholesterol crystals. The livedo reticularis may occur in the presence of fairly normal peripheral pulses, as these arteries are not occluded. Rarely, the livedo may be aggravated by standing and ameliorated by lying down.

In the case of a patient with absent pedal pulses, indicating distal arterial occlusion, atheroemboli cannot go to the toes because of occluded conduit vessels. Therefore, the diagnostic clue of blue toes will be absent.

An aortic source of atheroemboli may be sought with ultrasound evaluation of the abdominal aorta (looking especially for aneurysm) and TEE of the thoracic aorta. Ultrasound of the abdomen has been reported to have a specificity and positive predictive value of 100% for the diagnosis of abdominal aneurysm, whereas physical examination will detect only half of these lesions.[33] Computed tomography (CT) and magnetic resonance (MR) evaluations of the entire aorta and its branches may also be very valuable. TEE and MR have similar sensitivity for the detection of atheromas in the ascending and descending thoracic aorta, although TEE may more accurately measure plaque size in the aortic arch.[34]

The diagnosis is usually confirmed by skin or muscle biopsy, and, if necessary, renal biopsy. Cholesterol clefts are seen in these tissues, which may be accompanied by inflammation. More unusual presentations, such as lower GI bleeding, may require additional diagnostic testing (e.g., colonoscopy).

14.5.2 THROMBOEMBOLISM

Except in young patients, peripheral embolization or stroke should prompt consideration of the aorta as a thromboembolic source. The youngest reported patient with thromboembolism from an aortic plaque required an above-the-knee amputation at age 38, but he also had hypertension, hypercholesterolemia, and obesity (he subsequently developed emboli to his left arm and remaining leg).[13] However, the average age of patients with aortogenic thromboembolism is 71. The aorta should be especially high on the list in the absence of atrial fibrillation or another cardiac source of embolization (such as recent anterior MI). However, significant aortic plaque is common in patients with both of these entities (atrial fibrillation and MI), as well as in those with carotid artery disease. Therefore, there may be more than one potential source of embolization.

As with patients who have had atheroembolism, those with suspected thromboembolism from the aorta should undergo ultrasound imaging of the abdominal aorta and its branches. Currently TEE is the procedure of choice for the evaluation of the thoracic aorta for significant plaque, although CT and MR also produce excellent images.

An algorithm suggesting a staged evaluation in patients with peripheral embolic disease is shown in Figure 14.6.

14.6 TREATMENT

Treatment of patients with either atheroembolism or thromboembolism from the aorta is hampered by the lack of well-designed clinical trials from which to make evidence-based decisions. The information below comes from studies that are largely observational. Until better information is available, it is necessary to make therapeutic decisions based on clinical experience as well as our current understanding of the pathophysiology of these syndromes.

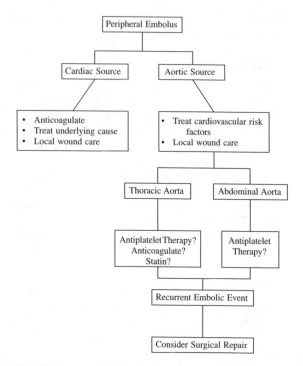

FIGURE 14.6 Suggested staged evaluation of patients with peripheral embolic disease.

14.6.1 ATHEROEMBOLISM

Although surgical treatment is usually advocated for patients with atheroembolism, Bartholomew and Olin[3] have emphasized a comprehensive three-pronged approach to the treatment of these patients: surgical removal of the source of atheromatous material if possible; symptomatic care directed toward the area(s) of end-organ damage; and lifestyle/medical management of the precipitating risk factors for atherosclerosis, when these can be identified.

As atherosclerosis is a diffuse process that often involves not only the aorta but also its branches, it may not be possible to identify an area of plaque that is the specific culprit. Nevertheless, with a combination of CT, MR, and ultrasound imaging (TEE for the thoracic aorta) a presumptive source is often found. Surgery for thoracic aortic plaque poses an especially high risk of complications (see below), and most of the patients reported in the literature have had a surgical approach to sources below the diaphragm. One of the largest recent series included 100 patients who were operated on over a 12-year period for lower-extremity, visceral, or nonthoracic outlet upper-extremity atheroemboli.[35] Imaging studies revealed occlusive aortoiliac disease in 47 patients, aortic aneurysms in 20 (the aneurysm need not be large: mean aneurysm size was only 3.5 cm), and suprarenal aortic thrombus in 12. The surgical procedures performed were aortic bypass in 52 patients, aortoiliac endarterectomy and patch in 11, femoral or popliteal endarterectomy and patch in 11, infrainguinal bypass in three, extra-anatomic reconstruction in six, graft revision in three, upper extremity bypass in 11, and upper extremity endarterectomy and patch in three. Others have reported ligation of the femoral artery(ies) accompanied by axillofemoral bypass. Thus, the surgical treatment of this syndrome requires a variety of approaches and an experienced operative team. Of primary importance is the identification of the source of embolization, without which it is difficult or impossible to plan a corrective operation.

Medical therapy in patients with atheroembolism is problematic, and no medical therapeutic approach has been shown to dramatically ameliorate the primary problem. A variety of pharmacologic interventions have been tried. The only regimen that is generally accepted is antiplatelet therapy (aspirin and dipyridamole),[36] although it must be emphasized that there are no data to support a direct beneficial effect once atheroemboli have occurred. Therapy with 3-hydroxy-3-methylglutaryl coenzyme A reductase inhibitors ("statins") is theoretically valuable in any patient with atherosclerosis, although data exist only for the prevention of MI and stroke, and there are only case reports of the use of these drugs for patients with atheroembolism.

Symptomatic and local lesion care are both very important in this syndrome. Attention must be paid to care of the toes and feet to prevent pressure necrosis and infection. Amputation may be necessary when gangrene ensues. Adequate pharmacologic pain relief is also vital.

As mentioned above in the section on pathophysiology, anticoagulation (warfarin or heparin) has been implicated in causing or worsening the atheroemboli syndrome. However, this idea is based only on observational reports. Although most often anticoagulation is stopped when a patient develops atheroemboli, in some patients (e.g., those with mechanical prosthetic heart valves, or pulmonary embolization), the best course of action may be to continue these therapies.

14.6.2   THROMBOEMBOLISM

14.6.2.1   Medical Therapy

Many physicians have been using warfarin to treat patients with significant aortic plaque and thromboembolism, and mobile aortic thrombi have been noted to disappear during anticoagulant therapy[37,38] or with the use of a thrombolytic agent.[39] However, there have been no randomized trials of warfarin in patients with this problem. Three studies do provide some evidence. In the first, 31 patients with mobile thrombi in the thoracic aorta on TEE were reviewed.[40] Embolic events were more common in those who were not treated with warfarin (by the referring physicians) (45% versus 5%). Strokes occurred in three of 11 patients not treated with warfarin, and in none of those on warfarin.

The second report is from the Stroke Prevention in Atrial Fibrillation Investigators Committee on Echocardiography.[18] This was a treatment trial for patients with "high-risk" nonvalvular atrial fibrillation (previous stroke, advanced age, hypertension), and not a trial in which patients with aortic plaque were randomized. However, the risk of stroke in 1 year in 134 patients with complex aortic plaque on TEE was reduced from 15.8% in those treated with fixed low-dose warfarin plus aspirin (international normalized ratio [INR], 1.2–1.5) to only 4% (three events) in those treated with adjusted dose warfarin (INR, 2–3). Thus, there was a 75% reduction in recurrent stroke in patients with aortic plaque who received "therapeutic-range" anticoagulation.

The third report was an observational study of 129 patients with emboli (cerebral and peripheral) who had significant aortic plaque on TEE.[41] Treatment with anticoagulation, aspirin, or ticlopidine was not random. There were significantly fewer recurrent emboli in patients who were treated with anticoagulants (none of 27, versus five events in 23 patients treated with antiplatelet agents). For patients with mobile thrombi, there was also a significant reduction in mortality on anticoagulants.

In spite of these observational data, a randomized trial that is powered to detect a significant benefit (or harm) from warfarin in patients with aortic plaque and thromboembolism will be necessary before this therapy can be widely accepted, especially in view of the theoretical (but unproven) risk of causing atheroemboli with this therapy. Similar studies to evaluate "statin" therapy are also necessary.

14.6.2.2   Surgical Therapy

There are case reports of successful removal of plaque and thrombus from the thoracic aorta in patients with multiple spontaneous emboli.[13] Because of this, one group attempted to reduce the high risk of stroke during heart surgery in patients with aortic plaque by performing this procedure (aortic arch endarterectomy with hypothermic circulatory arrest) as an adjunct to coronary artery bypass or valve surgery.[24] Unfortunately, this served to increase rather than decrease the already high intraoperative stroke rate in these patients (from 12% to 35%), and this procedure was abandoned. Surgery on the descending thoracic aorta (or thoracoabdominal aorta) also has a high operative rate of complications, especially paralysis caused by spinal cord ischemia. Thoracic aortic surgery to treat significant plaque and thrombi should be performed only as a last resort (in patients with critical, recurrent events, refractory to other treatment) and only in patients who are good operative risks (young patients

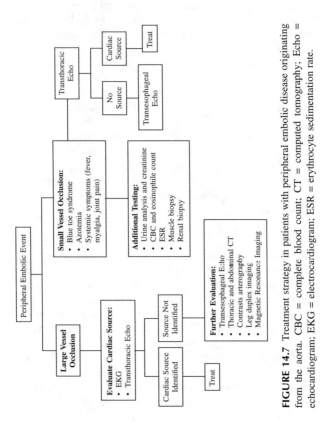

FIGURE 14.7 Treatment strategy in patients with peripheral embolic disease originating from the aorta. CBC = complete blood count; CT = computed tomography; Echo = echocardiogram; EKG = electrocardiogram; ESR = erythrocyte sedimentation rate.

without multisystem dysfunction). This latter caveat excludes the vast majority of patients with thromboembolism originating in the thoracic aorta. Surgery (abdominal aortic, iliac, or popliteal aneurysm resection) is indicated in patients with thromboembolism originating in the aneurysm.

An algorithm suggesting a treatment strategy in patients with peripheral embolic disease originating from the aorta is shown in Figure 14.7.

REFERENCES

1. Flory, C.M., Arterial occlusions produced by emboli from eroded aortic atheromatous plaques, *Am. J. Pathol.*, 21, 549, 1945.
2. Tunick, P.A. and Kronzon, I., Protruding atherosclerotic plaque in the aortic arch of patients with systemic embolization: a new finding seen by transesophageal echocardiography, *Am. Heart J.*, 120, 658, 1990.
3. Bartholomew, J.R. and Olin, J.W., Atheromatous embolization, in *Peripheral Vascular Diseases*, 2nd ed., Young, J.R., Olin, J.W., and Bartholomew, J.R., Eds., Mosby-Year Book, Inc., St. Louis, 1996, 261.
4. Kronzon, I. and Tunick, P.A., Aortic atheromas, in *Cardiogenic Embolism*, Daniel, W.G., Kronzon, I., and Mügge, A., Eds., Williams & Wilkins, Baltimore, 1995, 177.
5. Vigna, G.B., Bolzan, M., Romagnoni, F., et al., Lipids and other risk factors selected by discriminant analysis in symptomatic patients with supra-aortic and peripheral atherosclerosis, *Circulation*, 85, 2205, 1992.
6. Katz, E.S., Tunick, P.A., Rusinek, H., et al., Protruding aortic atheromas predict stroke in elderly patients undergoing cardiopulmonary bypass: experience with intraoperative transesophageal echocardiography, *J. Am. Coll. Cardiol.*, 20, 70, 1992.
7. Lye, W.C., Cheah, J.S., and Sinniah, R., Renal cholesterol embolic disease: case report and review of the literature, *Am. J. Nephrol.*, 13, 489, 1993.
8. Konecky, N., Malinow, M.R., Tunick, P.A., et al., Correlation between plasma homocyst(e)ine and aortic atherosclerosis, *Am. Heart J.*, 133, 534, 1997.

9. Martin Paredero, V., Vadillo, J., Diaz, J., et al., Fibrinogen and fibrinolysis in blood and in the arterial wall: its role in advanced atherosclerotic disease, *Cardiovasc. Surg.*, 6, 457, 1998.

10. Lederle, F.A., Johnson, G.R., Wilson, S.E., et al., Prevalence and associations of abdominal aortic aneurysm detected through screening. Aneurysm Detection and Management (ADAM) Veterans Affairs Cooperative Study Group. *Ann. Intern. Med.*, 126, 441, 1997.

11. Fine, M.J., Kapoor, W., and Falanga, V.. Cholesterol crystal embolization: a review of 221 cases in the English literature, *Angiology*, 38, 769, 1987.

12. Baumann, D.S., McGraw, D., Rubin, B.G., et al., An institutional experience with arterial atheroembolism, *Ann. Vasc. Surg.*, 8, 258, 1994.

13. Kvilekval, K.H., Yunis, J.P., Mason, R.A., et al., After the blue toe: prognosis of noncardiac arterial embolization in the lower extremities, *J. Vasc. Surg.*, 17, 328, 1993.

14. Tunick, P.A., Perez, J.L., and Kronzon, I., Protruding atheromas in the thoracic aorta and systemic embolization, *Ann. Intern. Med.*, 115, 423, 1991.

15. Tunick, P.A., Lackner, H., Katz, E.S., et al., Multiple emboli from a large aortic arch thrombus in a patient with thrombotic diathesis, *Am. Heart J.*, 124, 239, 1992.

16. Tunick, P.A., Rosenzweig, B.P., Katz, E.S., et al., High risk for vascular events in patients with protruding aortic atheromas: a prospective study, *J. Am. Coll. Cardiol.*, 23, 1085, 1994.

17. Amarenco, P., Cohen, A., Tzourio, C., et al., Atherosclerotic disease of the aortic arch and the risk of ischemic stroke, *N. Engl. J. Med.*, 331, 1474, 1994.

18. The Stroke Prevention in Atrial Fibrillation Investigators Committee on Echocardiography, Transesophageal echocardiography correlates of thromboembolism in high-risk patients with nonvalvular atrial fibrillation, *Ann. Intern. Med.*, 128, 639, 1998.

19. Montgomery, D.H., Ververis, J.J., McGorisk, G., et al., Natural history of severe atheromatous disease of the thoracic aorta: a transesophageal echocardiographic study. *J. Am. Coll. Cardiol.*, 27, 95, 1996.

20. Dávila-Román, V.G., Murphy, S.F., Nickerson, N.J., et al., Atherosclerosis of the ascending aorta is an independent predictor of long-term neurologic events and mortality, *J. Am. Coll. Cardiol.*, 33, 1308, 1999.

21. Blackshear, J.L., Zabalgoitia, M., Pennock, G., et al., Warfarin safety and efficacy in patients with thoracic aortic plaque and atrial fibrillation, SPAF TEE Investigators, *Am. J. Cardiol.*, 83, 453, 1999.

22. Karalis, D.G., Quinn, V., Victor, M.F., et al., Risk of catheter-related emboli in patients with atherosclerotic debris in the thoracic aorta, *Am. Heart J.*, 131, 1149, 1996.

23. Nitter Hauge, S. and Enge, I., Complication rates of selective percutaneous transfemoral coronary arteriography, a review of 1094 consecutive examinations, *Acta. Med. Scand.*, 200, 123, 1976.

24. Ramirez, G., O'Neill, W.M., Jr., Lambert, R., et al., Cholesterol embolization: a complication of angiography, *Arch. Intern. Med.*, 138, 1430, 1978.

25. Keeley, E.C. and Grines, C.L., Scraping of aortic debris by coronary guiding catheters, a prospective evaluation of 1000 cases, *J. Am. Coll. Cardiol.*, 32, 1861, 1998.

26. Stern, A., Tunick, P.A., Culliford, A.T., et al., Protruding aortic arch atheromas: risk of stroke during heart surgery with and without aortic arch endarterectomy, *Am. Heart J.*, 138, 746, 1999.

27. Feder, W. and Auerbach, R., "Purple toes": an uncommon sequela of oral coumarin drug therapy, *Ann. Intern. Med.*, 55, 911, 1961.

28. Blankenship, J.C., Butler, A.M., and Garbes, A., Prospective assessment of cholesterol embolization in patients with acute myocardial infarction treated with thrombolytic vs. conservative therapy, *Chest*, 107, 1995.

29. Davies, M.J., Richardson, P.D., Woolf, N., et al., Risk of thrombosis in human atherosclerotic plaques: role of extracellular lipid, macrophage, and smooth muscle cell content, *Br. Heart J.*, 69, 377, 1993.

30. Kuo, C.C., Gown, A.M., Benditt, E.P., et al., Detection of *Chlamydia pneumoniae* in aortic lesions of atherosclerosis by immunocytochemical stain, *Arterioscler. Thromb.*, 13, 1501, 1993.

31. Dubick, M.A., Keen, C.L., DiSilvestro, R.A., et al., Antioxidant enzyme activity in human abdominal aortic aneurysmal and occlusive disease, *Proc. Soc. Exp. Biol. Med.*, 220, 39, 1999.

32. Young, D.K., Burton, M.F., and Herman, J.H., Multiple cholesterol emboli syndrome simulating systemic necrotizing vasculitis, *J. Rheumatol.*, 13, 423, 1986.

33. Lederle, F.A., Walker, J.M., and Reinke, D.B., Selective screening for abdominal aortic aneurysms with physical examination and ultrasound, *Arch. Intern. Med.*, 148, 1753, 1988.

34. Kutz, S.M., Lee, V., Tunick, P.A., Krinsky, G., et al., Atheromas of the thoracic aorta: a comparison of transesophageal echocardiography and breath-hold gadolinium-enhanced 3-D magnetic resonance angiography, *J. Am. Soc. Echocardiogr.*, 12, 853, 1999.

35. Keen, R.R., McCarthy, W.J., Shireman, P.K., et al., Surgical management of atheroembolization, *J. Vasc. Surg.*, 21, 773, 1995.

36. Walden, R., Adar, R., and Mozes, M., Gangrene of the toes with normal peripheral pulses, *Ann. Surg.*, 185, 269, 1977.

37. Freedberg, R.S., Tunick, P.A., Culliford, A.T., et al., Disappearance of a large intra-aortic mass in a patient with prior systemic embolization, *Am. Heart J.*, 125, 1445, 1993.

38. Blackshear, J.L., Jahangir, A., Oldenburg, W.A., et al., Digital embolization from plaque-related thrombus in the thoracic aorta: identification with transesophageal echocardiography and resolution with warfarin therapy, *Mayo Clin. Proc.*, 68, 268, 1993.

39. Hausmann, D., Gulba, D., Bargheer, K., et al., Successful thrombolysis of an aortic arch thrombus in a patient after mesenteric embolism, *N. Engl. J. Med.*, 327, 500, 1992.

40. Dressler, F.A., Craig, W.R., Castello, R., et al., Mobile aortic atheroma and systemic emboli: efficacy of anticoagulation and influence of plaque morphology on recurrent stroke, *J. Am. Coll. Cardiol.*, 31, 134, 1998.

41. Ferrari, E., Vidal, R., Chevallier, T., et al., Atherosclerosis of the thoracic aorta and aortic debris as a marker of poor prognosis: benefit of oral anticoagulants, *J. Am. Coll. Cardiol.*, 33, 1317, 1999.

Section V

Vasculitis and Vasospasm

15 Thromboangiitis Obliterans (Buerger's Disease)

Jeffrey W. Olin

CONTENTS

15.1 Introduction 323
15.2 Epidemiology 324
    15.2.1 Buerger's Disease in Women....................................324
15.3 Etiology and Pathogenesis 325
15.4 Pathology..326
15.5 Clinical Features..327
    15.5.1 Laboratory and Arteriographic Findings 330
15.6 Therapy...331
15.7 Conclusions 335
References..335

15.1 INTRODUCTION

Thromboangiitis obliterans (TAO), or Buerger's disease, is a segmental inflammatory disease that most commonly affects small- and medium-sized arteries, veins, and nerves, especially in upper and lower extremities.[1] Von Winiwater first reported a case of TAO in 1879, but it was Leo Buerger's who quite accurately described the pathologic features in 11 amputated limbs in 1908.[2,3]

The pathologic hallmark of TAO is a highly inflammatory thrombus with relative sparing of the blood vessel wall. It is this feature, as well

0-8493-8413-3/01/$0.00+$1.50
© 2001 by CRC Press LLC

323

as the absence of serologic markers of acute inflammation and immunologic activation, that differentiates TAO from the necrotizing vasculitides. In early reports, TAO was almost exclusively found in young men; however, in the more recent Western literature TAO has become more prevalent in women. Most patients are heavy cigarette smokers, but other forms of tobacco use have also been reported in patients with TAO.

15.2 EPIDEMIOLOGY

Although Buerger's disease has worldwide distribution, it is more prevalent in the Middle, Near, and Far East regions than in North America and Western Europe.[4,5] At the Mayo Clinic, annual patient registration has increased, while the prevalence rate of patients with the diagnosis of Buerger's disease has steadily declined from 104 per 100,000 patient registrations in 1947 to 12.6 per 100,000 patient registrations in 1986.[5,6] Prevalence rates have varied from as low as 0.5% to 5.6% of all peripheral arterial disease patients in Western European countries as high as 45% to 63% in India, 16% to 66% in Korea and Japan, and 80% in Israel (Ashkenazim).[7]

15.2.1 BUERGER'S DISEASE IN WOMEN

The reported prevalence of Buerger's disease in women was 1% to 2% in most published series of cases before 1970. Reasons for the increasing prevalence are not known, but there are more women smokers now than in the past. A total of 26 of 112 (23%) patients with Buerger's disease from 1970 to 1987 at the Cleveland Clinic Foundation were women.[8] Of an additional 40 patients with Buerger's disease evaluated at this institution from 1988 to 1996, 30% were women.[9] Other series have shown a prevalence of TAO in women of 11% to 23%.[10,11]

15.3 ETIOLOGY AND PATHOGENESIS

The etiology of Buerger's disease is unknown. Although pathologically TAO is a vasculitis,[4,12] two major distinguishing features separate Buerger's disease from the other commonly encountered types of vasculitis. The pathologic hallmark of TAO is the presence of a highly cellular inflammatory thrombus with relative sparing of the blood vessel wall. In addition, serologic markers of acute inflammation and immunologic activation are absent, as are frequently measured autoantibodies.

Although genetic factors and hypercoagulability have been implicated in the pathogenesis of Buerger's disease, the role of these factors is minimal compared with cigarette smoking or other forms of tobacco use. Central to disease initiation and progression is tobacco use or exposure.[1]

There is an extremely strong association between heavy tobacco use and TAO.[8,10,13,14] TAO is more common in countries where the consumption of tobacco is large. There is a higher prevalence of TAO in India among individuals of low socioeconomic class who smoke *bidis* (homemade cigarettes with raw tobacco).[15] There have been occasional cases of TAO in users of smokeless tobacco or snuff.[16,17] Most investigators believe that current or past smoking is a requirement for the diagnosis of Buerger's disease. In addition, the progression and continued symptoms associated with TAO are closely linked with continued use of tobacco.[8,14] Although passive smoking (secondhand smoke) has not been shown to be associated with the onset of TAO, it may be an important factor in the continuation of symptoms in patients during the acute phase of Buerger's disease.

Because only a small number of smokers eventually develop TAO, other mechanisms must be involved in the pathogenesis. Perhaps tobacco acts as a trigger in individuals predisposed to develop TAO. Several investigators have examined the immunologic mechanisms in patients with TAO. Adar and colleagues demonstrated an increased cellular sensitivity to types I and III collagen (normal constituents of human arteries) in patients with TAO compared with patients with arteriosclerosis obliterans or healthy male control subjects.[18] Autoantibodies such as antinuclear antibody, rheumatoid factor, and anticardiolipin antibodies are usually negative.[14]

There has been considerable recent interest in the role of the endothelium in patients with TAO. In a study by Eichhorn and associates,[19] patients with active TAO had antiendothelial cell antibody titers that were significantly higher than a group of control subjects or patients with TAO in remission ($P <0.01$). Additional studies are required to further delineate the sensitivity and specificity of antiendothelial cell antibody titers in monitoring disease activity of patients with Buerger's disease. Makita et al. have clearly demonstrated that there is impaired endothelium-dependent vasorelaxation in the peripheral vasculature of patients with Buerger's disease.[20]

In summary, there is no single etiologic mechanism present in all patients with TAO. Tobacco seems to play a central role in both the initiation and continuance of the disease. Other etiologic factors, such as genetic predisposition, immunologic mechanisms, endothelial dysfunction, and abnormalities in coagulation, may play a role in some patients.

15.4   PATHOLOGY

An inflammatory thrombus that affects both the arteries and the veins is the characteristic pathology in Buerger's disease. The histopathology of the involved blood vessels in Buerger's disease varies according to the chronologic age of the disease. The acute phase of the disease is diagnostic and is most often demonstrated when a segment of superficial thrombophlebitis is biopsied. The hallmark of the acute phase lesion is an occlusive, highly cellular inflammatory thrombus. In the thrombus, polymorphonuclear leukocytes with karyorrhexis, the so-called microabscess, and one or more multinucleated giant cells may be present. There is relative sparing of the blood vessel wall. In the subacute (intermediate) phase of the disease, the pathology is suggestive of TAO. There is still significant inflammation in the thrombus, but the blood vessel wall has less inflammation. The chronic or end-stage lesion is nonspecific in that organized thrombus and fibrosis of the blood vessels are all that is present.[4,12,21-24] As noted elsewhere: "In all three stages the normal architecture of the vessel wall subjacent to the occlusive thrombus and including the internal elastic lamina remains essentially intact. These findings distinguish TAO from arteriosclerosis and from other systemic vasculitides in which there is usually more striking disruption of the internal elastic lamina and the media dispro-portionate to those attributable to aging alone."[1]

Buerger's disease has been demonstrated histologically in blood vessels in unusual locations. Although the disease most commonly affects the small- and medium-sized arteries and veins in the arms, hands, legs, and feet, it has been reported in many other vascular beds. Involvement of the cerebral arteries, coronary arteries, renal arteries, mesenteric arteries, aorta, pulmonary artery, and iliac arter-ies have occasionally been encountered, almost always in single-case reports.[25-29] Multiple organ involvement in TAO has also been observed.[30,31] When TAO occurs in unusual locations, the diagnosis should only be made when the histopathologic findings demonstrate the acute phase lesion.

15.5 CLINICAL FEATURES

Buerger's disease typically occurs in young male smokers, with onset of symptoms before the age of 40 to 45 years. However, there appears to be an increased prevalence of TAO in women.[8-10] Buerger's disease usually begins with ischemia of the distal small arteries and veins of the extremities. As the disease progresses, it may involve more prox-imal arteries. Large-artery involvement has been reported in TAO, but this is unusual and rarely occurs in the absence of small-vessel occlu-sive disease.[32]

A total of 152 patients with Buerger's disease were evaluated and treated between 1970 and 1996 at a single tertiary care referral center.[8,9] Of this group, 38 (25%) were women. The presenting clinical signs and symptoms are shown in Table 15.1. Superficial thrombophlebitis

TABLE 15.1
Thromboangiitis Obliterans: Presenting Signs and Symptoms

	N (%)
Intermittent claudication	70 (63)
Rest pain	91 (81)
Ischemic ulcers	
Upper extremity	24 (28)
Lower extremity	39 (36)
Both	22 (26)
Thrombophlebitis	43 (38)
Raynaud phenomenon	49 (44)
Sensory findings	77 (69)
Abnormal Allen test	71 (63)

From Olin, J. W., Young, J. R., Graor, R. A., Ruschhaupt, W. F., and Bartholomew, J. R., The changing clinical spectrum of thromboangiitis obliterans (Buerger's disease), *Circulation*, 82, IV-3, 1990. With permission.[8]

occurred in approximately 40% of patients with TAO.[8] The thrombophlebitis may be migratory and may parallel disease activity.

Foot or arch claudication could be the presenting manifestation and can be mistaken for an orthopedic problem, resulting in a delay before the correct diagnosis is made. As the disease progresses, patients may develop typical calf claudication, ischemic rest pain, ischemic ulcerations, or gangrene of the toes, feet, or fingers (Figure 15.1).

In patients with lower-extremity ulceration in whom Buerger's disease is a consideration, an Allen test should be performed to assess circulation in the hands and fingers.[33,34] An abnormal Allen test in a young smoker with lower-extremity ulcerations is highly suggestive of TAO, because it demonstrates small-vessel involvement in both the upper and lower extremities. However, it should be noted that an

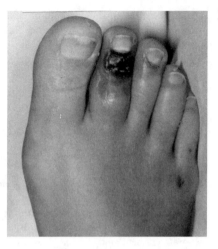

FIGURE 15.1 Typical ischemic ulcer on the dorsum of the second toe in a 28-year-old woman with Buerger's disease.

abnormal Allen test can also be present in other causes of small-vessel occlusive disease of the hands, such as scleroderma, CREST syndrome (characterized by calcinosis, Raynaud phenomenon, esophageal motility disorders, sclerodactyly, and telangiectasia), repetitive trauma (e.g., vibratory tool use, hypothenar hammer syndrome), emboli, hypercoagulable states (e.g., polycythemia vera, antiphospholipid antibody syndrome), and vasculitis.

Cold sensitivity is common and may be one of the earliest manifestations of TAO. This may be related to ischemia or to markedly increased muscle sympathetic nerve activity. Typical Raynaud phenomenon has been reported in approximately 40% of patients. The extremities of patients with Buerger's disease often have an erythematous or cyanotic appearance.

In Shionoya's series, more than one limb was always involved in Buerger's disease.[35] Two limbs were affected in 16% of patients, three limbs in 41%, and all four limbs in 43% of patients. Because of the likelihood of involvement of more than one limb, if an arteriogram is going to be obtained, it is advisable to image both upper and lower extremities in patients who clinically present with involvement of only one limb. It is common to see arteriographic abnormalities consistent with Buerger's disease in limbs that are not yet clinically involved.

15.5.1 Laboratory and Arteriographic Findings

There is no single laboratory test that will make the diagnosis of TAO except for a biopsy showing the acute phase lesion in a patient with compatible clinical features. A complete serologic profile to exclude other diseases that can mimic TAO should be obtained. These tests include the following: complete blood count with differential, liver function, renal function, fasting blood sugar, urinalysis, acute phase reactants (Westergren sedimentation rate and C-reactive protein), antinuclear antibody, rheumatoid factor, complement measurements, serologic markers for CREST syndrome and scleroderma (anti-centromere antibody and SCL70), and a complete hypercoagulability screen to include antiphospholipid antibodies.

A proximal source of emboli can be excluded by performing echocardiography (transthoracic or transesophageal) and arteriography. The angiographic features that are consistent with Buerger's disease are shown in Table 15.2 and Figure 15.2 We have found a diagnostic algorithm useful in helping to make the diagnosis of TAO (Figure 15.3).[1]

Arteriographically (and pathologically), TAO is a segmental disorder, demonstrating areas of diseased vessels interspersed with normal blood vessel segments. Corkscrew collaterals are not pathognomonic of Buerger's disease. The arteriographic appearance of Buerger's disease may be identical to that seen in patients with scleroderma, CREST syndrome, systemic lupus erythematosus, rheumatoid vasculitis, mixed connective tissue disease, and antiphospholipid antibody syndrome.

TABLE 15.2
Arteriographic Findings in Thromboangiitis Obliterans

Involvement of small- and medium-sized vessels
    Digital arteries of fingers and toes
    Palmer, plantar, tibial, peroneal, radial, and ulnar arteries
Segmental occlusive lesions
    Diseased arteries interspersed with normal-appearing
      arteries
More severe disease distally
Collateralization around areas of occlusion
    Corkscrew collateral
Normal proximal arteries
    No atherosclerosis
No source of embolus

However, the clinical and serological manifestations of these other immunologic diseases should help to differentiate them from TAO.

15.6 THERAPY

Although there are many therapies available for the treatment of TAO, most are just palliative (Table 15.3). The only therapy to prevent disease progression or limb amputation is complete discontinuation of cigarette smoking or use of tobacco in any form.[8,14] Even a small amount of tobacco exposure is enough to keep the disease active. Smokeless tobacco (chewing tobacco or snuff) has also been reported to cause Buerger's disease and to keep it active once it has already occurred.[16,17] Of 152 patients with Buerger's disease treated at our institution, 52 (43%) discontinued cigarette smoking.[8,9,14] If gangrene was not present at the time the patient discontinued smoking, amputation did not occur. Overall, 49 patients (94%) avoided amputation in the ex-smoking group (Figure 15.4).

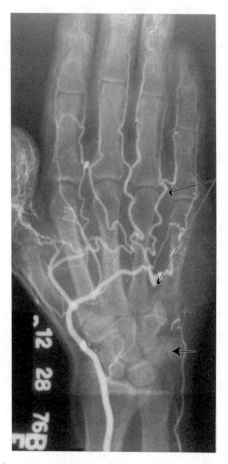

FIGURE 15.2 Angiographic features of a patient with Buerger's disease. Note a diminutive distal ulnar artery that occludes at the wrist (*arrowhead*). There are multiple digital occlusions and corkscrew collaterals (*arrow*).

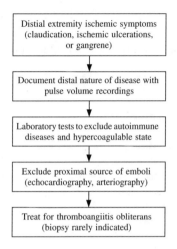

Distial extremity ischemic symptoms
(claudication, ischemic ulcerations,
or gangrene)

↓

Document distal nature of disease with
pulse volume recordings

↓

Laboratory tests to exclude autoimmune
diseases and hypercoagulable state

↓

Exclude proximal source of emboli
(echocardiography, arteriography)

↓

Treat for thromboangiitis obliterans
(biopsy rarely indicated)

FIGURE 15.3 Diagnostic algorithm for the diagnosis of thromboangiitis obliterans.

Because smoking cessation is so closely tied to disease activity and future amputation, it is extremely important for the physician to educate and counsel the patient on the importance of discontinuing the use of all tobacco products. Patients can be reassured that if they are able to discontinue tobacco use, the disease will remit and amputations will not occur as long as critical limb ischemia (gangrene and tissue loss) have not already occurred.

As mentioned previously, besides the discontinuation of cigarette smoking, all other forms of therapy are palliative. Intravenous iloprost (and, to a lesser extent, the oral form) have been shown to be effective in patients with active TAO.[36,37]

Good general vascular care is important in the treatment of all patients with severe ischemia. A reverse Trendelenburg (vascular) position should be used in patients who have severe ischemic rest pain. Good foot and hand care should be emphasized, and adequate narcotics should be made available during the period of severe ischemia. If

TABLE 15.3
Treatment of Thromboangiitis Obliterans

- Stop smoking or using tobacco in any form
- Avoid passive (secondhand) smoking, at least until ischemic ulcers are healed
- Treat local ischemic ulcerations and pain:
  - Foot care:
    1. Lubricate skin with lanolin-based cream
    2. Lamb's wool between toes
    3. Avoid trauma (i.e., use heel protectors, bed cradle)
  - Trial of calcium channel blockers, antiplatelet agents, or pentoxiffylline, or cilastozol
  - Iloprost (not currently available in U.S.)
  - Analgesics to control pain
  - Sympathectomy
  - Bypass surgery if anatomically feasible and patient has stopped smoking
  - Implantable spinal cord stimulator (last resort before amputation)
  - Gene therapy (investigational)
- Treat cellulitis with antibiotics and superficial phlebitis with non-steroidal anti-inflammatory drugs
- Amputate when all else fails

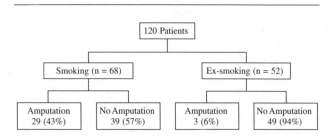

FIGURE 15.4 Smoking status related to amputation.

significant vasospasm is present, calcium-channel-blocking agents, such as nifedipine, nicardipine, or amlodipine, should be used.

Sympathectomy, surgical bypass, catheter-directed thrombolytic therapy, and intramuscular gene therapy with phVEGF165 (vascular endothelial growth factor)[38] have been used in some patients. The overall success of these techniques is not well defined.

15.7 CONCLUSIONS

Buerger's disease, or TAO, is a nonatherosclerotic, segmental, inflammatory disease that affects the small- and medium-sized arteries and veins in the lower and upper extremities. In some way, it is causally related to tobacco use. Discontinuation of tobacco is the mainstay of treatment. In those patients who successfully stop smoking, amputation almost never occurs.

REFERENCES

1. Olin, J.W. and Lie, J.T., Thromboangiitis obliterans (Buerger's disease), in *Vascular Medicine*, Loscalzo, J., Creager, M.A., and Dzau, V.J., Eds., Little, Brown and Co, Boston, 1996, 1033.

2. von Winiwater, F., Ueber eine eigenthumliche Form von Endarteritis und Endophlebitis mit Gangran des Fusses, *Arch. Klin. Chir.*, 23, 202, 1879.

3. Buerger's, L., Thromboangiitis obliterans: a study of the vascular lesions leading to presenile spontaneous gangrene, *Am. J. Med. Sci.*, 136, 567, 1908.

4. Lie, J.T., Thromboangiitis obliterans (Buerger's disease) revisited, *Pathol. Annu.*, 23, 257, 1988.

5. Lie, J.T., The rise and fall and resurgence of thromboangiitis obliterans (Buerger's disease), *Acta. Pathol. Jpn.*, 39, 153, 1989.

6. Lie, J.T., Thromboangiitis obliterans (Buerger's disease) in women, *Medicine*, 64, 65, 1987.

7. Cachovan, M., Epidemiologie und geographisches Verteilungsmuster der Thromboangiitis obliterans, in *Thromboangiitis Obliterans Morbus Winiwarter-Buerger's*, Heidrich, H., Ed., Georg Thieme, Stuttgart, 1988, 31.

8. Olin, J.W., Young, J.R., Graor, R.A., et al.,The changing clinical spectrum of thromboangiitis obliterans (Buerger's disease), *Circulation*, 82, IV-3, 1990.

9. Olin, J.W., Childs, M.B., Bartholomew, J.R.,et al., Anticardiolipin antibodies and homocysteine levels in patients with thromboangiitis obliterans, *Arthritis Rheum.*, 39, S-47, 1996.

10. Mills, J.L., Taylor, L.M., and Porter, J.K., Buerger's disease in the modern era, *Am. J. Surg.*, 154, 123, 1987.

11. Sasaki, S., Sakuma, M., Kunihara, T., et al., Current trends in thromboangiitis obliterans (Buerger's disease) in women, *Am. J. Surg.*, 177, 316, 1999.

12. Lie, J.T., Diagnostic histopathology of major systemic and pulmonary vasculitic syndromes, *Rheumatol. Clin. North Am.*, 16, 269, 1990.

13. Papa, M.Z. and Adar, R., A critical look at thromboangiitis obliterans (Buerger's disease), *Vasc. Surg.*, 5, 1, 1992.

14. Olin, J.W., Thromboangiitis obliterans (Buerger's disease), *Vascular Surgery*, 4th ed., Rutherford, R.B., Ed., W.B. Saunders, Philadelphia, 2000, 350.

15. Grove, W.J. and Stansby, G.P., Buerger's disease and cigarette smoking in Bangladesh, *Ann. R. Coll. Surg. Eng.*, 74, 115, 1992.

16. Joyce, J.W., Buerger's disease (thromboangiitis obliterans), *Rheum. Dis. Clin. North Am.*, 16, 463, 1990.

17. Lie, J.T., Thromboangiitis obliterans (Buerger's disease) and smokeless tobacco, *Arthritis Rheum.* 31, 812, 1988.

18. Adar, R., Papa, M.C., and Halperin, Z., Cellular sensitivity to thromboangiitis obliterans, *N. Engl. J. Med.*, 308, 1113, 1983.

19. Eichhorn, J., Sima, D., and Lindschau, C., Antiendothelial cell antibodies in thromboangiitis obliterans, *Am. J. Med. Sci.*, 315, 17, 1998.

20. Makita, S., Nakamura, M., Murakami, H., et al., Impaired endothelium dependent vasorelaxation in peripheral vasculature of patients with thromboangiitis obliterans (Buerger's disease), *Circulation*, 94, II-211, 1996.

21. Dible, J.H., *The Pathology of the Limb Ischaemia*, Oliver & Boyd, Edinburgh, 1966, 79.

22. Leu, H.J., Early inflammatory changes in thromboangiitis obliterans, *Pathol. Microbiol.*, 43, 151, 1975.
23. Leu, H.J., Thromboangiitis obliterans Buerger's, *Schweiz. Med. Woschenschr.*, 115, 1080, 1985
24. Shionoya, S., Leu, H.J, and Lie, J.T., Buerger's disease (thromboangiitis obliterans), in *Vascular Pathology*, Stehbens, W.E., and Lie, J.T., Eds., London, Chapman & Hall Medical, 657, 1995.
25. Deitch, E.A. and Sikkema, W.W., Intestinal manifestation of Buerger's disease, *Am. Surg.*, 47, 326, 1981.
26. Donatelli, F., Triggiani, M., and Nascimbene, S., Thromboangiitis obliterans of coronary and internal thoracic arteries in a young woman, *J. Thorac. Cardiovasc. Surg.*, 113, 800, 1997.
27. Rosen, N., Sommer, I., and Knobel, B., Intestinal Buerger's disease, *Arch. Pathol. Lab. Med.*, 109, 962, 1985.
28. Lie, J.T., Visceral intestinal Buerger's disease, *Int. J. Cardiol.*, 66, S249, 1998.
29. Michail, P.O., Filis, K.A., Delladetsima, J.K., et al.,Thromboangiitis obliterans (Buerger's disease) in visceral vessels confirmed by angiographic and histological findings, *Eur. J. Vasc. Endovasc. Surg.*, 16, 445, 1998.
30. Harten, P., Muller-Huelsbeck, S., Regensburger, D., et al., Multiple organ manifestations in thromboangiitis obliterans (Buerger's disease), *Angiology*, 47, 419, 1996.
31. Cebezas-Moya, R. and Dragstedt, L.R. III, An extreme example of Buerger's disease, *Arch. Surg.*, 101, 632, 1970.
32. Shionoya, S., Ban, I., Nakata, Y., et al.,Involvement of the iliac artery in Buerger's disease (pathogenesis and arterial reconstruction), *J. Cardiovasc. Surg. (Torino)*, 19, 69, 1978.
33. Allen, E.V., Thromboangiitis obliterans: Methods of diagnosis of chronic occlusive arterial lesions distal to the wrist with illustrative cases, *Am. J. Med. Sci.*, 178, 237, 1929.
34. Olin, J.W. and Lie, J.T., Thromboangiitis obliterans (Buerger's disease), in *Current Management of Hypertension and Vascular Disease*, Cooke, J.P. and Frohlich, E.D., Eds., St. Louis, Mosby Yearbook, 1992, 265.
35. Shionoya, S., Buerger's disease (thromboangiitis obliterans), in *Vascular Surgery*, Rutherford, R.B., Ed., W.B. Saunders, Philadelphia, 1989, 207.

36. Fiessinger, J.N. and Schafer, M., for the Thromboangiitis Obliterans Study Trial of iloprost vs. aspirin, treatment for critical limb ischemia of thromboangiitis obliterans, *Lancet*, 335, 555, 1990.

37. The European Thromboangiitis Obliterans Study Group, Oral iloprost in the treatment of thromboangiitis obliterans (Buerger's disease), a double-blind, randomized, placebo-controlled trial, *Eur. J. Vasc. Endovasc. Surg.*, 15,300, 1998.

38. Isner, J.M., Baumgartner, I., and Rauh, G., Treatment of thromboangiitis obliterans (Buerger's disease) by intramuscular gene transfer of vascular endothelial growth factor: preliminary clinical results, *J. Vasc. Surg.*, 28, 964, 1998.

16 Vasculitis

Emile R. Mohler III

CONTENTS

16.1 Introduction 339
16.2 Large-Vessel Vasculitis...340
    16.2.1   Giant-Cell Arteritides..340
            16.2.1.1 Temporal Arteritis 342
            16.2.1.2 Takayasu Arteritis 342
    16.2.2   Cogan Syndrome..344
16.3 Medium-Vessel Vasculitis 344
    16.3.1   Polyarteritis Nodosa..346
    16.3.2   Kawasaki Disease 347
16.4 Small-Vessel Vasculitis..348
    16.4.1   Churg-Strauss Syndrome 348
    16.4.2   Hypersensitivity Vasculitis................................350
    16.4.3   Wegener Granulomatosis 351
    16.4.4   Behçet Syndrome 353
References...358

16.1 INTRODUCTION

The term vasculitis describes pathologic inflammation and necrosis of blood vessels. Vasculitis can occur from an unknown cause (idiopathic) or be associated with an established disease (secondary). The etiology of the majority of vasculitides is thought to be either humoral or cellular immune-related injury. The inflammatory response may lead to narrowing or occlusion of vascular lumens and ischemia of tissue supplied by a particular vessel. Additionally, aneurysm and possible rupture may occur

0-8493-8413-3/01/$0.00+$1.50

in an involved vessel. Clinical "red flags" of vasculitis include fever of unknown origin, unexplained arthritis or myositis, suspicious rash (i.e., palpable purpura), mononeuritis multiplex, and glomerulonephritis. Specific classification is often difficult, however, because of overlapping pathologic features and clinical symptoms.[1] Difficulty in classification also occurs because the inciting antigen is unknown in the majority of cases. Generally, vasculitides are classified according to the vessel size and the histology of the inflammatory cell infiltrate.[2] The types of vasculitis presented in this chapter are categorized according to vessel size (Table 16.1).

16.2   LARGE-VESSEL VASCULITIS

Figure 16.1 presents an algorithm for diagnosis and treatment of patients with large-cell vasculitis.

16.2.1   GIANT-CELL ARTERITIDES

This group of vasculitides includes systemic giant cell or temporal arteritis and Takayasu arteritis.[3] Despite distinctive clinical patterns,

---

TABLE 16.1
Vasculitis Classification

- Large vessel
  - Temporal arteritis
  - Takayasu arteritis
- Medium vessel
  - Polyarteritis nodosa
  - Kawasaki disease
- Small vessel
  - Churg-Strauss syndrome
  - Hypersensitivity
  - Wegener granulomatosis
  - Behçet syndrome

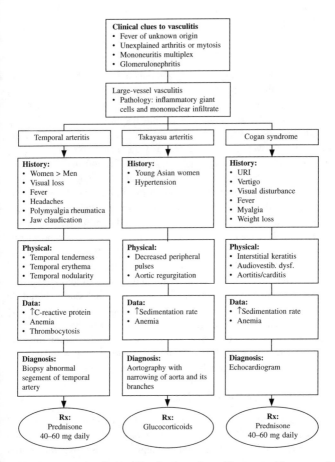

FIGURE 16.1 Treatment algorithm for the patient with suspected large-vessel vasculitis. Audiovestib. dysf. = audiovestibular dysfunction; Rx = treatment; URI = upper respiratory infection.

inflammatory giant cells and mononuclear infiltrates characterize both conditions.

16.2.1.1   Temporal Arteritis

This vasculitis typically occurs in patients older than 50 years of age, in women three times as frequently as men, and in whites more than other ethnic groups.[4] Branches of the carotid artery are often involved, but any large artery is susceptible. Clinical symptoms usually develop slowly and most characteristically manifest as tenderness, erythema, or nodularity over the temporal artery.[3] Other symptoms include fever, headaches, polymyalgia rheumatica, jaw claudication, and visual loss.[5] An important but uncommon cardiovascular complication is either aneurysm or stenosis of the aorta or its main branches. Thus, patients with temporal arteritis should be screened for abdominal aortic aneurysm. Laboratory findings include an elevated erythrocyte sedimentation rate, elevated C-reactive protein, anemia, and thrombocytosis. Diagnosis is suspected by biopsy of an abnormal segment of the temporal artery. Recent reports indicate that duplex Doppler ultrasound of the temporal arteries may be useful in diagnosis of temporal arteritis.[6] Treatment with prednisone (40 mg to 60 mg) daily should be initiated immediately after the diagnosis is made.[7] Corticosteroids can be slowly withdrawn after clinical and laboratory findings normalize. The cytokine interleukin-6 is elevated with disease symptoms and decreases with therapy.[8] There is a tendency for recurrence and patients should be monitored closely for disease recurrence after remission.

16.2.1.2   Takayasu Arteritis

This vasculitis is most commonly reported in young Asian women and primarily affects large vessels such as the aorta and its main branches.[9,10] From the pathologic inflammatory response, the arterial lumen is thickened and narrowed even to the point of critical stenosis. Cardiovascular symptoms include hypertension, decreased peripheral pulses, and aortic regurgitation.[11] Hypertension may be secondary to coarctation of the aorta or to renal artery stenosis. Diagnosis is made

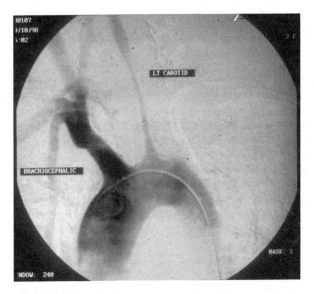

FIGURE 16.2 Image of aortic arch and great vessels demonstrating characteristic narrowing of Takayasu arteritis. (Angiographic photo by University of Minnesota Biomedical Graphics Department.)

by aortography and typically demonstrates narrowing of affected arteries with a well-developed collateral circulation (Figure 16.2).[10] The erythrocyte sedimentation rate, as a marker for disease activity, is not considered reliable by some clinicians.[12] Glucocorticoids are considered the first line of therapy, with the addition of cytotoxic agents for steroid-resistant patients.[12] The response to therapy can be monitored by ultrasonography or magnetic resonance imaging (MRI). Invasive vascular procedures such as angioplasty, stent placement, and bypass surgery are reserved for patients refractory to medical management. Indications for invasive intervention include: (1) hypertension from critical renal artery stenosis, (2) clinical features of cerebrovascular ischemia, (3) extremity ischemia limiting normal daily activities, and (4) cardiac ischemia from coronary artery stenosis.[12]

16.2.2 COGAN SYNDROME

This is a rare disease of young adults that is predominantly associated with interstitial keratitis and audiovestibular symptoms.[13] However, up to 15% of patients can suffer from vasculitis, usually manifested as aortitis or carditis. The majority of patients have a preceding upper respiratory infection, accompanied by eye and ear manifestations.[14] This syndrome is named after the ophthalmologist who described the ocular symptoms of interstitial keratitis, which can include decreased visual acuity, photophobia, and lacrimation. Uveitis, optic neuritis, and scleritis may also occur in conjunction with the other ocular findings. Audiovestibular dysfunction may also occur in close temporal associ-ation with interstitial keratitis. Patients may suffer acute Ménière dis-ease–like episodes with symptoms of vertigo, nausea, vomiting, and tinnitus. Somatic complaints may include fever, myalgia, fatigue, or weight loss.[15] The ocular and audiovestibular manifestations are likely mediated by organ-specific autoimmunity and not necessarily a con-sequence of vasculitis.

Pathologic findings of aortitis typically include a mixed infiltrate of neutrophils and mononuclear cells with disruption of the elastic lamina and vessel wall necrosis. Patients may develop aortic valve regurgitation (approximately 10%) due to inflammation involving the valve cusps.[15] In addition to aortic involvement, medium and small arteries may become inflamed and develop scar tissue.

Early use of corticosteroids is advocated to ameliorate the ocular and audiovestibular symptoms. Patients may require a hearing aid or cochlear implants because of sensorineural hearing loss. The symp-toms of vasculitis are usually controlled with high-dose steroids, but there are reports of patients requiring aortic valve replacement owing to severe aortic regurgitation.[15]

16.3 MEDIUM-VESSEL VASCULITIS

Figure 16.3 presents a diagnosis and treatment algorithm for medium-vessel vasculitis.

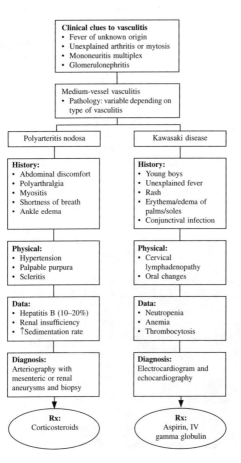

FIGURE 16.3 Treatment algorithm for the patient with suspected medium-vessel vasculitis. IV = intravenous; Rx = treatment.

16.3.1   POLYARTERITIS NODOSA

Kussmaul and Maier first described this vasculitic condition in 1866. Polyarteritis nodosa (PAN) typically presents as a disseminated necrotizing vasculitis involving medium-sized and small muscular arteries. A variety of clinical features may be observed due to frequent multiorgan involvement.[16] The most common are glomerulonephritis, mesenteric ischemia, polyarthralgia, and overlap connective tissue disease (i.e., polymyositis). Other features may include palpable purpura, new-onset hypertension, renal dysfunction, congestive heart failure, and scleritis. Hepatitis B infection is reported in approximately 10% to 20% of patients with PAN.[17-19] The initial arterial injury is believed to begin in the intima and progress to focal transmural inflammatory necrosis.[20] Inflammatory destruction of the media may lead to aneurysmal development (Figure 16.4). Aneurysmal rupture is a reported source of morbidity and mor-

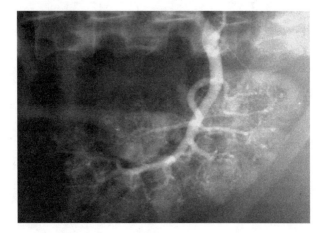

FIGURE 16.4 Angiogram of mesenteric arteries with characteristic aneurysm seen with polyarteritis nodosa. (Photo by University of Minnesota Biomedical Graphics Department.)

tality. The diagnosis is usually made by arteriographic documentation of mesenteric or renal artery aneurysms and is supplemented with biopsy of clinically involved tissue. Treatment of polyarteritis nodosa includes corticosteroids and the addition of cyclophosphamide in severe cases.[21-23]

16.3.2 KAWASAKI DISEASE

This vasculitic disease predominantly affects boys and was first described by Tomisaku Kawasaki in 1967.[24] Kawasaki disease, also known as mucocutaneous lymph node syndrome, can involve the large, medium, or small arteries but is most notable for coronary artery involvement. A mononuclear infiltrate with endothelial cell proliferation, elastic laminar disruption, and vessel-wall necrosis is characteristic of the arterial disease. Patients usually have unexplained fever for 5 or more days accompanied by at least four of the five following physical findings:

1. rash
2. peripheral extremity changes manifest as erythema or edema of palms/soles (acute phase) and periungual desquamation (convalescent phase)
3. bilateral conjunctival infection
4. oral mucous membrane changes (fissured lips, injected pharynx, strawberry tongue)
5. cervical lymphadenopathy

Some of the findings of Kawasaki disease can appear similar to those found with β-hemolytic streptococcal infection and measles.[25]

Laboratory findings can include anemia, neutropenia, and elevated platelet count. Electrocardiographic monitoring is important, as carditis occurs in up to 50% of patients.[26] Echocardiography is useful in diagnosing coronary artery aneurysms, which can occur within 2 weeks of disease onset.[27] Ruptured coronary aneurysms are rare but myocardial infarction can result from coronary artery thrombosis.[28,29] Treatment includes aspirin—80 mg/kg/day to 100 mg/kg/day for 2 weeks along with a single high-dose intravenous γ-globulin infusion of 2 g/kg given within the first 10 days of illness.[27,30] If echocardiography is normal at

8 weeks, then salicylates are discontinued, but if the echocardiogram is abnormal, salicylates should be continued for at least 1 year.

16.4   SMALL-VESSEL VASCULITIS

Figure 16.5 presents an algorithm for diagnosis and treatment of small-vessel vasculitis.

16.4.1   CHURG-STRAUSS SYNDROME

This syndrome, also known as allergic angiitis and granulomatosis, was initially described in 1951 and usually involves the small muscular arteries but also can involve medium-sized arteries.[31,32] The disease presentation usually includes eosinophilia and extravascular granulomas occurring in patients with a history of allergic rhinitis, asthma, or both.[32] However, the disease presentation can be variable and without some of the above findings.

The mean age of onset is 38 years, with a male predominance, and typically presents in three phases.[33] The initial phase is an allergic response manifested by either allergic rhinitis or asthma. The second phase involves blood eosinophilia with or without transient pulmonary infiltrates. Loffler syndrome can present similarly during this phase, and this diagnosis is often considered. The third phase involves systemic necrotizing vasculitis.

The asthmatic condition frequently remits during the onset of vasculitis, but can occur later in the disease. Approximately 75% of patients have pulmonary infiltrates that can appear as patchy peripheral infiltrates, hilar shadows, and even large pulmonary nodules.[34] At least 50% of patients have upper respiratory symptoms including allergic rhinitis and polyposis. Skin manifestations can include purpura with leukocytoclastic vasculitis. Granulomatous nodules may also develop on the skin. Some patients may experience diarrhea secondary to eosinophilia infiltration of the bowel wall, with resultant bleeding and nodular masses that may cause gastrointestinal obstruction.[35] Bowel ischemia with perforation, bleeding, or colitis is reported and may be heralded

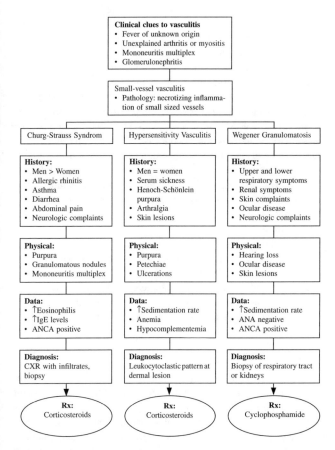

FIGURE 16.5 Treatment algorithm for the patient with suspected small-vessel vasculitis. ANA = antinuclear antibodies; ANCA = antineutrophil cyoplasmic antibodies; CXR = chest X-ray; IgE = immunoglobulin E; Rx = treatment.

by abdominal pain. The nervous system abnormalities that accompany Churg-Strauss can mirror those of PAN and include mononeuritis multiplex, symmetric peripheral neuropathy, ischemic optic neuritis, and cranial nerve palsies.[33] Cardiac involvement may result in pericarditis or myocardial infarction. Patients may also experience urinary tract involvement or focal segmental glomerulonephritis.

Characteristic laboratory findings include fluctuating levels of eosinophils and an increase in immunoglobulin (Ig) E levels. In addition, antibodies to myeloperoxidase with positive antineutrophil cytoplasmic antibodies (ANCA) can occur.[36] A strong correlation between disease activity and eosinophil count is reported.[33] The diagnosis of Churg-Strauss disease includes the clinical presentation, chest radiograph, laboratory studies, and pathologic specimen. Several diseases can mimic Churg-Strauss. The differential diagnosis includes Wegener's granulomatosis (usually has more destructive airway component without asthma), Löffler syndrome, sarcoidosis, and allergic bronchopulmonary asperigillosis.

Churg-Strauss vasculitis usually responds to corticosteroid administration.[33,34] The majority of patients entering remission have a mean survival of approximately 10 years. The mortality from this condition is usually secondary to pulmonary and cardiac failure. Patients experiencing fulminating vasculitis should be given immunosuppressive drugs if corticosteroids have not proven successful.

16.4.2   HYPERSENSITIVITY VASCULITIS

The hypersensitivity vasculitides are vasculitic diseases that were reported under a variety of names including cutaneous necrotizing vasculitis, allergic vasculitis, and leukocytoclastic vasculitis.[37] These diseases characteristically have inflammation of small vessels (especially venules) with leukocytoclasis (nuclear debris) and cutaneous skin involvement.[37] The clinical syndromes include serum sickness, drug hypersensitivity reactions, Henoch-Schönlein purpura, mixed cryoglobulinemia, and urticarial vasculitis (hypocomplementemic vasculitis).[38] The pathologic findings are necrotizing inflammation of vessels less than 1 mm in diameter accompanied by polymorpho-nuclear cells or, less frequently, lymphocytes.[39] The onset of hypersensitivity vasculitis is usually abrupt and can occur in all age groups with an equal predominance in men and women. The cutaneous signs of hypersensivity vasculitis can include palpable purpura (classic finding), petechiae, vesicles, urticaria, papules, pustules, necrotic ulcerations, and nodules.[37] The skin lesions usually appear in groups and are symmetrically distributed on dependent areas. The resolution of lesions may take up to 4 weeks, and hyperpigmentation or scars sometimes occur. Patients may develop arthralgias or arthritis. The knees are most frequently involved, followed by ankles, wrists, or elbows. Muscular or nervous involvement can also occur as usually associated with connective tissue diseases or cryoglobulinemia. Gastrointestinal involvement suggests Henoch-Schönlein purpura[40] or vasculitis secondary to inflammatory bowel disease. Renal involvement can also occur and should be suspected if patients suffer from hematuria. The laboratory findings may include an elevated erythrocyte sedimentation rate with leukocytosis, eosinophilia, anemia, heme-positive stool, hematuria, proteinuria, cryoglobulinemia, and hypocomplementemia as well as abnormal liver or renal tests. IgA-containing immune complexes are characteristically found with Henoch-Schönlein purpura.[41,42]

Patients presenting with symptoms of hypersensitivity vasculitis should be carefully evaluated for underlying systemic illness or exposure for an offending agent. The diagnosis is confirmed by the presence of a leukocytoclastic pattern involving small vessels at the site of a dermal lesion. The treatment involves removal of the offending agent or treatment of an associated systemic illness. A spontaneous resolution of symptoms is common, although some patients may require long-term treatment with corticosteroids for control of disease.

16.4.3 WEGENER GRANULOMATOSIS

The etiology of this vasculitis is unknown and characteristically involves a necrotizing granulomatous process of the respiratory tract along with glomerulonephritis. This disease occurs primarily in young and middle-aged persons, with a slight male predominance.[43,44] Pathologic findings can include necrotizing vasculitis of small arteries and veins, necrotizing granulomata, and glomerulonephritis. The vascular lesions usually have fibrinoid necrosis, with vessels at different stages of inflammation and healing. The kidney lesions are most commonly focal segmental glomerulonephritis. This condition is usually distinguished from PAN by an infiltration of predominantly mononuclear cells as well as frequent involvement of the small veins. Most patients develop both upper and lower respiratory tract involvement, although some patients with pulmonary infiltrates may be asymptomatic.[43-45] In addition to respiratory and renal disease manifestations, patients may also develop cutaneous lesions, ocular disease, peripheral and central nervous system involvement, and cardiovascular inflammation (i.e., carditis). Laboratory findings can include elevated erythrocyte sedimentation rate, leukocytosis, thrombocytosis, and anemia of chronic disease. Most patients (approximately 93%) with diffuse, active disease have a positive ANCA test but a negative antinuclear antibody test.[46-48] Antibodies are directed against proteinase-3, myeloperoxidase, and, occasionally, human leukocyte elastase.[49]

Initial evaluation should include a chest radiograph and urinalysis in addition to blood tests.[50] The differential diagnosis includes other vasculitides, especially systemic lupus erythematosus. Other disorders that should be considered include cholesterol atheroemboli, infective endocarditis, malignancies, fibromuscular dysplasia, and radiation fibrosis. The diagnosis is confirmed with a tissue biopsy of the respiratory tract or kidneys.[50] The lung is the most likely tissue to show classic pathologic findings on biopsy. The decision to treat is not usually made solely on the basis of a positive ANCA but also in conjunction with biopsy findings. Most patients respond to treatment with cyclophosphamide in conjunction with steroids. If left untreated, the prognosis of Wegener granulomatosis is poor, with 90% of patients dying within 2 years due to respiratory or renal failure. Patients that initially require dialysis due to renal failure may recover enough to come off dialysis.[51,52]

16.4.4 Behçet Syndrome

Behçet syndrome is a rare multisystem inflammatory disorder characterized by recurrent oral aphthous ulcers, genital ulcers, uveitis, and skin lesions.[53,54] Patients commonly have synovitis and meningioencephalitis. The etiology of Behçet syndrome is unknown, but clusters of cases are reported along the ancient Silk Road, which extends from eastern Asia to the Mediterranean Basin. The highest prevalence of this syndrome is in the eastern Mediterranean region, especially Turkey, but also in Japan. There is an increased prevalence of the human leukocyte antigen (HLA)-B51 allele that matches the disease distribution along the Silk Road and in Japan, but not among Caucasian patients who live in Western countries. Microbial infection is implicated in development of Behçet's disease, as herpes simplex virus DNA and serum antibodies against the virus were noted in a higher proportion of patients with disease than in controls. Other possible viruses include *Parvovirus* B19 and hepatitis C virus. However, none of these infectious agents has been definitively proven to cause the autoimmune response.

The pathophysiology involves an autoimmune response that can result in vascular injury. The vasa vasorum can be affected by vasculitis in large vessels. Aneurysms and occlusions of large arteries can result in morbid complications. There are reports of cerebrovascular accidents, claudication, and renal vascular hypertension secondary to arteritis or thrombosis. In addition, recurrent thrombophlebitis of both superficial and deep veins can occur and may manifest as fever. Neurologic involvement may include cerebral venous thrombosis.

Diagnosis is made on the basis of criteria proposed by the International Study Group for Behçet's Disease (Table 16.2).[53] Valvular and coronary disease can occur in some patients. Neutrophil and lymphocyte function is abnormal, and this is thought responsible for the host

TABLE 16.2
Criteria for the Diagnosis of Behçet Disease[a]

Finding	Definition
Recurrent oral ulceration	Minor apthous or herpetiform ulcers, observed by physician or patient, that have recurred ≥3 times over a 12-mo period
Recurrent genital ulceration	Apthous ulceration or scarring observed by physician or patient
Eye lesions	Anterior uveitis, posterior uveitis, or cells in the vitreous body on slit-lamp examination; or retinal vasculitis detected by ophthalmologist
Skin lesions	Erythema nodosum observed by physician or patient, pseudofolliculitis, or papulopustular lesions; or acneiform nodules observed by physician in a postadolescent patient who is not receiving corticosteroids
Positive pathology test	Test interpreted as positive by physician at 24–48 hr

[a] Criteria of the International Study Group for Behçet's Disease. For diagnosis to be made, patient must have recurrent oral ulceration plus ≥2 of the other findings in the absence of other clinical explanations.

From Sakane, T., Takeno, M., Suzuki, N., and Inaba, G., Behçet's disease. *N. Engl. J. Med.*, 341, 1284, 1999. With permission.[54]

of immunologic abnormalities that can occur.[55] Useful imaging studies to detect vascular lesions include computed tomography, MRI, angiography, and ventilation-perfusion scintigraphy. Treatment of this disease depends on the clinical manifestations (Table 16.3).[54] Unfortunately, treatment of Behçet vasculitis with immunosuppressive agents is not as successful as with other vasculitides. Other potential remedies include estradiol, dapsone, colchicine, cyclosporin, and levamisole.[54]

TABLE 16.3
Treatment for Behçet Disease

Treatment	Dose	Used as First-Line Therapy
Topical corticosteroids		
Triamcinolone acetonide ointment	3 times daily topically	Oral ulcers
Betamethasone ointment	3 times daily topically	Genital ulcers
Betamethasone drops	1–2 drops 3 times daily topically	Anterior uveitis, retinal vasculitis
Dexamethasone	1.0–1.5 mg injected below Tenon capsule for an ocular attack	Retinal vasculitis
Systemic corticosteroids		
Prednisolone	20–100 mg/day orally	GI lesions, acute meningoencephalitis, chronic progressive CNS lesions, arteritis
Methylprednisolone	1,000 mg/day for 3 days IV	Acute meningoencephalitis, chronic progressive CNS lesions, arteritis
Tropicamide drops	1–2 drops once or twice daily topically	Anterior uveitis

(continued)

TABLE 16.3 (CONTINUED)
Treatment for Behçet Disease

Treatment	Dose	Used as First-Line Therapy
Tetracycline	250 mg in water solution once a day topically	
Colchicine	0.5–1.5 mg/day orally	Oral ulcers,[a] genital ulcers,[a] pseudofolliculitis,[a] erythema nodosum, anterior uveitis, retinal vasculitis
Thalidomide	100–300 mg/day orally	
Dapsone	100 mg/day orally	
Pentoxifylline	300 mg/day orally	
Azathioprine	100 mg/day orally	
Chlorambucil	5 mg/day orally	
Cyclophosphamide	50–100 mg/day orally 700–1,000 mg/mo IV	
Methotrexate	7.5–15 mg/wk orally	
Cyclosporine[b]	5 mg/day per kg body weight orally	Retinal vasculitis[a]

Interferon-α	5 million U/day IM or SC	Arthritis
Indomethacin	50–75 mg/day orally	GI lesions
Sulfasalazine	1–3 g/day orally	
Warfarin[c]	2–10 mg/day orally	Venous thrombosis
Heparin[c]	5,000–20,000 U/day SC	Venous thrombosis
Aspirin[d]	50–100 mg/day orally	Arteritis, venous thrombosis
Dipyridamole	300 mg/day orally	Arteritis, venous thrombosis
Surgery	—	—

CNS = central nervous system; GI = gastrointestinal; IM = intramuscular; IV = intravenous; SC = subcutaneous.

[a] Efficacy of this drug for this use has been reported in controlled clinical trials.

[b] Contraindicated in patients with acute meningoencephalitis or chronic progressive CNS lesions.

[c] Use with caution in patients with pulmonary vascular lesions.

[d] Low-dose aspirin is used as an antiplatelet agent.

From Sakane, T., Takeno, M., Suzuki, N., and Inaba, G., Behçet's disease. *N. Engl. J. Med.*, 341, 1284, 1999. With permission.[54]

REFERENCES

1. Rao, J.K., Allen, N.B., and Pincus, T., Limitations of the 1990 American College of Rheumatology classification criteria in the diagnosis of vasculitis, *Ann. Intern. Med.*, 129, 345, 1998.
2. Hunder, G.G., Arend, W.P., Bloch, D.A., et al., The American College of Rheumatology 1990 criteria for the classification of vasculitis: introduction, *Arthritis Rheum.*, 33, 1065, 1990.
3. Hunder, G.G., Bloch, D.A., Michel, B.A., et al., The American College of Rheumatology 1990 criteria for the classification of giant cell arteritis, *Arthritis Rheum.*, 33, 1122, 1990.
4. Huston, K.A., Hunder, G.G., Lie, J.T., et al., Temporal arteritis: a 25-year epidemiologic, clinical, and pathologic study, *Ann. Intern. Med.*, 88, 162, 1978.
5. Hunder, G.G., Giant cell arteritis in polymyalgia rheumatica, *Am. J. Med.*, 102, 514, 1997.
6. Hunder, G.G., and Weyand, C.M., Sonography in giant-cell arteritis, *N. Engl. J. Med.*, 337, 1385, 1997.
7. Hellmann, D.B., Immunopathogenesis, diagnosis, and treatment of giant cell arteritis, temporal arteritis, polymyalgia rheumatica, and Takayasu's arteritis, *Curr. Opin. Rheumatol.*, 5, 25, 1993.
8. Roche, N.E., Fulbright, J.W., Wagner, A.D., et al., Correlation of interleukin-6 production and disease activity in polymyalgia rheumatica and giant cell arteritis, *Arthritis Rheum.*, 36, 1286, 1993.
9. Nakao, K., Ikeda, M., Kimata, S., et al., Takayasu's arteritis, clinical report of 84 cases and immunological studies of seven cases, *Circulation*, 35, 1141, 1967.
10. Arend, W.P., Michel, B.A., Bloch, D.A., et al., The American College of Rheumatology 1990 criteria for the classification of Takayasu arteritis, *Arthritis Rheum.*, 33, 1129, 1990.
11. Ishikawa, K., Diagnostic approach and proposed criteria for the clinical diagnosis of Takayasu's arteriopathy, *J. Am. Coll. Cardiol.*, 12, 964, 1988.
12. Kerr, G.S., Hallahan, C.W., Giordano, J., et al., Takayasu arteritis, *Ann. Intern. Med.*, 120, 919, 1994.
13. Cheson, B.D., Bluming, A.Z., and Alroy, J., Cogan's syndrome: a systemic vasculitis, *Am. J. Med.*, 60, 549, 1976.

14. Haynes, B.F., Kaiser-Kupfer, M.I., Mason, P., et al., Cogan syndrome: studies in 13 patients, long-term follow-up, and a review of the literature, *Medicine*, 59, 426, 1980.

15. Vollertsen, R.S., McDonald, T.J., Younge, B.R., et al., Cogan's syndrome: 18 cases and a review of the literature, *Mayo Clin. Proc.*, 61, 344, 1986.

16. Lightfoot, R.W.J., Michel, B.A., Bloch, D.A., et al., The American College of Rheumatology 1990 criteria for the classification of polyarteritis nodosa, *Arthritis Rheum.*, 33, 1088, 1990.

17. Sergent, J.S., Lockshin, M.D., Christian, C.L., et al., Vasculitis with hepatitis B antigenemia: long-term observation in nine patients, *Medicine* 55, 1, 1976.

18. Duffy, J., Lidsky, M.D., Sharp, J.T., et al., Polyarthritis, polyarteritis and hepatitis B, *Medicine*, 55, 19, 1976.

19. Marcellin, P., Calmus, Y., Takahashi, H., et al., Latent hepatitis B virus (HBV) infection in systemic necrotizing vasculitis, *Clin. Exp. Rheumatol.*, 9, 23, 1991.

20. D'Agati, V., Chander, P., Nash, M., et al., Idiopathic microscopic polyarteritis nodosa: ultrastructural observations on the renal vascular and glomerular lesions, *Am. J. Kidney Dis.*, 7, 95, 1986.

21. Fauci, A.S., Katz, P., Haynes, B.F., et al., Cyclophosphamide therapy of severe systemic necrotizing vasculitis, *N. Engl. J. Med.*, 301, 235, 1979.

22. Guillevin, L. and Lhote, F., Treatment of polyarteritis nodosa and microscopic polyangiitis, *Arthritis Rheum.*, 41, 2100, 1998.

23. Guillevin, L., Treatment of classic polyarteritis nodosa in 1999 (editorial), *Nephrol. Dial. Transplant.*, 14, 2077, 1999.

24. Kawasaki, T., Acute febrile mucocutaneous syndrome with lymphoid involvement with specific desquamation of the fingers and toes in children (in Japanese), *Arerugi* (Japanese Journal of Allergology), 16, 178, 1967.

25. Burns, J.C., Mason, W.H., Glode, M.P., et al., Clinical and epidemiologic characteristics of patients referred for evaluation of possible Kawasaki disease, United States Multicenter Kawasaki Disease Study Group, *J. Pediatr.*, 118, 680, 1991.

26. Hiraishi, S., Yashiro, K., Oguchi, K., et al., Clinical course of cardiovascular involvement in the mucocutaneous lymph node syndrome, relation between clinical signs of carditis and development of coronary arterial aneurysm, *Am. J. Cardiol.*, 47, 323, 1981.

27. Newburger, J.W., Takahashi, M., Burns, J.C., et al., The treatment of Kawasaki syndrome with intravenous gamma globulin, *N. Engl. J. Med.*, 315, 341, 1986.

28. Tatara, K. and Kusakawa, S., Long-term prognosis of giant coronary aneurysms in Kawasaki disease, *Prog. Clin. Biol. Res.*, 250, 579, 1987.

29. Kato, H., Ichinose, E., Yoshioka, F., et al., Fate of coronary aneurysms in Kawasaki disease: serial coronary angiography and long-term follow-up study, *Am. J. Cardiol.*, 49, 1758, 1982.

30. Newburger, J.W., Takahashi, M., Beiser, A.S., et al., A single intravenous infusion of gamma globulin as compared with four infusions in the treatment of acute Kawasaki syndrome, *N. Engl. J. Med.*, 324, 1633, 1991.

31. Churg, J. and Strauss, L., Allergic granulomatosis, allergic angiitis and periarteritis nodosa, *Am. J. Pathol.*, 27, 277, 1951.

32. Masi, A.T., Hunder, G.G., Lie, J.T., et al., The American College of Rheumatology 1990 criteria for the classification of Churg-Strauss syndrome (allergic granulomatosis and angiitis), *Arthritis Rheum.*, 33, 1094, 1990.

33. Lanham, J.G., Elkon, K.B., Pusey, C.D., et al., Systemic vasculitis with asthma and eosinophilia: a clinical approach to the Churg-Strauss syndrome, *Medicine*, 63, 65, 1984.

34. Chumbley, L.C., Harrison, E.G.J., and DeRemee, R.A., Allergic granulomatosis and angiitis (Churg-Strauss syndrome), Report and analysis of 30 cases, *Mayo Clin. Proc.*, 52, 477, 1977.

35. Abell, M.R., Limond, RV., Blamey, W.E., et al., Allergic granulomatosis with massive gastric involvement, *N. Engl. J. Med.*, 282, 665, 1970.

36. Cohen, T.J., Limburg, P.C., Elema, J.D., et al., Detection of autoantibodies against myeloid lysosomal enzymes: a useful adjunct to classification of patients with biopsy-proven necrotizing arteritis, *Am. J. Med.*, 91, 59, 1991.

37. Calabrese, L.H., Michel, B.A., Bloch, D.A., et al., The American College of Rheumatology 1990 criteria for the classification of hypersensitivity vasculitis, *Arthritis Rheum.*, 33, 1108, 1990.

38. McCombs, R.P., Systemic "allergic" vasculitis, Clinical and pathological relationships, *JAMA*, 194, 1059, 1965.

39. Soter, N.A., Mihm, M.C.J., Gigli, I., et al., Two distinct cellular patterns in cutaneous necrotizing angiitis, *J. Invest. Dermatol.*, 66, 344, 1976.

40. Kauffmann, R.H., Herrmann, W.A., Meyer, C.J., et al., Circulating IgA-immune complexes in Henoch-Schönlein purpura, a longitudinal study of their relationship to disease activity and vascular deposition of IgA, *Am. J. Med.*, 69, 859, 1980.

41. Trygstad, C.W. and Stiehm, ER., Elevated serum IgA globulin in anaphylactoid purpura, *Pediatrics*, 47, 1023, 1971.

42. Mills, J.A., Michel, B.A., Bloch, D.A., et al., The American College of Rheumatology 1990 criteria for the classification of Henoch-Schönlein purpura, *Arthritis Rheum.*, 33, 1114, 1990.

43. Fauci, A.S., Haynes, B.F., Katz, P., et al., Wegener's granulomatosis: prospective clinical and therapeutic experience with 85 patients for 21 years, *Ann. Intern. Med.*, 98, 76, 1983.

44. Hoffman, G.S., Kerr, G.S., Leavitt, R.Y., et al., Wegener granulomatosis: an analysis of 158 patients, *Ann. Intern. Med.*, 116, 488, 1992.

45. Leavitt, R.Y., Fauci, A.S., Bloch, D.A., et al., The American College of Rheumatology 1990 criteria for the classification of Wegener's granulomatosis, *Arthritis Rheum.*, 33, 1101, 1990.

46. Cohen, T.J., van der Woude, F.J., Fauci, A.S., et al., Association between active Wegener's granulomatosis and anticytoplasmic antibodies, *Arch. Intern. Med.*, 149, 2461, 1989.

47. Nolle, B., Specks, U., Ludemann, J., et al., Anticytoplasmic autoantibodies: their immunodiagnostic value in Wegener granulomatosis, *Ann. Intern. Med.*, 111, 28, 1989.

48. Specks, U., Wheatley, C.L., McDonald, T.J., et al., Anticytoplasmic autoantibodies in the diagnosis and follow-up of Wegener's granulomatosis, *Mayo Clin. Proc.*, 64, 28, 1989.

49. Muller, K.A., Kallenberg, C.G., and Tervaert, J.W., Monocyte activation in patients with Wegener's granulomatosis, *Ann. Rheum. Dis.*, 58, 237, 1999.

50. Israel, H.L. and Patchefsky, A.S., Wegener's granulomatosis of lung: diagnosis and treatment, experience with 12 cases, *Ann. Intern. Med.*, 74, 881, 1971.

51. Glassock, R.J., Intensive plasma exchange in crescentic glomerulonephritis: help or no help?, *Am. J. Kidney Dis.*, 20, 270, 1992.

52. Nachman, P.H., Hogan, S.L., Jennette, J.C., et al., Treatment response and relapse in antineutrophil cytoplasmic autoantibody-associated microscopic polyangiitis and glomerulonephritis, *J. Am. Soc. Nephrol.*, 7, 33, 1996.

53. International Study Group for Behçet's Disease, Criteria for diagnosis of Behçet's disease, *Lancet*, 335, 1078, 1990.

54. Sakane, T., Takeno, M., Suzuki, N., et al., Behçet's disease, *N. Engl. J. Med.*, 341, 1284, 1999.

55. Ehrlich, G.E., Vasculitis in Behçet's disease, *Int. Rev. Immunol.*, 14, 81, 1997.

17 Raynaud Phenomenon

Jay D. Coffman

CONTENTS

17.1 Clinical Presentation and Natural History 364
17.2 Epidemiology 365
17.3 Pathophysiology 366
17.4 Diagnosis and Evaluation..368
    17.4.1 Secondary Causes of Raynaud Phenomenon 371
        17.4.1.1 Connective Tissue Diseases 372
        17.4.1.2 Carpal Tunnel Syndrome 373
        17.4.1.3 Thoracic Outlet Syndrome.......................373
        17.4.1.4 Traumatic Vasospastic Disease 373
        17.4.1.5 Drugs 374
        17.4.1.6 Obstructive Arterial Disease 374
17.5 Treatment...375
    17.5.1 Calcium Channel Blockers 377
    17.5.2 Sympatholytic Agents 378
    17.5.3 Nitroglycerin Preparations 379
    17.5.4 Angiotensin Inhibitors 380
    17.5.5 Thyroid Preparations..380
    17.5.6 Prostaglandins 381
    17.5.7 Sympathectomy..381
References...382

17.1 CLINICAL PRESENTATION AND NATURAL HISTORY

Raynaud phenomenon is the occurrence of episodic attacks of well-demarcated blanching (dead white finger) or blue discoloration of one or more digits.[1,2] The attacks are confined to the fingers and toes; the hands and feet are not involved. Vasospastic attacks occur on exposure to cold or sometimes with emotional upsets. During an attack, the digit becomes white, or sometimes yellow, and numb; the pallor may then be replaced by cyanosis due to slow blood flow, and finally the digit turns red during a hyperemic phase. During the latter phase, there may be a throbbing pain. Raynaud phenomenon is termed primary (or idiopathic) when no underlying cause is present, or secondary when caused by an underlying disease, drug, or inciting event.

In several large studies, approximately 60% of patients with the primary phenomenon had attacks only in the fingers, 40% in the fingers and toes, and less than 1% only in the toes. Many patients present with vasospastic attacks in only one or two fingers but, with time, more fingers and even the toes may become involved. Thumbs are often spared. The digit may be involved in part or in whole. Studies vary in reporting how many of the three color changes are usually present, but, in the author's experience, pallor alone is the most common presentation.

The prognosis for patients with primary Raynaud phenomenon is good. In a study of 307 patients who had the phenomenon for an average of 17 years, 38% reported no change in symptoms, 36% improved, 16% were worse, and 10% no longer had symptoms. Sclerodactyly disappeared in 19 of 27 patients and was unchanged in seven patients; it developed in 3.3% overall. Only 0.4% (two patients) had digital amputations for ulcers. Of the 44 patients who moved to a warmer climate, more than 50% improved.

In several studies that observed patients for approximately 7 years after the onset of vasospastic attacks, those considered to have primary Raynaud phenomenon developed a secondary disease, usually scleroderma or the CREST syndrome (calcinosis, Raynaud phenomenon, esophageal dysfunction, sclerodactyly, telangiectasias) variety, in 0%

to 8%. Even having a positive antinuclear antibody test did not predict the development of a secondary disease.

17.2 EPIDEMIOLOGY

There are few good studies of the prevalence of Raynaud phenomenon in the general population and no study of its incidence. The diagnosis of Raynaud phenomenon is entirely clinical, because it is difficult to induce attacks and there are no diagnostic tests. In England, one of the first studies reported that 25% of men and 30% of women described finger changes consistent with Raynaud phenomenon (n = 122 subjects, mostly medical students and nurses). A later study in England estimated that among 520 patients in a general practice, 8.3% of men and 17.6% of women had symptoms consistent with vasospastic attack.[3] This study did not question subjects about blue color changes. In Denmark, 22% of 67 healthy female physical therapists were considered to have the phenomenon. The largest survey of 1,752 randomly selected subjects found that 4.6% reported symptoms consistent with Raynaud phenomenon in the warm climate of South Carolina. These same investigators then compared the prevalence of the phenomenon in South Carolina with a much cooler climate in France.[4] They found the prevalence to be much higher (16.8%) in the cooler climate than in the warmer climate (5%). In this study, subjects were shown colored pictures of fingers with vasospastic attack; therefore, the reports of disease prevalence may be more exact. The prevalence of primary compared with secondary Raynaud phenomenon could not be ascertained from these studies, but the presence of dysphagia and the use of vibratory tools were common in the South Carolina study, suggesting a secondary cause. One study has reported that 89% of patients had the primary and 11% had the secondary phenomenon.[5]

Onset of primary Raynaud phenomenon usually occurs between the ages of 11 and 45, although it has been reported in younger and older patients. Among 474 female patients, the average age was 31 years[6]; the oldest patient was 68. In another study of 100 patients, 81% had onset of the disease at 11 to 40 years of age. In a series of

100 male patients, the phenomenon appeared before age 40 in 73%, with an age range of 5 to 63 years.

Two studies have reported that approximately 77% of patients with primary Raynaud phenomenon were female. An equal distribution of Raynaud phenomenon (primary and secondary) was found among women and men in a large study in South Carolina. They also reported an equal distribution of the phenomenon among blacks and whites.

17.3 PATHOPHYSIOLOGY

Digital artery vasospasm has been shown to be the cause of the pallor phase of Raynaud phenomenon. The involved digits become numb owing to the cessation of blood flow. During the cyanotic phase, blood flow is very slow, which allows the hemoglobin to desaturate. When the vessels reopen, a red, reactive hyperemia phase occurs. The cause of digital artery vasospasm is unknown. In some secondary causes of Raynaud phenomenon, the vessel wall may be thickened, allowing a normal sympathetic stimulus to obliterate the vessel lumen. If there is a proximal arterial obstruction, the distal blood vessel will have a low distending pressure and a normal sympathetic stimulus may lead to vessel closure. In primary Raynaud phenomenon, arteriograms are usually normal and digital artery pathology has not been demonstrated.

Primary Raynaud phenomenon has been explained by two theories.[1,2] The first attributes it to overactivity of the sympathetic nervous system, whereas the second considers that there is an abnormal sensitivity of the digital arteries to cold stimuli.

Evidence for overactivity of the sympathetic nervous system in Raynaud phenomenon includes the following:

- Sympathectomy may stop vasospastic attacks in the toes.
- Emotional stimuli may induce attacks.
- Hand blood flow is normal with heating.
- Increased catecholamines may be found in wrist venous blood.
- Exaggerated vasoconstrictor responses may occur with postural changes.

However, local cooling of one hand does not increase sympathetic vasoconstriction in the opposite hand, patients have normal central thermoregulatory responses, measurements of cutaneous sympathetic nerve activity to the hand are normal, and there are normal plasma and urinary catecholamines in patients with the primary phenomenon and with scleroderma.

Abnormal sensitivity of digital blood vessels to cold is supported by the following:

1. Local cooling produces ischemic attacks in single fingers and in sympathetically denervated fingers.
2. Local ischemic cold stimulus causes a loss of digital systolic blood pressure.
3. Patients with primary Raynaud phenomenon have an increased sensitivity to stimulation of the α_2-adrenoceptors. Increased levels of platelet α_2-adrenoceptors by binding capacity and affinity studies has been found in patients with the primary phenomenon compared with control subjects and patients with secondary Raynaud phenomenon.

Other theories implicate platelets and their products, such as serotonin, increased free radical activity, endothelial products, inflammatory and immune responses, increased plasma and blood viscosity, and decreased fibrinolysis. Most of these findings are a consequence and not a cause of the phenomenon. Hereditary or familial factors, a central nervous system abnormality of vascular control, endothelin-1, calcitonin gene-related peptide, and a generalized defect in vascular function have been implicated in vasospastic attacks. A significant correlation with variant angina pectoris and migraine headaches has been described in patients with Raynaud phenomenon. Vasospasm has also been described in other vascular beds in patients with scleroderma and vasospastic attacks. Patients with primary Raynaud phenomenon have low systemic and digital artery systolic blood pressure. Therefore, pressure on the digits plus a cold stimulus commonly induces vasospastic attacks. Pressure on the digits on a cold steering wheel or holding cold drinks are two very common causes of attacks.

In summary, vasospastic attacks in primary Raynaud phenomenon may be caused by a combination of factors, including a local sensitivity of the digital arteries to cold involving the α_2-adrenoceptors, low digital artery intravascular pressure, reflex sympathetic vasoconstriction, and external pressure on the digit.

17.4   DIAGNOSIS AND EVALUATION

If the patient describes episodic attacks of white or blue color changes of the digits on exposure to cold, the diagnosis is not difficult. If color changes are well demarcated, the diagnosis is substantiated. It is important for prognosis and treatment of the patient to attempt to distinguish primary from secondary Raynaud phenomenon (Table 17.1).

The history must include questions regarding symptoms of connective tissue disease (e.g., arthralgias, arthritis, dysphagia, heartburn, butterfly rash on the face, pleurisy, epilepsy, tender muscles); trauma to the hands or fingers, including vibration exposure; positional symptoms in the arms; drug usage (see Table 17.2); symptoms of arterial disease of the limbs (i.e., intermittent claudication, rest pain), blood

---

TABLE 17.1
Criteria for Diagnosis of Primary Raynaud Phenomenon

1. Vasospastic attacks confined to the digits on cold exposure
2. Bilateral involvement of extremities
3. Absence of gangrene or limited to the fingertip skin
4. No underlying disease, medication, or occupation that could be responsible for vasospastic attacks
5. History of symptoms for at least 2 years
6. Normal sedimentation rate
7. Absence of antinuclear antibodies
8. Normal nailfold capillaries

---

dyscrasias (i.e., fatigue, purpura), and hypothyroidism (lethargy, constipation, nonpitting edema). In primary Raynaud phenomenon, the history is usually negative.

The physical exam is normal in primary Raynaud phenomenon. Absent pulses or signs of connective tissue disease are important and may lead to the underlying etiology of secondary causes. The carpal tunnel and thoracic outlet maneuvers should be performed.

Nailfold capillary microscopy of the fingers may aid in the diagnosis.[7] In primary Raynaud phenomenon, the capillaries are normal, and they may be normal in the secondary phenomenon. In some patients with scleroderma, the capillary loops are enlarged and tortuous and there may be avascular areas. This pattern may also be seen in mixed connective tissue and dermatomyositis. Abnormal capillary loops and a prominent subpapillary venous plexus can occur in systemic lupus erythematosus (SLE). Bushy capillary formations may occur in mixed connective tissue disease.

Objective tests for the diagnosis of Raynaud phenomenon are lacking. Provocation of vasospastic attacks by immersing the hand in cold water, holding a cold tray or iron pipe, or blowing cold air on the fingers with or without body cooling has not usually been successful in primary Raynaud phenomenon. Skin temperature recovery after a cold challenge and digital blood pressure also give inconsistent results. One method that does help to document Raynaud phenomenon is digital systolic pressure measurements after a 5-minute occlusion of the circulation with progressive cooling temperatures. In one study, a relative digital systolic pressure (digital systolic pressure divided by brachial systolic pressure) of less than 70% at local finger cooling temperatures of 15°C and 10°C had a sensitivity of 97.1% in differentiating scleroderma Raynaud phenomenon from the primary phenomenon.[8] This test was also sensitive to differentiate primary Raynaud phenomenon from normal subjects. Other investigators have not found this test to be sensitive. Not many laboratories are equipped to perform this labor-intensive, time-consuming test.

Laboratory blood tests may be helpful in diagnosing some secondary forms of Raynaud phenomenon. In primary Raynaud phenomenon, all tests are normal or negative. Antinuclear antibodies usually indicate the presence of a connective tissue disease, but they also occur in vinyl chloride disease. Anticentromere antibodies are seen in the CREST syndrome. In systemic sclerosis, anti–SCL-70 may be present. A homogeneous pattern of antinuclear antibodies with antibodies to deoxyribonucleic acid is often present in SLE. One study reported that measuring antinuclear antibodies by immunofluorescence and immunoblotting had a positive predictive value of 65% and 71% and a negative predictive value of 93% and 83%, respectively, for diagnosing connective tissue diseases.[9] Immunoblotting was best for diagnosing scleroderma, the CREST syndrome, and mixed connective tissue disease. Even with the presence of an elevated level of antinuclear antibodies, patients with Raynaud phenomenon may not develop other signs and symptoms for many years.

The erythrocyte sedimentation rate is normal in patients with primary and many secondary causes of Raynaud phenomenon. It may be normal in as many as one third of patients with scleroderma.

Patients with Raynaud phenomenon may complain of heartburn, regurgitation, or dysphagia. Although some studies have measured normal esophageal motility in primary Raynaud phenomenon, others have reported esophageal abnormalities. More than two thirds of patients with scleroderma have abnormal peristalis of the lower two thirds of the esophagus and a low esophageal sphincter pressure. Patients with SLE and mixed connective tissue disease may also have esophageal dysfunction.

Using the criteria shown in Table 17.1, about 90% of patients with Raynaud phenomenon can be classified as primary or secondary. A cost-effective workup for patients includes a history, complete physical examination, complete blood count, sedimentation rate, urinalysis, and chest radiography. If the history, physical exam, and laboratory tests are normal, patients can be assured they most likely have the primary, benign disease. Men, persons with the onset of attacks after age 40, and those with severe disease or trophic changes of the digits should have a more extensive workup.

17.4.1 SECONDARY CAUSES OF RAYNAUD PHENOMENON

Secondary causes of Raynaud phenomenon are presented in Table 17.2.

TABLE 17.2
Secondary Causes of Raynaud Phenomenon

Connective tissue diseases
    Systemic lupus erythematosus
    Mixed connective tissue disease
    Sjögren syndrome
    Rheumatoid arthritis
    Polymyositis, dermatomyositis
Carpal tunnel syndrome
Traumatic vasospastic disease
Thoracic outlet syndrome
Drugs
    βadrenergic receptor blocking agents
    Ergot preparations
    Vinblastine and bleomycin
    Methysergide
    Amphetamines
    Imipramine
    Bromocriptine
    Cyclosporine
    Clonidine
Hypothenar hammer syndrome
Obstructive arterial disease
    Thromboangiitis obliterans
    Arteriosclerosis obliterans
    Arterial emboli

(continued)

TABLE 17.2 (CONTINUED)
Secondary Causes of Raynaud Phenomenon

Blood abnormalities
   Cryoproteinemias
Cold agglutinins
Polycythemia
Vasculitis
   Hepatitis B antigemia
Hypothyroidism
Arteriovenous fistula
Neoplasms
Reflex sympathetic dystrophy
Vinyl chloride disease
Primary biliary cirrhosis

17.4.1.1   Connective Tissue Diseases

Approximately 90% of patients with scleroderma or mixed connective tissue disease, one third of patients with SLE or polymyositis, and some patients with rheumatoid arthritis and Sjögren syndrome have Raynaud phenomenon. It is often difficult to rule out a diagnosis of scleroderma despite using the above strict criteria for diagnosis of the primary phenomenon; all criteria may be absent even though scleroderma eventually develops. However, a long history of Raynaud phenomenon with no other symptoms or signs precedes the more benign form of scleroderma, whereas diffuse scleroderma usually develops within a year of the onset of vasospastic attacks. In scleroderma, Raynaud phenomenon is usually severe, with the more common occurrence of digital ulcerations, gangrene, and sclerodactyly. There are often occlusions of the ulnar and digital arteries; in rare cases, there may be occlusion of the radial artery.

17.4.1.2 Carpal Tunnel Syndrome

Carpal tunnel syndrome may manifest Raynaud phenomenon 6 to 12 months before other symptoms. The common causes are occupational (keyboard operators), pregnancy, arthritis, and fractures or dislocations, but any disease causing edema or infiltration of the carpal tunnel may lead to symptoms. Symptoms result from compression of the median nerve in the carpal tunnel and are usually bilateral. The vasospastic attacks may or may not be relieved by decompression of the entrapped nerve after the diagnosis is made by nerve conduction studies.

17.4.1.3 Thoracic Outlet Syndrome

Raynaud phenomenon is especially common in the hyperabduction syndrome. The nerves or blood vessels in the thoracic outlet may be compressed by cervical ribs, the scalenus anticus muscle, between the first rib and clavicle, or by the pectoralis minor tendon. Vasospastic attacks are produced by cold or emotions as in the primary phenomenon. One or both hands may be involved. Attacks may be caused by irritation of the sympathetic nerves. Some patients have emboli to the digital arteries from thrombi in an aneurysm of the subclavian artery distal to the point of compression. Diagnosis is difficult to make except by thoracic outlet maneuvers. Nerve conduction studies are often normal. Exercises to build up the shoulder muscles are the best treatment; surgery is usually only successful when the nerve conduction studies are abnormal.

17.4.1.4 Traumatic Vasospastic Disease

Raynaud phenomenon can be caused by the use of any vibrating tool, but especially chain saws, pneumatic hammers, and brush saws. A very high proportion of chain-saw and brush-saw workers develop the phenomenon, usually after 6,000 to 7,000 hours of exposure. Blanching and numbness of the fingers occur but pain and cyanosis are uncommon. There are protective measures now in place limiting the number of hours of daily vibratory exposure. Vasospastic attacks are alleviated when the patient stops using the tools but do not always completely disappear.

Hammering with the palm of the hand, practicing karate, and using walkers or bowling balls may cause ulnar artery occlusion or aneurysms at the wrist. Digital artery occlusions may be present, probably from emboli from thrombus in the aneurysm. Raynaud phenomenon may develop in the affected hand. Pallor and cyanosis occur, but there is no red, reactive hyperemia phase. Resection of the thrombosed or aneurysmal vessel or bypass surgery is the usual treatment; sympathectomy has also been successful.

17.4.1.5 Drugs

Both selective and nonselective β-adrenoceptor blockers may induce Raynaud phenomenon in both sexes. The mechanism has been postulated to be unopposed α-adrenoceptor vasoconstriction, central cardiovascular depressant effects with increased peripheral sympathetic vasoconstriction, or a decreased cardiac output or blood volume with reflex vasoconstriction. However, administration of β-adrenoceptor blockers does not aggravate the vasospastic attacks in patients who already have Raynaud phenomenon. Ergotamine preparations can cause Raynaud phenomenon by stimulation of α-adrenoceptors. It occurs from excess use of the drugs, usually more than 10 mg a week. Heparin is the treatment of choice until the vessels relax in approximately 3 days, but intra-arterial or intravenous nitroprusside and oral nifedipine have been used. Other drugs reported to cause Raynaud phenomenon are listed in Table 17.2. Treatment of drug-induced Raynaud phenomenon is withdrawal of the medication, when possible. Vasospastic attacks often persist after treatment with vinblastine and bleomycin is completed.

17.4.1.6 Obstructive Arterial Disease

Raynaud phenomenon is a manifestation of thromboangiitis obliterans in over 50% of patients with TAO. It is very difficult to treat, but sympathectomy may help. Vasospastic attacks may occur in the toes of the extremity affected by arteriosclerosis obliterans. Only pallor or cyanosis occurs. Surgical bypass of the arterial obstruction cures the problem. Raynaud phenomenon may also occur in the fingers or toes after an arterial embolus.

17.5 TREATMENT

Figure 17.1 presents a treatment algorithm for Raynaud phenomenon. Most patients with primary Raynaud phenomenon do not consult a physician. Medical advice is usually sought for reassurance that there is no serious underlying disease. Patients should be assured that they have a benign disease that does not lead to loss of digits or limbs. Conservative therapy should be attempted before drug therapy is considered. Hands and feet must be kept warm and dry; mittens should be used instead of gloves because the fingers provide heat to each other. Situations that induce vasospastic attacks should be avoided. Attacks usually involve a cold environment plus pressure on the digits. Grasping a cold steering wheel, holding cold drinks, and picking up frozen food are examples. Patients must also wear warm clothes because digital blood vessels will constrict when cold is applied to almost any area of the body owing to sympathetic nervous system reflexes to save body heat. Moving to a warm climate may be helpful, but air conditioning or sudden small temperature drops may still precipitate attacks. If the patient's hands are dry, a moisturizing cream should be applied frequently to prevent cracking of the skin and ensuing infections. If patients must be exposed to cold, a variety of hand or foot warmers is available. Chemical heat packets are the most useful and last 6 to 8 hours when activated. Warmers can be carried in pockets or slipped into mittens and shoes. Tobacco smoking should be avoided because it causes cutaneous vasoconstriction.

If the patient has mild to moderate disease and desires active therapy, Pavlovian conditioning or biofeedback can be tried. Conditioning requires that patients immerse their hands in 43° C water for 30 minutes while their lightly clothed bodies are exposed to 0° temperature.[10] Sessions take place daily for 3 weeks. Treated patients have

Treatment of Raynaud Phenomenon

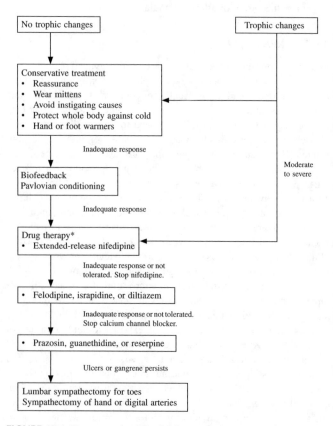

FIGURE 17.1 Treatment algorithm for Raynaud phenomenon. *Use of combination drugs with different actions has not been studied.

shown a rise in digital temperature on cold exposure compared with untreated patients. Subjective benefit may be maintained for 1 year. Many types of biofeedback have been studied. Some have used digital temperature feedback or muscle relaxation with frontalis electromyographic feedback. Some patients have been able to raise their skin temperature, and symptoms may improve moderately to markedly. Finger-temperature increases have not always correlated with the decreased frequency of vasospastic attacks. Patients with connective tissue diseases often can raise their finger temperatures more than patients with the primary phenomenon.

If vasospastic attacks interfere with work or daily activities, or if digital ulcers or gangrene develops, drug therapy should be considered. Pharmacologic agents may decrease the frequency, severity, and duration of vasospastic attacks but do not correct the underlying abnormality. They may be effective in primary and secondary Raynaud phenomenon. Most medications have side effects, some of which are tolerable, but others are not.

17.5.1 CALCIUM CHANNEL BLOCKERS

Calcium channel blockers selectively block the movement of calcium ions in the slow channels leading to decreased smooth muscle contractility. Nifedipine has also been shown to block α_2-adrenoceptors in *in vitro* studies. Several of these drugs are potent peripheral vasodilators, especially the dihydropyridines.

Nifedipine is the best studied of these drugs and has been shown to decrease the number and severity of vasospastic attacks in primary and secondary Raynaud phenomenon, although patients with the primary condition may receive the most benefit.[11] Digital ulcers have been reported to heal in patients with scleroderma. Children have shown as much benefit as adults. Adverse reactions to nifedipine are transient or continual headaches, lightheadedness, palpitations, flushing, leg edema, and gum hyperplasia. About two thirds of patients report subjective benefit. Most studies have been performed with the short-acting preparation, but the extended-release preparations have been shown to be effective, with fewer side effects. Patients should be started on the extended-release 30 mg preparation, which can be increased to 60 mg or 90 mg if needed. Most patients require 60 mg daily.

Another potent peripheral vasodilator, felodipine, has been shown to be of benefit in two small studies. In one of these studies, it compared favorably to nifedipine. Side effects are palpitations, faintness, ankle swelling, and headaches. A daily dose of 5 mg to 10 mg is recommended.

Israpidine, also a strong vasodilator, has been shown to decrease the frequency and severity of vasospastic attacks in an open-label study. Side effects include leg edema, dizziness, flushing, fatigue, and abdominal discomfort. The recommended daily dose is 5 mg to 20 mg.

Diltiazem significantly decreased the frequency, duration, and severity of vasospastic attacks in patients with primary or secondary Raynaud phenomenon in three placebo-controlled studies. It benefited about two thirds of patients. However, one study found no effect of this drug in patients with secondary Raynaud phenomenon. Side effects are not as frequent as with nifedipine and include headache, flushing, nausea, ankle edema, and lightheadedness. The usual dose has been 30 mg to 120 mg 3 times a day. There are no studies with the extended-release preparations.

17.5.2 SYMPATHOLYTIC AGENTS

Prazosin is a specific α_1-adrenoceptor antagonist that has been shown to decrease the frequency and duration of attacks in patients with primary or secondary Raynaud phenomenon in several studies. One study reported that improvement lessened with prolonged treatment.[12] About two thirds of patients have an overall good but moderate response. Side effects include nausea, headache, palpitations, lightheadedness, fatigue, leg edema, and diarrhea. A daily dosage of 2 mg to 8 mg is recommended, usually in divided doses. Because syncope has been reported with the first dose, 1 mg should be given at bedtime.

Reserpine depletes norepinephrine from arterial walls and has been used in the treatment of Raynaud phenomenon. Reserpine has been shown to increase the capillary blood flow in fingertips of patients with primary or secondary Raynaud phenomenon in both warm and cool environments.[13] Several uncontrolled studies have shown that oral reserpine may benefit some patients. Patients with primary and secondary Raynaud phenomenon have responded. The recommended oral dose of reserpine is 0.25 mg to 1.0 mg daily. The smaller dose should be started and then increased weekly until there is relief of symptoms or nasal congestion or bradycardia develops. Bradycardia, postural hypotension symptoms, dyspepsia, fluid retention, lethargy, and depression are possible side effects. Reserpine should not be used in patients with depression or a history of depression.

Guanethidine interferes with the release of norepinephrine at the sympathetic neuroeffector junction. It has been shown to increase finger capillary blood flow during body cooling in patients with scleroderma. No controlled studies of guanethidine in patients with Raynaud phenomenon have been performed, but investigators have reported it to be of value. Recommended doses are 10 mg to 50 mg daily, starting with the smallest dose and increasing the dose weekly until relief of symptoms or development of side effects. The most common side effects are symptoms of postural hypotension, diarrhea, and impotence.

17.5.3   NITROGLYCERIN PREPARATIONS

Nitroglycerin ointment has been used in the treatment of Raynaud phenomenon for many years. Study results have been varied. Nitroglycerin is a direct-acting vasodilator that has a greater action on the venous than the arterial circulation, although it increased fingertip blood flow in normal subjects to a greater extent than nitroprusside when given intra-arterially. In a study of patients with secondary Raynaud phenomenon, 1% nitroglycerin ointment, compared with lanolin placebo, decreased the number and severity of vasospastic attacks and ulcers healed. All 17 patients in this study were on maximally tolerated doses of sympatholytic agents. Nitropatches were reported to be of benefit in one study, but were ineffective in another. Recommended doses are 2% nitroglycerin ointment (7.5 mg to 30 mg) twice a day, or 5 cm^2 nitropatches.

17.5.4   ANGIOTENSIN INHIBITORS

Captopril and other angiotensin-converting enzyme inhibitors block
the angiotensin I to angiotensin II reaction and also inhibit kininase
II, which allows the vasodilator bradykinin to accumulate. An original
report of two patients with scleroderma treated with large doses of
captopril (600 mg daily) to control their blood pressure found that their
fingers became warm and digital ulcers healed. Two uncontrolled studies
of smaller doses of captopril reported improvement in vasospastic
attacks in some patients with primary or secondary Raynaud phenomenon. A recent analysis of the studies of angiotensin-converting
enzyme inhibitors concluded that there is little evidence that they are
effective treatment.[14]

Losartin, a drug that blocks the angiotensin receptor has been the
subject of one small study of patients with primary Raynaud phenomenon. There was a significant decrease in the frequency and severity
of vasospastic attacks compared with placebo treatment. More studies
are needed. The recommended daily dose of losartin is 50 mg to 100
mg. Side effects are few, but muscle cramps, dizziness, or insomnia
may occur.

17.5.5   THYROID PREPARATIONS

As early as 1960, triiodothyroxine was reported to alleviate vasospastic
attacks in euthyroid patients with primary Raynaud phenomenon. In
a more recent study, 60 µg to 80 µg of triiodothyroxine daily decreased
the frequency, duration, and severity of vasospastic attacks in 18
patients with secondary Raynaud phenomenon compared with placebo. However, there was a high incidence of palpitations and
increases in pulse rate and pulse pressure at this dose. The investigators
recommended that smaller doses should be studied. In patients with
hypothyroidism, thyroid replacement therapy may alleviate the vasospastic attacks.

17.5.6   PROSTAGLANDINS

Prostaglandins can induce vasodilation and inhibit platelet aggregation. Small studies of intravenous prostaglandin E_1 have shown promise for the treatment of Raynaud phenomenon, but a multicenter study found no benefit in patients with the primary or secondary phenomenon compared with placebo. Studies of prostacyclin (PGI_2) and its analog, iloprost, are more promising and report long-term benefits after daily infusions for 3 weeks. One study compared intravenous iloprost with oral nifedipine and found significant improvement with both drugs.[15] Side effects of hypotension, headache, facial flushing, abdominal pain, nausea, vomiting, and diarrhea occurred only during the iloprost infusions, whereas the side effects of nifedipine continued. Improvement with iloprost lasted several weeks. Prostaglandins are not available for this indication in the United States.

17.5.7   SYMPATHECTOMY

Sympathectomy of the upper extremities has been performed to alleviate vasospastic attacks in patients with Raynaud phenomenon. Although reports claim that 50% to 60% of patients are improved, vasospastic attacks often recur at the same frequency and intensity in 6 months to 2 years.[16] Return of sympathetic vasoconstrictor activity has been attributed to incomplete denervation, reinnervation, or denervation hypersensitivity. Several surgical approaches have been used, including endoscopy. Both pre- and postganglionic resection have been tried with little difference in results. This treatment cannot be recommended for primary or secondary Raynaud phenomenon. Complications of surgery include pleural effusion, hemothorax, pneumothorax, neuralgia, wound sepsis and hematomas, atrial fibrillation, and Horner syndrome.

In contrast to cervicothoracic sympathectomy, lumbar sympathectomy is very successful treatment for Raynaud phenomenon of the toes. Cures are common and results are usually permanent. More than 80% of patients show improvement. Complications of the surgery are neuralgia and wound hematoma or sepsis. There may be excess sweating of the upper body.

Resection of portions of thrombosed digital arteries and vein bypasses of arterial obstructions have been performed with beneficial results in some patients with severe ischemia or ulcers. It may be that these operations also produce sympathectomy of the arteries. Digital artery sympathectomy has also improved digital ischemia and cold intolerance.

REFERENCES

1. Coffman, J.D., *Raynaud's Phenomenon*, Oxford University Press, New York, 1989.
2. Coffman, J.D., Raynaud's phenomenon, an update, *Hypertension*, 17, 593, 1991.
3. Heslop, J., Coggon, D., and Acheson, E.D., The prevalence of intermittent digital ischemia (Raynaud's phenomenon) in a general practice, *J. Coll. Gen. Pract.*, 33, 85, 1983.
4. Maricq, H.R., Carpentier, P., Weinrich, M.C., et al., Geographic variation in the prevalence of Raynaud's phenomenon: Charleston, SC, USA, vs. Tarentaise, Savoire, France, *J. Rheumatol.*, 20, 70, 1993.
5. Riera, G., Vilardell, M., Vaqué, J., et al., Prevalence of Raynaud's phenomenon in a healthy Spanish population, *J. Rheumatol.*, 20, 66, 1993.
6. Gifford, R.W., Jr. and Hines, E.A., Jr., Raynaud's disease among women and girls, *Circulation*, 16, 1012, 1957.
7. Maricq, H.R., LeRoy, E.C., D'Angelo, W.A., et al., Diagnostic potential of *in vivo* capillary microscopy in scleroderma and related disorders, *Arthritis Rheum.*, 23, 183, 1980.
8. Maricq, H.R., Weinrich, M.C., Valter, I., et al., Digital vascular responses to cooling in subjects with cold sensitivity, primary Raynaud's phenomenon, or scleroderma spectrum disorders, *J. Rheumatol.*, 23, 2068, 1996.
9. Wollersheim, H., Thien, T.H., Hoet, M.H., et al., The diagnostic value of several immunological tests for anti-nuclear disease in patients presenting with Raynaud's phenomenon, *Eur. J. Clin. Invest.*, 19, 535, 1989.

10. Jobe, J.B., Sampson, J.B., Roberts, D.E., et al., Induced vasodilation as treatment for Raynaud's disease, *Ann. Intern. Med.*, 97, 706, 1982.

11. Smith, C.D. and McKendry, R.V.R., Controlled trial of nifedipine in the treatment of Raynaud's phenomenon, *Lancet*, ii, 1299, 1982.

12. Nielsen, SL., Vithing, K., and Rasmussen, K., Prazosin treatment of primary Raynaud's phenomenon, *Eur. J. Clin. Pharmacol.*, 24, 421, 1983.

13. Coffman, J.D. and Cohen, A.S., Total and capillary fingertip blood flow in Raynaud's phenomenon, *N. Engl. J. Med.*, 285, 259,1971.

14. Challenor, V.F., Angiotensin converting enzyme inhibitors in Raynaud's phenomenon, *Drug*, 48, 864, 1994.

15. Rademaker, M., Cooke, E.D., Almond, N.E., et al. Comparison of intravenous infusions of iloprost and oral nifedipine in treatment of Raynaud's phenomenon in patients with systemic sclerosis: a double blind randomized study, *BMJ*, 298, 561, 1989.

16. Baddeley, R.M., The place of upper dorsal sympathectomy in the treatment of primary Raynaud's disease, *Br. J. Surg.*, 52, 426, 1965.

Section VI

Less Common Vascular Diseases and Syndromes

18 Unusual Vascular Diseases of the Extremities

Jeffrey W. Olin

CONTENTS

18.1 Introduction 388
18.2 Popliteal Artery Entrapment Syndrome 388
    18.2.1 Clinical Presentation 391
    18.2.2 Treatment 392
18.3 Cystic Adventitial Disease 395
18.4 Fibromuscular Dysplasia of the Extremities 398
18.5 Arterial Calcification Diseases 400
    18.5.1 Mönckeberg Arteriosclerosis 400
    18.5.2 Idiopathic Infantile Arterial Calcification.................401
    18.5.3 Arterial Calcification Associated with Chronic
              Renal Failure 401
18.6 Ergotism 403
18.7 Livedo Reticularis 403
    18.7.1 Treatment 404
18.8 Acrocyanosis 405
18.9 Pernio (Chilblains) 405
    18.9.1 Clinical Manifestations 406
    18.9.2 Treatment 407
18.10 Erythromelalgia...407
References..409

0-8493-8413-3/01/$0.00+$1.50

18.1   INTRODUCTION

Claudication is the most common symptom indicating arterial insufficiency of the lower extremities. The most common cause of claudication is atherosclerosis. However, when claudication occurs in a younger individual in whom the suspicion of atherosclerosis is low, other causes of exercise-induced leg discomfort should be considered. Some of these disorders are: thromboembolism, thromboangiitis obliterans (TAO, or Buerger's disease; see Chapter 15), popliteal artery entrapment syndrome (PAES), cystic adventitial disease, fibromuscular dysplasia, ergotamine ingestion, popliteal artery aneurysm, vasculitis (see Chapter 16), and connective tissue diseases. The scope of this chapter precludes discussion of all of these disorders; therefore, only the more common and important causes are discussed. Other less common types of vascular disease are also described.

18.2   POPLITEAL ARTERY ENTRAPMENT SYNDROME

Entrapment of the popliteal artery is often encountered in younger individuals, although it can occur in all age groups. Although entrapment can occur at a number of sites (axillary, brachial, celiac, common femoral, and superficial femoral arteries), the most common site is the popliteal artery.

Popliteal artery entrapment was first described in 1879 by T.P. Anderson Stuart, focusing on an amputated gangrenous limb.[1] He described the abnormal pathology of the popliteal artery as it deviated medially around the medial head of the gastrocnemius muscle rather than coursing between the heads of the muscle. The involved muscle rose much higher on the femoral condyle than usual, allowing space for the artery to pass. Other anatomic variations have been described over the years. In 1965, Love and Whelan labeled this disease PAES.[2]

Popliteal artery entrapment has generally been regarded as a congenital aberration. Most frequently, the medial head of the gastrocnemius muscle has been the compressing structure, although involvement of a concomitant compressive popliteal muscle or band may also occur.[3] Iatrogenic entrapment after placement of bypass grafts has also been described. This technical error usually has been the result of placing the graft medial to the medial head of the gastrocnemius muscle.

Different classification schemes for PAES have been based on anatomic or angiographic characteristics. However, there are so many different anomalies in muscle, arterial, venous, and neural structures, it is virtually impossible to create a simple classification for these disorders. The normal anatomy is shown in Figure 18.1 and the most common types of anomalies are shown in Figures 18.2 to 18.4.[4]

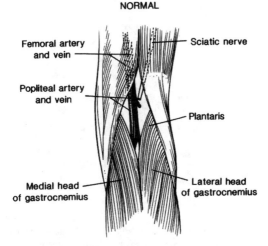

NORMAL

Femoral artery and vein

Sciatic nerve

Popliteal artery and vein

Plantaris

Medial head of gastrocnemius

Lateral head of gastrocnemius

FIGURE 18.1 Normal anatomic relation (posterior view) of the right popliteal space. (From Insua, J.A., Young, J.R., and Humphries, A.W., Popliteal artery entrapment syndrome, *Arch. Surg.*, 101 ,771, 1970. Copyrighted 1970, American Medical Association. With permission.[4])

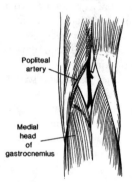

FIGURE 18.2 Type I anomaly. The popliteal artery deviates medially around the medial head of the gastrocnemius muscle that arises close to its normal location. (From Insua, J.A., Young, J.R., and Humphries, A.W., Popliteal artery entrapment syndrome, *Arch. Surg.*, 101, 771, 1970. Copyrighted 1970, American Medical Association. With permission.[4])

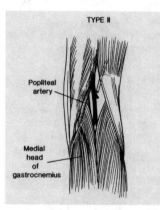

FIGURE 18.3 Type II anomaly. The medial head of the gastrocnemius muscle arises more laterally on the femoral condyle, with a separation between the artery and vein. The artery may be minimally displaced on the arteriogram. (From Insua, J.A., Young, J.R., and Humphries, A.W., Popliteal artery entrapment syndrome, *Arch. Surg.*, 101, 771, 1970. Copyrighted 1970, American Medical Association. With permission.[4])

TYPE III

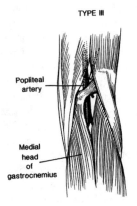

Popliteal
artery

Medial
head
of
gastrocnemius

FIGURE 18.4 Type III anomaly. The popliteal artery is entrapped by a lateral slip of the medial gastrocnemius muscle. The artery takes a normal course. (From Insua, J.A., Young, J.R., and Humphries, A.W., Popliteal artery entrapment syndrome, *Arch. Surg.*, 101, 771, 1970. Copyrighted 1970, American Medical Association. With permission.[4])

18.2.1 CLINICAL PRESENTATION

Most commonly, a healthy, "athletic-type" male notes typical claudication symptoms in the absence of evidence of premature atherosclerosis. It is not unusual for the onset of the claudication to be sudden. Patients may also describe nocturnal cramps, numbness, paresthesias, focal ischemia in the distal digits, worsening of symptoms with knee flexion, or the sudden development of a cold leg. Symptoms are, in a large part, dependent on the degree of stenosis and the presence of collateral flow. Acute thrombosis, distal embolization, or rupture of the artery can also occur if entrapment leads to poststenotic dilation and aneurysm formation.

Males are involved predominantly by a 15:1 ratio over females. Patient age at the time of diagnosis has ranged from 12 to 64 years, with 60% being younger than 30 years of age. Bilateral popliteal artery involvement has been found in 22% to 67% of individuals.

Palpation of the arteries in the involved limb is the cornerstone of the initial evaluation. The timing and the quality of the pulse may suggest the level of disease, the extent of involvement, and the presence of aneurysm. The disappearance of the pulse with passive dorsiflexion of the foot or active plantar flexion against resistance may suggest the diagnosis.[5] In patients with pulses that are difficult to palpate, duplex ultrasound increases the diagnostic yield. Pulse volume recordings may be helpful in making the diagnosis of PAES. A baseline waveform and blood pressure is established with the patient in the supine position. The foot is then put through flexion maneuvers, and changes in the flow tracing can be evaluated. Finally, the addition of stress testing with treadmill walking can precipitate symptoms and document the physiologic and functional alterations in blood flow.[6]

Confirmatory evidence for PAES can be provided by computed tomography (CT) or magnetic resonance imaging (MRI).[7,8] CT scanning can clearly delineate soft tissue, vascular, and bony structures much better than ultrasound. The relation between the popliteal artery and vein, the architecture of the local osseous prominences, and the presence of underlying muscle can be documented. Furthermore, both popliteal spaces can be evaluated at the same time. Clinically, this is also useful in differentiating cystic adventitial disease of the popliteal artery from PAES.

Arteriography remains a useful adjunct to CT or MRI. A characteristic finding is medial deviation of the artery in the popliteal region, although the course of the artery may be normal (Figure 18.5). Poststenotic dilation, aneurysms, and mid-popliteal artery occlusion (Figure 18.6) are other findings that may be present.[8] Other entities that may cause mid-popliteal arterial occlusion include cystic adventitial disease, thrombosed popliteal artery aneurysm, and atherosclerosis. The arteriogram is helpful to the surgeon to fully delineate the anatomy before surgical repair.

18.2.2 TREATMENT

Once the diagnosis of PAES is made, surgical intervention is warranted regardless of symptoms. Surgical repair prevents thrombotic and

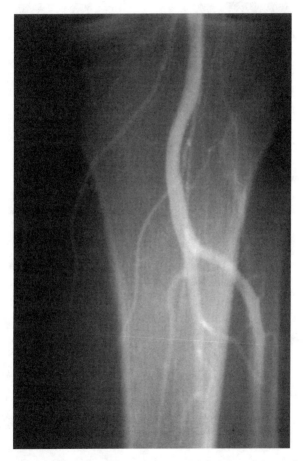

FIGURE 18.5 Arteriogram demonstrating medial deviation of the popliteal artery. This can be seen in a type I anomaly and in a type IV anomaly (popliteus muscle or fibrous band compresses the popliteal artery).

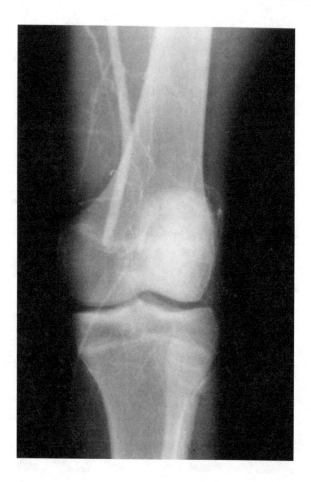

FIGURE 18.6 Popliteal artery occlusion in a patient with popliteal artery entrapment syndrome.

embolic complications, which can be quite serious. If the artery is already thrombosed, or if emboli have occurred, the surgical procedure can be preceded by attempting catheter-directed thrombolytic therapy. The surgical approach is made either through a medial or posterior incision. The medial approach is generally used in standard bypass surgery. However, the posterior approach offers a distinct advantage in the ability to visualize many of these anatomic variants. Transection of the offending structure is mandatory, as the artery needs to be freely mobilized. The condition of the underlying vessel dictates the need for thrombectomy, resection, patch angioplasty, or bypass procedure. Aneurysms need to be treated with excision or bypass and ligation. Excellent long-term results have been achieved by using a saphenous vein interposition graft.

18.3 CYSTIC ADVENTITIAL DISEASE

Cystic adventitial disease most commonly affects the popliteal artery, although it can be associated with other upper- or lower-extremity vessels.[9,10] Although the first reported case of cystic adventitial disease occurred in 1946,[11] by 1970 approximately 40 cases had been reported in the world literature, with most of them involving the popliteal artery and causing either stenosis or occlusion of the affected vessel.[12] Most patients with cystic adventitial disease are men, with a mean age of 42 years.[13]

The cyst arises in the outer tunica media or subadventitial layer with cyst expansion into the adventitia of the vessel wall. The rate of growth is unknown, but once the intracystic pressure exceeds that in the lumen of the vessel, stenosis (70%) or occlusion (30%) results. The exact pathophysiologic mechanism for the development of cystic adventitial disease is unknown. However, cystic adventitial disease is an isolated lesion, devoid of a systemic process.

Analysis of pathologic specimens reveals a cyst arising from the subadventitial layer or the outer tunica media layer of the vessel. The cyst is usually filled with clear fluid, although it can be hemorrhagic (currant jelly appearance) or even yellow in color. Mucoprotein and mucopolysaccharides, hyaluronic acid, and hydroxyproline have been reported as the major cystic components. The mechanism for the fluid accumulation in the cyst is unknown.

Claudication in a younger individual in the absence of atherosclerotic risk factors should heighten the clinical suspicion of cystic adventitial disease. Typically, symptoms develop over several months and can wax and wane.[14] The degree of artery narrowing, as well as the degree of collateralization, dictates the severity of claudication. In the presence of stenosis, distal pulses are frequently present, but may disappear upon flexion of the knee joint (Ishikawa sign).[10] A systolic bruit in the popliteal artery may be present. Occlusion of the involved artery usually appears with absent distal pulses, but distal ischemia at rest or neurologic deficit secondary to ischemia is a rare finding.

Pulse volume recordings may show the characteristic drop in blood pressure and change in waveform configuration at the affected level. These changes may not be evident at rest but can be brought out by exercise. Duplex ultrasound can be helpful in recognizing the presence of a perivascular cystic structure. Ultrasound can demonstrate hypoechoic spaces that may be septated, whereas Doppler imaging can show turbulence and an elevated velocity of blood flow in the area of stenosis.[16] CT scanning can provide direct evidence of adjacent masses, muscle insertions, and the course of the artery.[14,16] On CT, the cystic contents show no enhancement and the relative attenuation value is between those of water and muscle, thus clearly delineating the soft tissue structures.

Arteriography is a very useful diagnostic test, especially when lateral and anterior–posterior projections are performed. The arteriographic appearance is most frequently that of a scimitar, hourglass, or flute embouchure configuration but can also appear as an M-shaped or triangular filling defect (Figure 18.7).[10]

Treatment options differ on the basis of whether the artery is stenotic or occluded.[10] In the past, most cases were diagnosed at the time of surgery, after the artery had occluded. However, with increased awareness of the disease and with excellent noninvasive diagnostic studies available, early diagnosis allows greater treatment options. In

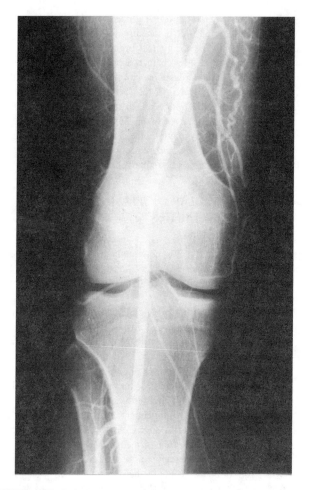

FIGURE 18.7 Typical angiographic appearance of cystic adventitial disease. Note scimitar appearance caused by the cyst compressing the popliteal artery.

the stenotic lesion, ultrasound or CT-guided needle aspiration of the cyst has been attempted, but the recurrence rate is high.[17] Needle aspiration, which may be the logical initial therapy in the stenotic lesion, may improve the flow characteristics of the involved vessel. Percutaneous balloon angioplasty has not proven to be a viable alternative.[18] If the artery is occluded, intra-arterial thrombolysis should be considered as the initial procedure to restore lumen patency. The underlying lesion can then be corrected. Surgical therapy that includes evacuation with vein or synthetic patch, or simple aspiration has an overall success rate of 85% compared with a success rate of 91% in patients undergoing surgical revascularization.

18.4 FIBROMUSCULAR DYSPLASIA OF THE EXTREMITIES

Fibromuscular dysplasia (FMD) is an uncommon, noninflammatory disease of the arteries. FMD most commonly involves the renal arteries (60% to 75%) but has been described in almost every arterial bed, including the cervicocranial (25% to 30%), visceral (9%), and extremity arteries (5%).[14,19–22]

Most types of FMD occur predominantly in females.[19] Clinical suspicion of FMD should be raised when a young woman develops hypertension. In 24% of patients with FMD there is involvement in more than one vascular territory.[21]

The angiographic appearance is often quite suggestive of FMD, but some forms of FMD (i.e., intimal fibroplasia) can mimic a large artery vasculitis such as giant-cell arteritis or Takayasu arteritis. Diagnosis is best made with histologic confirmation, but this is rarely available. Therefore, the classic angiographic features and a lack of systemic manifestations are often all that is needed to make a correct diagnosis. The typical angiographic appearance of medial fibroplasia is that of a string of beads, where the beads are larger than the normal caliber of the native artery. Intimal disease is characterized as either long, smooth narrowing, or a concentric-like band around the artery.[19,20] The appearance of concomitant atherosclerosis may make the diagnosis more difficult, particularly in the older age groups; however, classic intimal or medial changes on arteriography are highly suggestive of FMD.[23] Lesions of FMD typically arise in the middle or distal arterial segments, sparing orificial or bifurcation sites typical of atherosclerotic disease.[19,20]

The histologic classification system of renal artery FMD proposed by Harrison and McCormack is also used for extrarenal FMD.[24] These authors separated FMD into subtypes according to the layers of vessel wall involved. The classification includes intimal fibroplasia, medial hyperplasia, medial fibroplasia, perimedial fibroplasia, and periarterial fibroplasia. Whether spontaneous dissection is a complication of FMD or whether it is a separate category of FMD remains controversial. The pathogenesis of FMD is not known.

The differential diagnosis of FMD should include vasospasm, arterial hypoplasia, and vasculitis. In the presence of arterial dilations, other considerations include aneurysmal disease, pseudoaneurysm, or atherosclerosis with poststenotic dilation. Disease conditions that have been associated with FMD include coarctation of the aorta, neurofibromatosis, pheochromocytoma, Ehlers-Danlos syndrome type IV,[25] and Alport syndrome.

FMD has been described in all of the peripheral arteries of the extremities (iliac, superficial femoral, popliteal, tibial, subclavian, axillary, radial, and ulnar). These lesions are typically asymptomatic, but can produce signs and symptoms such as a difference in blood pressure, paresthesias, claudication, or critical limb ischemia (CLI).[26] FMD should be considered in the differential diagnosis in all young patients with claudication.

Most studies of FMD in the extremities demonstrate a female predominance. Vasculitis, TAO, aneurysmal disease, or atherosclerosis can masquerade as FMD. The symptomatic population has generally been older than 50 years of age, but complications of aneurysmal disease have been reported in the very young. Older patients may have had predominantly asymptomatic FMD, but when the atherosclerotic process is superimposed on FMD, symptoms may arise. Most cases of FMD have been diagnosed angiographically. Intimal fibroplasia seems to be the most frequent histologic subtype seen in peripheral FMD, although medial and perimedial fibroplasias have been described.[27–29]

The appropriate interventional therapy may be different, depending on the site, extent, and distal manifestations of the disease. Therapy should be reserved for symptomatic disease. Successful therapies reported in the past include graduated intraluminal dilation, surgical bypass or resection, and sympathetic blockade or transection. If intervention is indicated, percutaneous balloon angioplasty is now considered the procedure of choice.[19,20] Surgical bypass is rarely required for this condition.

18.5   ARTERIAL CALCIFICATION DISEASES

A heterogenous group of diseases (Mönckeberg arteriosclerosis or medial calcinosis, idiopathic infantile arterial calcification, and arterial calcification associated with chronic renal failure) share a common feature of arterial calcification.

18.5.1   Mönckeberg Arteriosclerosis

In 1903, Mönckeberg described a condition of extensive calcification involving the tunica media of the large and medium-sized arteries. This calcification can involve the lower extremities and the visceral and upper-extremity vessels. The actual mechanism leading to calcification is unknown, but calcium, phosphate, and parathyroid hormone levels are usually normal. The dense medial calcinosis produces a rigid conduit without encroachment on the vessel lumen. Therefore, end-organ ischemia is not a complication.[30] Mönckeberg arteriosclerosis is distinctly different from the intimal and medial calcification seen with atherosclerosis, where plaque progression leads to luminal narrowing and, ultimately, ischemia. Calcification in atherosclerosis is diffuse and frequently affects orificial and bifurcation arterial sites.

Patients with diabetes tend to have a higher incidence of medial arterial calcification.[31] Corticosteroids and immunosuppressant therapies have also been implicated in stimulating calcification. Histologic examination of affected arteries shows fibrotic and calcified replacement of the tunica media. The internal and external elastic lamina may be involved in the fibrotic process, whereas the intima is normal in pure Mönckeberg arteriosclerosis.[30] The intimal changes of atherosclerosis can be superimposed on the medial disruption of Mönckeberg arteriosclerosis. This is usually present in patients over 50 years of age, who may have had asymptomatic medial calcification for years.

Diagnosis of Mönckeberg arteriosclerosis is usually made by the classic radiographic appearance on plain radiograms. These changes are described as ringlike calcifications against a finely granular background.

18.5.2 IDIOPATHIC INFANTILE ARTERIAL CALCIFICATION

Idiopathic infantile arterial calcification has been reported in fewer than 100 cases.[32] Diagnosis has been made by postmortem examination in most cases, but as awareness of the condition broadens, premortem and even prepartum diagnoses have been made. Most newborns and infants who develop cardiac or respiratory dysfunction, with myocardial ischemia being the primary mode of death, do so early in life. Marked intimal proliferation sets this disease apart from the other calcification disorders, especially with the aggressive and progressive nature of the disease process. Calcification may affect all of the vessels, including the heart, brain, mesentery, and extremities.

Treatment has consisted of strict blood pressure control with calcium channel blockers or angiotensin-converting enzyme inhibitors. Although most patients die at an early age, diphosphonates combined with a low-calcium diet have been shown to cause regression of the vessel calcification in some patients.

18.5.3 ARTERIAL CALCIFICATION ASSOCIATED WITH CHRONIC RENAL FAILURE

Arterial disease is common in patients with chronic renal insufficiency, especially if diabetes is also present. The prevalence of arterial calcification is substantially greater in the dialysis population as compared with subjects with normal renal function. At least one third of dialysis patients have arterial calcification, and this number escalates to 90% of diabetic dialysis patients.[33]

Atherosclerosis usually does not occur in the distal portion of the arms or hands. An exception to this rule occurs in patients with chronic renal failure, especially those with diabetes who undergo chronic dialysis treatment or who have undergone renal transplantation. The exact pathogenesis of this involvement of the arms and hands is unknown, but it cannot be solely explained on the basis of calcium–phosphorus imbalance or hyperparathyroidism. Accelerated atherosclerosis seems to be a more likely explanation, with an associated progressive systemic intimal proliferation. The smaller-caliber vessels are most affected by the intimal proliferation; therefore an acral distribution to the ischemia ensues. Usually, there is calcification of the media. These patients can present in a dramatic fashion, with progressive gangrene of the fingers eventually leading to multiple amputations and, occasionally, loss of the entire hand.[34] There is no known treatment for this complication.

Another severe form of calcification in end-stage renal disease patients is called systemic calcinosis, metastatic calcification, or calciphylaxis. This infrequent soft tissue and arterial deposition of calcium phosphate complex (hydroxyapatite) is a result of a high calcium–phosphorus product (greater than 60 to 70).[35] Precipitation occurs in the connective tissue of organs such as the skin, lungs, kidneys, stomach, heart, and arteries. Most patients have elevated parathyroid hormone levels. Factors that exacerbate this calcification process include vitamin D, calcium carbonate, corticosteroids, immunosuppressants, and blood product therapies.[35]

The goal of treatment is to lower the calcium phosphate product and remove any aggravating factors. Parathyroidectomy has been performed with successful reversal of the calcification process in some patients. A vigilant approach should also be taken to control infectious and septic complications, as this is a frequent complicating feature. Early reports suggest that hyperbaric oxygen may be of help in some patients.

18.6 ERGOTISM

Ergotamine preparations are often used to treat migraine headaches. The effect of these drugs on the vascular system, causing intense vasoconstriction leading to severe pain and burning of the extremities (thus the name Saint Anthony fire), has been known for centuries. Excessive use of ergotamine preparations can produce CLI.[36] If this is not recognized in time, it can lead to limb loss. The angiographic appearance is that of normal proximal vessels, with a gradual tapering of vessels until ultimately no vessels are seen. It is not uncommon to see a total absence of blood vessels from the knee distally.

A careful history for the presence of migraine headaches will alert the clinician to the possibility of ergotamine use. If the patient denies ergotamine use, and no other plausible cause of lower-extremity ischemia exists, ergotamine blood levels should be obtained. We cite a patient who denied the use of ergotamine preparations and was willing to undergo bilateral above-knee amputations. When her room was searched, dozens of ergotamine suppositories were found.

In addition to lower-extremity ischemia, ergotamine has been associated with stroke, myocardial infarction, ischemic bowel, and upper-extremity ischemia. The cornerstone of treatment is to stop the use of all ergotamine preparations. To reverse the intense vasoconstriction associated with these agents, intravenous sodium nitroprusside and oral calcium channel blockers are quite effective. Although not commonly encountered, ergotamine abuse requires a high index of suspicion. Once the diagnosis is made, treatment is usually quite effective.

18.7 LIVEDO RETICULARIS

Livedo reticularis is characterized by a reticular, fishnet, or lacy pattern on the skin, most often of the lower extremities. However, any part of the body can be involved. The reticular pattern is red or blue in color and is caused by deoxygenated blood in the surrounding horizontally arranged venous plexus.[37]

Primary or benign livedo reticularis occurs most commonly in young women. Ulceration generally does not occur with primary livedo reticularis. The primary form may be due to vasomotor instability or hyperreactivity of the dermal blood vessels. The condition is intensified by cold exposure and may occur in association with Raynaud phenomenon or disease.

Secondary livedo reticularis occurs in association with atheromatous embolization (see Chapter 14), polyarteritis nodosa, systemic lupus erythematosus (SLE), leukocytoclastic vasculitis, connective tissue diseases, amantadine hydrochloride, various neurologic or endocrine diseases, and in patients receiving large doses of pressors such as epinephrine, norepinephrine, and dopamine. Livedo reticularis is one of the many skin manifestations of the antiphospholipid antibody syndrome. In Sneddon syndrome there is the combination of livedo racemosa (a variant of livedo reticularis) and small-vessel ischemic disease of the brain, producing transient ischemic attack or stroke. Approximately 50% of patients with Sneddon syndrome have elevated anticardiolipin antibodies.

In livedoid vasculopathy or livedoid vasculitis, there is extensive livedo reticularis surrounding an ischemic-appearing ulceration. These ulcers may be located on the anterior or posterior portion of the lower leg and are extremely painful. Pathologically, there is thrombosis of the microvasculature with little or no active inflammatory component

18.7.1 TREATMENT

The treatment of livedo depends on the underlying disease. The benign variety often needs no treatment other than measures to keep the body part as warm as possible. Therapy should be directed at the underlying cause in patients with secondary livedo reticularis. Small doses of tissue plasminogen activator (10 mg intravenously daily for 14 days) may be very effective in treating the ulcerations associated with livedoid vasculopathy.[38]

18.8   ACROCYANOSIS

A persistent blue or cyanotic discoloration of the digits is present in patients with acrocyanosis.[37] This disorder occurs most commonly in the hands but may involve other parts of the body. Acrocyanosis may worsen with exposure to cold and improve with rewarming of the limb. The primary form is a benign condition that is mainly a cosmetic problem for patients. Acrocyanosis may also be seen in patients with connective tissue diseases, TAO (Buerger's disease), and diseases associated with central cyanosis.

The pathophysiologic abnormality in acrocyanosis is not clear. Some authors suggest that there is vasospasm in the cutaneous arteries and arterioles. There may be an abnormal vascular response to the cold, because with body heating or hand rewarming the color returns to normal.

The overall prognosis is excellent, and tissue loss or ulceration generally does not occur. Patients should be advised to keep their extremities warm. Sympathetic inhibiting drugs, α-blocking agents, or calcium channel blockers may be helpful.

18.9   PERNIO (CHILBLAINS)

Pernio produces localized inflammatory lesions of the skin as a result of abnormal response to the cold. Pernio is most common in temperate humid climates of northwestern Europe and in the northern United States.

Pernio develops in susceptible individuals who are exposed to nonfreezing cold. Pathologic changes in the dermis and subcutaneous tissue include edema of the papillodermis, vasculitis characterized by perivascular infiltration (with lymphocytes) of the arterioles and venules of the dermis, thickening and edema of the blood vessel walls, fat necrosis, and chronic inflammatory reaction with giant-cell formation.

18.9.1 CLINICAL MANIFESTATIONS

Pernio most commonly occurs in young women between the ages of 15 and 30, but can occur in older individuals or in children. Acute pernio can develop 12 to 24 hours after exposure to the cold. Single or multiple erythematous, purplish, edematous lesions appear, accompanied by intense itching or burning. These lesions may have a yellowish or brownish discoloration and may be associated with some flaking. There may be violet or yellow-brown blisters and shallow ulcers on the toes and dorsum of the foot that burn and itch (Figure 18.8).[39] The arterial circulation is normal on physical examination and in the noninvasive vascular laboratory. Chronic pernio occurs when repeated exposure to the cold results in the persistence of lesions with

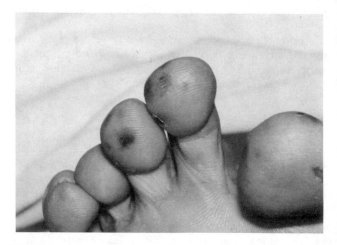

FIGURE 18.8 Yellow-brown discoloration with shallow ulcers in a patient with chronic pernio. (From Olin, J.W., and Arrabi, W., Vascular diseases related to extremes in environmental temperature, in *Peripheral Vascular Diseases*, 2nd ed., Young, J.R., Olin, J.W., and Bartholomew, J.R., Eds., C.V. Mosby Co., St. Louis, 1996, 613. With permission.[39])

subsequent scarring and atrophy. Characteristically, the lesions begin in the fall or winter and disappear in the spring or early summer. In advanced cases, the seasonal variation may disappear and chronic occlusive vascular disease may develop.

The differential diagnosis of pernio includes recurrent, erythematous, nodular, and ulcerative lesions such as erythema induratum, nodular vasculitis, erythema nodosum, and cold panniculitis. Skin lesions of pernio may look similar to skin manifestations of atheromatous embolization (see Chapter 14). This may present a significant diagnostic problem in the older patient, and an arteriogram may be necessary to help clarify the diagnosis.

18.9.2 TREATMENT

Prevention is the best of form of therapy. Cold exposure should be minimized as much as possible. Suitable clothing protecting the patient from cold is the cornerstone of therapy. In a double-blind, placebo-controlled, randomized trial followed by a long-term open trial, nifedipine was shown to reduce the pain associated with the lesions and speed the healing process.[40] Severe itching may be treated with local application of an antipruritic agent.

18.10 ERYTHROMELALGIA

The term erythromelalgia is derived from the combination of three Greek words: *erythros*, meaning "red"; *melos*, meaning "extremity"; and *algos*, meaning "pain"—literally, red, painful extremities. Erythromelalgia can be classified as the primary or idiopathic form, which may be nonfamilial or familial. The secondary form is associated with other diseases, most commonly myeloproliferative disorders such as polycythemia vera and essential thrombocythemia. Erythromelalgia may precede the clinical appearance of myeloproliferative disorders by several years. Therefore, patients with erythromelalgia who are past age 30 should be monitored periodically with blood counts. Other diseases are associated with secondary erythromelalgia (e.g., hypertension, diabetes, rheumatoid arthritis, gout, spinal cord disease, multiple sclerosis, SLE, cutaneous vasculitis, and viral infection) as are various drugs (i.e., nifedipine, nicardipine, verapamil, bromocriptine, and pergolide).

The underlying pathophysiology of erythromelalgia is not known. The histology varies from normal (in the primary form) to arterial occlusion with thrombus formation (in patients with myelo-proliferative diseases).

Erythromelalgia is characterized by the clinical triad of erythema, burning pain, and increased temperature, usually of the extremities. The feet, and especially the soles, are more commonly involved than the hands. Peripheral pulses are generally normal in the primary type and variable in the secondary form. A warm environment, exercise, and dependency tend to exacerbate symptoms. Patients seek relief by exposing the affected extremity to a cooler environment such as placing it in ice water, walking on a cold floor barefoot, running the air conditioner year round, or strapping ice packs to the feet. Symptoms of erythromelalgia can be so severe that the patient may consider suicide to obtain relief.

Diagnosis of erythromelalgia is based on all of the following criteria:

- Erythema
- Severe burning pain
- Increased skin temperature over the affected region
- Precipitation by warm environment
- Relief by a cool environment
- Exclusion of other diseases that can mimic erythromelalgia

Other causes of painful erythematous extremities include reflex sympathetic dystrophy, atherosclerotic peripheral arterial disease, and TAO (Buerger's disease).

Treatment of erythromelalgia is often difficult and frustrating for patient and physician alike. In cases of secondary erythromelalgia, treatment of the underlying disease (phlebotomy in patients with poly-cythemia vera and normalization of the platelet count in patients with thrombocythemia) may relieve the symptoms.

It is critical that patients avoid cold injury to the skin of the affected extremity. Repeated cold exposure can lead to further injury of the skin and the circulation. Ice packs and immersion in ice water should definitely be avoided.

Aspirin is the most effective modality available, particularly for patients with erythromelalgia secondary to myeloproliferative disorders. Other drugs that have been used with varying degrees of success include methysergide, ephedrine, nonsteroidal, anti-inflammatory drugs, phenoxybenzamine, nitroglycerin, sodium nitroprusside, and corticosteroids. Nonsteroidal drugs, in particular, can offer relief of burning pain and obviate the need for stronger pain medications. Surgical sympathectomy has been tried and produced various short-term results, but it is not effective as long-term therapy.

REFERENCES

1. Stuart, T.P.A., Note on a variation in the course of the popliteal artery, *J. Anat. Physiol.*, 13, 162, 1879.
2. Love, J.W. and Whelan, T.J., Popliteal artery entrapment syndrome, *Am. J. Surg.*, 109, 620, 1965.
3. Collins, P.S., McDonald, P.T., and Lim, R.C., Popliteal artery entrapment: an evolving syndrome, *J. Vasc. Surg.*, 10, 484, 1989.
4. Insua, J.A., Young, J.R., and Humphries, A.W., Popliteal artery entrapment syndrome, *Arch. Surg.*, 1970, 101, 771.
5. Hamming, J.J. and Vink, M., Obstruction of the popliteal artery at an early age, *J. Cardiovasc. Surg. (Torino)*, 6, 516, 1965.
6. McDonald, P.T., Easterbrook, J.A., and Rich, N.M., Popliteal artery entrapment syndrome: clinical noninvasive and angiographic diagnosis, *Am. J. Surg.*, 139, 318, 1980.
7. Rizzo, R.J., Flinn, W.R., and Yao, J.S., Computed tomography for evaluation of arterial disease in the popliteal fossa, *J. Vasc. Surg.*, 11, 112, 1990.
8. Fowl, R.J. and Kepmczinski, R.F., in *Vascular Surgery*, 5th ed., Rutherford, R.B., Ed., W.B. Saunders Co., Philadelphia, 2000, 1087.
9. Levien, L.J. and Bergan, J.J., Adventitial cystic disease of the popliteal artery, in *Vascular Surgery*, 5th ed., Rutherford, R.B., W.B. Saunders Co., Philadelphia, 2000, 1079.

10. Ishikawa, K., Cystic adventitial disease of the popliteal artery and of other stem vessels in the extremities, *Jpn. J. Surg.*, 17, 221, 1987.

11. Atkins, H.J.B. and Key, J.A., A case of myxomatous tumour arising in the adventitia of the left external iliac artery, *Br. J. Surg.*, 34, 426, 1946.

12. Haid, S.P., Conn, J., Jr., and Bergan, J.J., Cystic adventitial disease of the popliteal artery, *Arch. Surg.*, 101, 765, 1970.

13. Flanigan, D.P., Burnham, S.J., Goodreau, J.J.,et al., Summary of cases of adventitial cystic disease of the popliteal artery, *Ann. Surg.*, 189, 165, 1979.

14. Gray, B.H., Young, J.R., and Olin, J.W., Miscellaneous arterial diseases, in *Peripheral Vascular Diseases*, 2nd ed., Young, J.R., Olin, J.W., and Bartholomew, J.R., Eds., C.V. Mosby Co., St. Louis, 1996, 425.

15. Bunker, S.R., Lauten, G.J., and Hutton, J.E., Jr., Cystic adventitial disease of the popliteal artery, *Am. J. Roentgenol*, 136, 1209, 1981.

16. Jasinski, R.W., Masselink, B.A., and Partridge, R.W., Adventitial cystic disease of the popliteal artery, *Radiology*, 163, 153, 1987.

17. Wilbur, A.C., and Spigos, D.G., Adventitial cyst of the popliteal artery: CT-guided percutaneous aspiration, *J. Comput. Assist. Tomogr.*, 10, 161, 1986.

18. Fox, R.L., Kahn, M., and Adler, J., Adventitial cystic disease of the popliteal artery: failure of percutaneous transluminal angioplasty as a therapeutic modality, *J. Vasc. Surg.*, 2 ,464, 1985.

19. Begelman, S. and Olin, J.W., Fibromuscular dysplasia, *Curr. Opin. Rheumatol.*, 12, 41, 2000.

20. Begelman, S. and Olin, J.W., Non-atherosclerotic arterial disease of the extracranial cerebrovasculature, *Semin. Vasc. Surg.*, 13, 153, 2000.

21. Luscher, T.F., Lie, J.T., and Stanson, A.W., Arterial fibromuscular dysplasia, *Mayo Clin. Proc.*, 62, 931, 1987.

22. Iwai, T., Konno, S., and Hiejima, K., Fibromuscular dysplasia in the extremities, *J. Cardiovasc. Surg.*, 26, 496, 1985.

23. McCormack, L.J., Poutasse, E.F., and Meaney, T.F., A pathologic-arteriographic correlation of renal arterial disease, *Am. Heart J.*, 72, 188, 1966.

24. Harrison, E.G., Jr. and McCormack, L.J., Pathologic classification of renal arterial disease in renovascular hypertension, *Mayo Clin. Proc.*, 46, 161, 1971.

25. Schievink, W.I. and Limburg, M., Angiographic abnormalities mimicking fibromuscular dysplasia in a patient with Ehlers-Danlos syndrome, type IV, *Neurosurgery*, 25, 482, 1989.

26. Walter, J.F., Stanley, J.C., and Mehigan, J.T., External iliac artery fibrodysplasia, *Am. J. Roentgenol.*, 131, 125, 1978.

27. Esfahani, F., Rooholamini, S.A., Azadeh, B., et al., Arterial fibrodysplasia: a regional cause of peripheral occlusive vascular disease, *Angiology*, 40,108, 1989.

28. Stinnett, D.M., Graham, J.M., and Edwards, W.D., Fibromuscular dysplasia and thrombosed aneurysm of the popliteal artery in a child, *J. Vasc. Surg.*, 5, 769, 1987.

29. van den Dungen, J.J.A.M., Boontje, A.H., and Oosterhuis, J.W., Femoropopliteal arterial fibrodysplasia, *Br. J. Surg.*, 77, 396, 1990.

30. Lachman, A.S., Spray, T., and Kerwin, D.M., Medial calcinosis of Mönckeberg, *Am. J. Med.*, 63, 615, 1977.

31. Goebel, F.D. and Fuessl, H.S., Mönckeberg's sclerosis after sympathetic denervation in diabetic and non-diabetic subjects, *Diabetologia*, 24, 347, 1983.

32. Juul, S., Ledbetter, D., Wight, T.N., and Woodrum, D., New insights into idiopathic infantile arterial calcinosis, *Am. J. Dis. Child*, 144, 229, 1990.

33. Meema, H.E., Oreopoulos, D.G., and deVeber, G.A., Arterial calcifications in severe chronic renal disease and their relationship to dialysis treatment, renal transplant and parathyroidectomy, *Radiology*, 121, 315, 1976.

34. Wilkinson, S.P., Stewart, W.K., Parham, D.M., et al., Symmetric gangrene of the extremities in late renal failure: a case report and review of the literature, *Q. J. Med.*, 67, 319, 1988.

35. Conn, J., Jr., Krumlovsky, F.A., Del Greco, F., et al., Calciphylaxis: etiology of progressive vascular calcification and gangrene?, *Ann. Surg.*, 177,206, 1973.

36. Garcia, G.D., Goff, J.M., Jr., and Hadro, N.C., Chronic ergot toxicity: a rare cause of lower extremity ischemia, *J. Vasc. Surg.*, 31, 1245, 2000.

37. Olin, J.W., Other peripheral arterial diseases, in *Cecil Textbook of Medicine*, Goldman, L. and Bennett, J.C., Eds., W.B. Saunders Co., Philadelphia, 2000, 362.

38. Klein, K.L. and Pittelkow, M.R., Tissue plasminogen activator for the treatment of livedoid vasculitis, *Mayo Clin. Proc.*, 67, 1004, 1992.

39. Olin, J.W. and Arrabi, W., Vascular diseases related to extremes in environmental temperature, in *Peripheral Vascular Diseases*, 2nd ed., Young, J.R., Olin, J.W., and Bartholomew, J.R., Eds., C.V. Mosby Co., St. Louis, 1996, 613.

40. Dowd, P.M., Rustin, M.H.A., and Lanigan, S., Nifedipine in the treatment of chilblains, *Br. Med. J*, 293, 923, 1986.

41. Kalgaard, O.M., Seem, E., and Kvernebo, K., Erythromelalgia: a clinical study in 87 cases, *J. Intern. Med.*, 242 ,191, 1997.

19 Compression Syndromes of the Thoracic Outlet

J. Ernesto Molina

CONTENTS

19.1 Introduction 413
19.2 Subclavian Vein Compression..415
    19.2.1 Effort Thrombosis of the Subclavian Vein 417
    19.2.2 Diagnosis...419
    19.2.3 Treatment 420
    19.2.4 Other Causes of Subclavian Vein Obstruction 424
    19.2.5 Treatments to Avoid..425
19.3 Arterial Compression 425
19.4 Neurogenic Thoracic Outlet Syndrome 427
    19.4.1 Etiology...428
    19.4.2 Diagnosis...429
    19.4.3 Other Tests 431
    19.4.4 Treatment 431
19.5 Conclusions 432
References...433

19.1 INTRODUCTION

Thoracic outlet syndrome comprises several situations entailing compression of vascular structures and nerves. The structures that pass through the thoracic outlet are the subclavian vein, the subclavian

0-8493-8413-3/01/$0.00+$1.50
© 2001 by CRC Press LLC

artery, and, coming from the brachial plexus, the bundle of nerves that supply the upper extremity. Although the brachial plexus originates in the cervical spine, the nerves travel through muscle bundles that insert on top of the first rib and course down into the arm.

Figure 19.1 shows the anatomic arrangement of these structures that travel across separate channels over the first rib. The channel through which the subclavian vein travels, being the most anterior

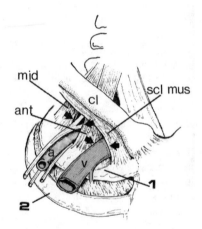

FIGURE 19.1 Anatomy of the thoracic outlet. The subclavian vein (*v*) enters the chest between the subclavius tendon muscle (*scl mus*) and the anterior scalene muscle (*ant*). The first rib (*1*) forms the floor of the tunnel. Arrows and the dotted line indicate the site where the pinching occurs. The subclavian artery runs between the anterior scalene muscle (*ant*) and the medial scalene muscle (*mid*). The nerve trunks of the brachial plexus accompany the artery in the same tunnel. Arrows indicate the level at which compression or pinching of the nerves and the artery occurs. The clavicle (*cl*) and the subclavius muscle (*scl mus*) form the roof of this channel. The second rib (*2*) does not participate in the compression syndrome. The upper insertion of the scalene muscle is located in the cervical spine transverse processes shown in the upper part of the figure.

structure of the thoracic outlet, is formed by the clavicle and the subclavian muscle on top (it inserts in the head of the first rib), the anterior scalene tendon in the back, and the first rib at the bottom.

The subclavian artery, behind the vein, travels through a wider tunnel formed by the anterior scalene tendon anteriorly, the clavicle at the top, the first rib in the inferior aspect, and the medial scalene muscle posteriorly. The brachial plexus, with its multiple branches, travels between the fibers of the anterior and medial scalene muscles, which insert in the superior aspect of the first rib. The syndrome that results from the compression of the subclavian vein is clearly defined clinically and corroborated by radiographic studies. The syndrome that results from compression of the subclavian artery can be suspected by physical exam and confirmed by radiologic tests; it is often associated with compression of the brachial plexus branches. Despite the many attempts to use laboratory testing, compression of the brachial plexus has remained a clinical diagnosis. The clinician often is confronted with a wide variety of symptoms attributed to nerve compression. On occasion, diagnosis is further complicated by what is called a cervical rib, seen by radiographic exam as a fully developed rib (attached to the seventh cervical vertebrae posteriorly and to the first rib anteriorly), or as a partially developed rib (visualized radiographically only as a stump that extends with a strong fibrous tendon across the neck to insert in the first rib). In another unusual anomaly, the first rib is fused with a cervical rib or with the second rib, constituting a very wide, large, sharp bony structure and leading to compression of the vascular as well as the neurogenic structures. When the subclavian vein is compressed in the anterior portion of the thoracic outlet, it is usually not associated with any compression of the artery or the nerves. Therefore, this feature clearly separates the syndromes of venous obstruction from the arterial–neurogenic type.

This chapter presents a description of each entity, the clinical picture, and the recommended treatment.

19.2   SUBCLAVIAN VEIN COMPRESSION

Compression of the subclavian vein at the thoracic outlet may occur acutely as a result of a sudden effort with the arm (e.g., from lifting heavy weights, pushing heavy objects, or carrying them with the arm in a down position, with the arm at shoulder level, or above the head). This is known as Paget-Schroetter syndrome, or effort thrombosis of the subclavian vein. A chronic process can occur without great exertion (e.g., just from repetitively moving the arm over the head). It can also occur in persons with a body habitus in which the chest is depressed or sunken in relation to hunched shoulders. Repetitive or continuous compression of the vein between the first rib and the tendons of the subclavius muscle and the anterior scalene gradually leads to fibrosis and stricture of the vein at that level (Figure 19.2). This type of compression can occur in people who do secretarial work, type, or use the computer keyboard for many hours every day. Further damage to the vein can usually be prevented by correcting

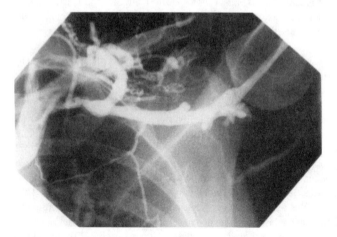

FIGURE 19.2 Chronic recurring obstruction of the subclavian vein in a 38-year-old woman who habitually carried heavy objects with her arm in the down position for several years. Subclavian vein is shown in this venogram coming from the left arm (which is elevated) down to the very narrow point of stenosis on the left side of the picture. Beyond that point the subclavian vein looks perfectly normal.

the body habitus with straps or elastic devices that pull the shoulders back and keep the back straight.

The symptoms of intermittent or partial compression of the subclavian vein[1–4] are usually edema of the hands and fingers as well as engorgement of the veins in the hand or forearm. The person usually experiences some type of tightening sensation in the hands and fingers caused by edema and often notes that rings cannot be removed from the fingers at the end of the day. In more severe situations, the hand becomes discolored (bluish), and a throbbing tightening pain is felt in the hands, forearms, and sometimes the arm. This pain is usually relieved by raising the arm over the head and straightening the back, which opens the subclavian vein and allows the stagnant blood in the arm to empty or drain. These symptoms can go on for quite some time, even years. If no corrective measures are taken, the vein will eventually stricture down to a minimal opening. Once this happens, the trigger of any sudden movement or effort can cause the vein to thrombose acutely. The dramatic clinical picture of subclavian vein effort thrombosis thus develops. [2, 5–9]

19.2.1 Effort Thrombosis of the Subclavian Vein

When compression of the vein occurs suddenly as the result of an unusual physical movement of the arms, the person develops acute damage of the subclavian vein at the thoracic outlet. The endothelium is injured, leading to immediate thrombosis of the vein at that level and extending rapidly toward the arm distally. This sequence of events (Figure 19.3), known as Paget-Schroetter syndrome, or effort thrombosis of the subclavian and axillary veins, can happen to any person even without any abnormal anatomic predisposition for compression of the vein. Lifting a heavy weight with the arms down along the body can cause this syndrome. So can a sudden pull of the arm to support the body weight during a fall or a climbing maneuver. Young people are usually affected by this syndrome, because they frequently are physically active in sports. Baseball pitching, swimming, weight lifting, tennis playing, climbing, and other activities involving sudden movements with the arm may cause damage to the

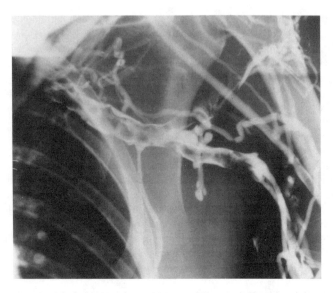

FIGURE 19.3 Acute thrombosis of the subclavian vein (Paget-Schroetter syndrome). The figure shows total occlusion of the subclavian vein (*left*). The vein itself is filled with clots extending distally toward the arm, which is being held in the down position.

intima of the vein and trigger the full-blown picture of subclavian vein effort thrombosis.

The person suffering from this acute event feels a sudden sharp pain in the area of the subclavian region along the shoulder and into the arm. Within minutes, severe edema and congestion of the affected arm occurs, with bluish discoloration and engorgement of the veins that extend from the shoulder level down to the fingers. Because the thrombosis of the vein extends distally or peripherally into the arm (and not centrally toward the heart), other veins draining into the axillary vein thrombose as well, leading to edema of the axillary area and anterior portion of the chest wall. The veins coming from the neck are usually engorged. Some supraclavicular edema may be present as well. The acute picture requires immediate care: the person should be seen and treated on an emergency basis.

As explained in section 19.2.4, it is important that the patient be cared for immediately to prevent further extension of the thrombus into the arm, which would cause damage and fibrosis of the entire arm's venous network. The process, if not treated properly and within a short time, leads to irreversible damage of the vein to such a degree that total obliteration with fibrosis may extend not only to the subclavian vein, but into the axillary and even the brachial vein. Once the veins fibrose and obliterate, nothing can be done, leaving the patient permanently disabled.[7,10] Each time such a patient tries to undertake any type of physical activity with the affected arm, it will invariably become edematous and painful within minutes. The matter is not so crucial for someone who is bedridden or confined to a hospital, or for anyone who is not expected to make any type of physical effort with the arm. Eventually, the edema may disappear or significantly decrease, and as long as patients are not involved with any type of activity, they may tolerate this situation. However, for the young or active individual who expects to recover and return to a demanding sport or occupation, treatment must be prompt and effective to restore functionality.[6,7]

Persons whose occupations involve carrying relatively heavy objects with the arms down are also at risk of developing a chronic obstruction of the subclavian vein by the compressive mechanism explained above. Even if they do not develop full-blown thrombosis, the vein may become extremely narrow. Symptoms will recur in the arm as long as the person continues that specific activity.

19.2.2 Diagnosis

When subclavian vein stenosis, compression, or thrombosis is suspected, the test of choice is the duplex ultrasound exam. It provides both anatomic and hemodynamic information in a noninvasive manner, making possible a direct diagnosis of thrombosis, stenosis, and collateral circulation. It permits sensitive spectral wave for analogies.[11,12]

We use Grayscale duplex and color Doppler sonography to evaluate all vessels. It is important to do the test bilaterally, because some subtle abnormalities can be appreciated only by comparison with the contralateral spectra. Any institution must have a standard protocol for accurate and consistent evaluation of the upper-extremity veins. All vessels are imaged in the transverse plain for localization and in the longitudinal plain for Doppler interrogation.

Indirect signs of pathology include dampening wave forms, decreased velocities, loss of transmitted pulsatility, and respiratory phasicity distal to the stenosis or occlusion (Figure 19.4).

Once the diagnosis is established with ultrasonography, the next step is venography for prompt and proper treatment, as well as for assessment of the obstructive problem.

19.2.3 TREATMENT

In a nonemergency situation, if signs of stricture or stenosis are visualized in the vein by ultrasound, but no acute thrombosis exists, the patient should be referred for a venogram. It will establish the location, exact configuration, and length of any stricture. A surgical consultation should be requested to evaluate possibilities to relieve the obstruction. The patient usually does not have to be anticoagulated at this stage if only chronic changes are present.

But with acute thrombosis of the subclavian vein, the situation is quite different. The patient needs to be hospitalized immediately. Venography must be done to evaluate the extension of the clot. A therapeutic plan must be implemented involving the use of thrombolytic agents (Figure 19.5) to dissolve the clot in the axillary or subclavian vein until total resolution is obtained. The author's therapeutic plan has been in place at the University of Minnesota for many years.[6,7] We recommend that, as soon as the entire clot is lysed— which usually takes less than 24 hours — surgery must follow.[7] The operation involves decompression of the vein from the surrounding structures of the thoracic outlet and patch widening of the stenotic segment of the vein using autologous vein. Normal flow through the

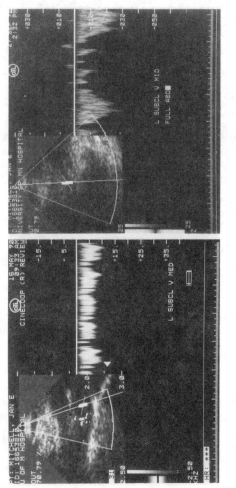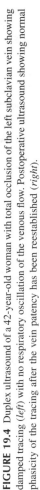

FIGURE 19.4 Duplex ultrasound of a 42-year-old woman with total occlusion of the left subclavian vein showing damped tracing (*left*) with no respiratory oscillation of the venous flow. Postoperative ultrasound showing normal phasicity of the tracing after the vein patency has been reestablished (*right*).

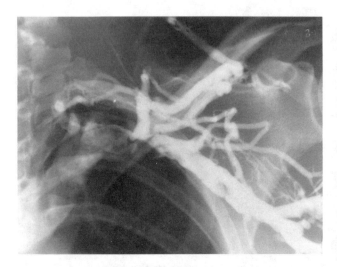

FIGURE 19.5 Patient with Paget-Schroetter syndrome after undergoing thrombolytic therapy. All clots have been dissolved, and the subclavian vein as well as its collaterals can be clearly outlined. The vein is totally occluded (*left*). The patient subsequently underwent surgery to open the obstructed site.

vein is thus reestablished and further thrombosis distally is prevented. The patient is anticoagulated for a total of 8 weeks. After that, if a Doppler ultrasound exam confirms the patency of the vein, the anticoagulation regimen is discontinued, and the patient can resume normal activities.

In general, all patients who develop this syndrome must undergo surgery as the only treatment of choice. Decompression of the thoracic outlet entails resection of the following structures: the first rib needs to be removed to open the channel in its inferior portion. The subclavius tendon is resected, because it inserts in the first rib anteriorly and pinches the vein anteriorly and superiorly against the first rib (Figure 19.1). The anterior scalene muscle tendon must be removed as well; doing so frees up the entire channel where the subclavian vein runs into the chest. The first rib is usually resected at its mid portion, behind the level of the subclavian artery course. Thus, future compression of the artery when the bone heals will be prevented. The entire operation is done in an extrapleural manner. In other words, the chest cavity is not entered. The technique has been detailed elsewhere.[6,7,13] Once the vein is free of all the surrounding tissues, it is pulled gently into the field and the site of the stricture identified. The vein is now opened lengthwise and the stricture is patched, usually using a piece of autologous greater saphenous vein. The patch is laid over this stricture segment to widen the diameter of the vein.

Postoperatively, the patient is kept on anticoagulants for about 2 months until the vein completely heals. Coumadin®* is usually prescribed to maintain an international normalized ratio between 2 and 3. An antiplatelet agent is added, usually clopidogrel (Plavix ®**) at the usual dose of 75 mg/day. Plavix is preferred over aspirin or persantin because it has been found more effective and free of gastrointestinal side effects. At the end of 2 months, an ultrasound is again obtained to evaluate the flow of the vein. The patient is taken off the anticoagulants permanently. No further care is necessary, and normal physical activities can be resumed. There is no fear of the thrombosis recurring, because the vein is completely free. No constricting structures are around the vein, and even if the person renews heavy physical activity, the mechanism of compression has been eliminated.

The obstructed segment of the vein typically is less than 2 cm long; therefore, the patch is small. However, if the process has been going on for more than a week, up to 20% of patients may have a stricture of the entire subclavian vein, even extending into the innominate trunk. In that case, exposing the vein is more difficult through the standard incision. To cope with this problem, the author has previously described a technique[14] in which the sternum is entered at the manubrium level, and the entire innominate vein can be exposed for patching or replaced with a vascular homograft.

---

* Registered trademark of DuPont Pharma, Wilmington, Delaware.
** Registered trademark of Sanofi Pharmaceuticals Inc., New York, New York.

19.2.4   OTHER CAUSES OF SUBCLAVIAN VEIN OBSTRUCTION

Severe obstruction, fibrosis, and obliteration of the vein can occur with invasive procedures or with transvenous device implantation. Among the potential mechanisms of obstruction are the following:

- Prolonged implantation of central venous catheters for chemotherapeutic purposes or antibiotic administration.[14,15] If the catheter remains in the vein for weeks or months, it will likely damage the endothelium of the vein and fibrose the vessel to a smaller size. If, for any reason, the patient is involved in activity causing pinching of the vein, this may become occluded at any time.
- Insertion of pacemaker transvenous leads (usually two), particularly in children, or in adult patients whose previous pacemaker leads had not been removed. New leads inserted in the same vein may lead to total occlusion of the vein or cause severe stenosis, particularly in small persons.[15,16]
- Implantation of transvenous defibrillator leads. These leads have the same potential for occlusion of the vein as do pacemaker leads.[16] Defibrillator leads usually are larger in diameter, and frequently more than one is needed to obtain proper function. Replacing or removing these leads to reestablish patency of the veins can be quite challenging and difficult. Therefore, when transvenous leads are inserted, care must be taken to ensure proper diameter of the vein and eliminate any obstructions. The vein situation should be assessed preoperatively with a Doppler ultrasound exam.
- Dialysis catheters used for chronic hemodialysis. Such catheters often cause strictures and obstructions of the subclavian vein.[15,17,18] A very complicated problem could ensue, because some of these patients have arteriovenous fistulas for dialysis in the same arm where the obstruction occurs. The fistula may thrombose if the stricture or the obstruction of the subclavian vein is not eliminated.

19.2.5 TREATMENTS TO AVOID

New procedures have been developed that, although invasive, avoid surgical incisions. Among them are percutaneous procedures. Attempts have been made to open an obstructed vein by using balloon angioplasty or by placing of stents, instead of performing surgery. Implant of stents should never be attempted in anybody who has not had the thoracic outlet decompressed first. In other words, stents should not be used instead of surgery. Balloon angioplasty alone will only lead to further damage of the vein endothelium already compromised by the extrinsic compression between the first rib, the subclavius tendon, and the scalene muscle tendon. Stent placement, in an attempt to maintain the proper caliber of the vein, is contraindicated if the patient has not had decompressive surgery of the vein first.[19] If a stent is placed in this narrow segment of the vein without decompressing the channel through which the vein runs will invariably cause collapse of the stent as soon as the patient raises the arm. The compressive mechanism is still present and will work like a vise as it squeezes the vein and the stent.[20] Balloon angioplasty and stent placement are only appropriate—and then actually quite successful—when the thoracic outlet has already been decompressed (operated) and the vein develops a stricture despite the patching maneuver or decompression alone. In that case, when there is no extrinsic compression of the vein, balloon angioplasty of the strictured segment and stent placement are quite effective and, in fact, recommended. If the patient suffers from terminal illness and surgery cannot be tolerated, the treatment should be restricted to anticoagulant therapy only. Stenting of the subclavian vein will not provide any palliation, even for a few days.

19.3 ARTERIAL COMPRESSION

Most of the classic literature on thoracic outlet syndromes focuses on the compression of the subclavian artery, for which several maneuvers that are used during the physical examination and evaluation have been described. The patient with suspected arterial compression of the thoracic outlet usually complains of numbness, tingling, and coldness of the hand when the arm is abducted to 90° or over the head. This maneuver usually blanches the arm and the hand; the pulse is lost by palpation (but is usually restored when the arm comes down). Several so-called provocative tests are used. In the Adson test, described in 1951, the patient is instructed to take and hold a deep breath, extend the neck fully, and turn the head toward the affected side. Obliteration or decrease of the radial pulse suggests compression. Another test is the costal clavicular test (military position), in which the shoulders are drawn down and back. Changes in the radial pulse with reduction of symptoms indicate compression. Still another test is the hyperabduction (Allen) test, in which the patient raises the arm over the head 180°; usually, the pulse disappears.

Although these tests help suggest compression, more objective tests are necessary. Some have been developed during the past few years. The Doppler ultrasound exam is accurate and noninvasive. If done properly with the correct maneuvers,[11,12] it shows if compression exists and to what degree the vessel is involved. It will also demonstrate whether intrinsic stenosis exists, whether an aneurysm is present, and whether other obstructions downstream may be present.

If there is a question about whether the subclavian artery is abnormal or whether an aneurysm exists, the patient should be referred for an angiography or magnetic resonance arteriogram study that will precisely outline the pathology of the arterial compression. Rarely or never is the artery compression simultaneously associated with vein obstruction. In more than 200 operative cases, this author has never found any instance of a subclavian venous obstruction coexisting with arterial compression. The mechanism of compression is different because of the anatomic location of the vessels.[21,22]

The coexistence of arterial and neurogenic compression of the brachial plexus trunks is more common than venous compression with accompanying neurogenic symptoms. In our own series, we found that about 38% of patients with compression of the brachial plexus trunks have compression of the subclavian artery by ultrasound exam as well.[26] The number of patients who had a cervical rib in the entire group is very low (6%). A chest radiograph, always a routine in the evaluation of these patients, should be sufficient to verify the presence or absence of a congenital cervical rib. Although this extra rib always compresses both structures, nerves and artery, the more severe symptoms usually come from compression of the nerve trunks. Considering the patients with cervical rib alone, compression of the arterial or venous system at the thoracic outlet occurs in 50% of them by ultrasound examination. Symptomatic patients who have arterial compression (objectively verified by ultrasound) should be referred to surgery without any hesitation. It is the only treatment that will solve the problem permanently. With more than 50 patients with arterial compression (documented by ultrasound), only one had a subclavian artery aneurysm at the thoracic outlet that required repair (namely, interposition of a graft using an infra- and supraclavicular approach). If only arterial compression is demonstrated, the operation is done exactly the same as for neurogenic compression alone, i.e., complete excision of the first rib with the scalene tendons to assure cure of the neurogenic and vascular symptoms. When the first rib is removed in its entirety along with the anterior and medial scalene muscles, the subclavian artery is completely released of any type of impingement.

19.4 NEUROGENIC THORACIC OUTLET SYNDROME

Compression of the brachial plexus trunks is the most common condition that leads to symptoms among patients with thoracic outlet syndrome. An extensive volume of literature describes the pain, numbness, and tingling of the fingers that occur when the brachial plexus is compressed at that level. However, the clinical picture of neurogenic compression of the brachial plexus has been too often associated with arterial compression. If the pulse in the radial artery persists while the examining physician implements abduction of the arm or any of the tests to elicit symptoms, the diagnosis of neurogenic thoracic outlet compression is often dismissed. This is an incorrect concept. Neurogenic compression may exist without vascular compression.[2] If, in addition, an electromyographic (EMG) test is negative, neurogenic compression is erroneously ruled out. Patients with neurogenic thoracic outlet syndrome have pain almost 100% of the time. Numbness in the arm, forearm, or down to the fingers is present in 85%, and a tingling sensation in the fingers in 85%. In 9%, weakness of the thenar area of the hand is experienced, with a clinical history of dropping objects and, in more severe cases, atrophy of the thenar area and interosseal muscles. The EMG, which in the past was given a significant role as the diagnostic tool,[23,24] has been found by me and others[2,25] to be practically useless. In more than 100 patients diagnosed in our clinic, only 2% had positive EMGs. Patients with a positive EMG usually already have permanent, severe damage of the nerve trunks, but they are a minority. In the large majority (98%) with compression of the brachial plexus, the EMG is invariably negative. Therefore, as Leffert[2] stated a few years ago, "Despite many attempts to simplify and make the diagnosis a matter of objective laboratory testing, it remains a clinical one."

19.4.1 ETIOLOGY

The syndrome can occur in a variety of situations, most commonly in certain occupations or sports. A large number of patients (usually women), though they do not undertake vigorous physical exertion, may have the postural habit of a sunken chest with shoulders hunched forward (this is often the case with typists, computer workers, and secretaries). Sports like cross-country skiing, with its strong forward movement in front of the body at 90°, may lead to this syndrome. Restaurant workers who carry large trays with one hand at the shoulder level, or people who lift a heavy weight to shoulder level or higher, are also prone to this problem. Another cause is trauma that has been inflicted on the superior aspect of the shoulder over the trapezius area. Finally, the possibility of a congenital cervical rib must be explored in children or young adults who complain of numbness or tiredness of their arms while doing sports or routine schoolwork. The anatomy of a cervical rib shows a wide spectrum of abnormalities, including fusion of the cervical rib with the first rib or strong fibrous tendons

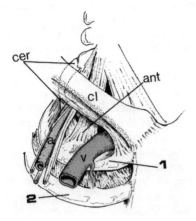

FIGURE 19.6 Anatomy of a neurogenic and arterial compression thoracic outlet syndrome due to cervical rib (*cer*). The abnormal rib is attached to the cervical spine posteriorly and its anterior end extends as a strong ligament inserting on the top of the first rib, creating a sharp angle for the subclavian artery (*a*) and a narrow channel for the brachial plexus branches to pass between this ligament and the anterior scalene muscle (*ant*). The artery makes a sharp bend going over this ligament before heading toward the arm. The clavicle (*cl*) forms the roof of this channel and the first rib (*1*) constitutes the floor of the channel. The fibers of the medial scalene muscle can be seen behind the insertion of the cervical rib ligament. The second rib (*2*) does not participate in the compression syndrome.

extending from the tip of the bony cervical rib to the superior aspect of the first rib anteriorly (Figure 19.6). Occasionally, the first rib is fused with the second rib and the cervical rib, causing severe symptoms that could easily be diagnosed by radiographic exams.

19.4.2 DIAGNOSIS

The clinical evaluation is of utmost importance because there is no objective test to diagnose compression of the brachial plexus trunks. The typical provocative tests (as earlier) involve the following:

- Lateral arm abduction to 90° to 180°. The patient with thoracic outlet syndrome does not have any limitation to raising the arm over the head. If such limitation exists, it should alert the physician to other conditions or to an intrinsic abnormality of the shoulder joint.
- Anterior arm abduction to 90° ("driving position").
- Anterior arm abduction reaching up above the eye level. Symptoms can also be elicited by having the patient lie down in a lateral decubitus position. Symptoms usually appear promptly in the arm that is down.

The patient frequently has a history of progressive disability and severity of symptoms. It is useful to ask patients to compare their present condition with the year before the consultation to determine whether they could engage in more physical activity than at present.

Some young people with severe symptoms of neurogenic compression are even unable to type or do regular homework with the arms at desk level. Any type of activity with their arms moving over their head (e.g., swimming, tennis, and baseball) will invariably make the symptoms worse. Some relief can be found by bringing the arm down along the body for a few minutes. If the compression of the nerve has been present for a long time, degeneration of the nerve trunks can occur. At that point, the EMG test becomes positive. However, it is unwise to wait until then, because atrophy of the muscles may become irreversible even after the brachial plexus is decompressed.

Maneuvers that relieve some of the symptoms in these patients include bringing the arm down along the body or lying down in a dorsal decubitus position with the arms kept along the body. The military position (shoulders pulled back) also relieves the compression to the brachial plexus. In contrast to vascular compression, the military position makes it worse.

Symptoms of which patients may complain, although they usually are not related to thoracic outlet syndrome, include: shoulder pain, high neck pain, or back pain going down toward the waistline. If these symptoms exist, they are probably caused by something other than thoracic outlet syndrome. The physician should request a workup for the cervical spine or for the shoulder joint. Orthopedic or neurosurgery consultations are in order. Use of the EMG, though suggested by various authors in the past, is not worthwhile. It is also a very uncomfortable test for the patient. Frequently, if the EMG report is negative, thoracic outlet syndrome is erroneously ruled out. As Leffert[2] states, "This misinterpretation has been a recurrent problem in patients who have often been subjected to multiple evaluations and then confined to a diagnostic limbo because of the misinterpretation of the value of these tests."

Neurogenic thoracic outlet syndrome needs to be differentiated from cervical radiculopathy, carpal tunnel syndrome, ulnar neuropathy, and apical or supraclavicular fossa lesions such as lung tumors or metastatic tumors in the apex of the chest, especially in adults. Brachial neuritis and reflex sympathetic dystrophy are other possibilities, though less likely.

19.4.3 OTHER TESTS

The only other test of importance for patients with symptoms of neurogenic thoracic outlet syndrome is Doppler ultrasound, as mentioned in the previous section. It will rule out or rule in arterial compression. If vascular compression exists along with neurogenic symptoms, there is clear justification to refer the patient to surgery. Tests often requested in trying to diagnose neurogenic compression include: magnetic resonance imaging, computed tomography scan, arteriogram, and EMG. None of these tests are necessary or useful in the diagnosing of neurogenic thoracic syndrome. They are justified only when the clinical assessment and plain chest radiography and ultrasound fail to provide the proper diagnosis for these patients. They should not be used as first-line tests.

Most patients with neurogenic thoracic syndrome are women (73% in our experience), with equal distribution by handedness (50% for right-handed patients, 50% for left-handed patients).

19.4.4 TREATMENT

Conservative management of neurogenic thoracic outlet syndrome has been recommended and implemented with various degrees of success. Correcting the postural habits of the patient long-term may be helpful, as long as no cervical rib or other anatomic abnormality exists. But usually, the patient benefits only for a short time. In the end, surgery becomes a strong option either because the postural corrections fail or the patient finds it hard to continue with them. Many surgical procedures have been proposed throughout the years, including scalenotomy and cervical rib resection (alone or with concomitant first rib resection). The approach to accomplish decompression has varied considerably through the years. The transaxillary approach, introduced in the 1960s by Roos,[26] became quite popular throughout the 1970s and 1980s and even at present. However, when done alone, it is often insufficient and leads to a significant rate of complications.[29] The supraclavicular approach proposed by Stoney is favored by some surgeons.[27] Other techniques, like the posterior approach initially proposed by Clagett[28] and then described by Ferguson[4] and Urschel[23] has also been applied with varying success, mostly in reoperations for recurrence of symptoms, but it is a more formidable procedure involving division of multiple back muscles that, in the author's opinion, is unnecessary. All these procedures are not equal. To decompress the brachial plexus, the first rib needs to be removed along with the tendons that insert on it. The operation must be considered a definitive procedure that will prevent reoperation later. The syndrome may recur because the operation was not done completely, or because it was too limited to achieve complete decompression of the thoracic outlet structures. The procedure that combines transaxillary, anterior, and posterior approaches in the same session, introduced in 1998,[25] is my operation of choice. Details of this technique have been fully described elsewhere.[25]

19.5   CONCLUSIONS

An algorithm of diagnosis and care for thoracic outlet problems is shown in Figure 19.7. Compressive syndromes of the thoracic outlet can be effectively treated with specific surgical interventions involving a hospital stay of 3 to 4 days. Subclavian vein compression, which is

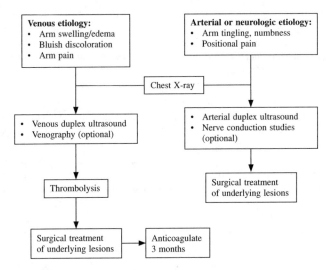

FIGURE 19.7 Algorithm of compressive syndromes of the thoracic outlet.

anterior in the thoracic outlet space, is usually handled by an anterior approach using a subclavicular incision. This operation is not aimed at decompressing the thoracic outlet posteriorly. Rather, it is meant to solve the compression of the subclavian vein and to allow the surgeon to widen this vein if needed. If the patient has arterial or neurogenic compression, the operation should use a combined approach with both a transaxillary incision and a posterior incision to remove the first rib with all three scalene muscles, thus completely relieving the compression of artery and brachial plexus trunks.

REFERENCES

1. McCleery, R.S., Kesterson, J.E., and Kirtley, J.A., Subclavius and anterior scalene muscle compression as a cause of intermittent obstruction of the subclavian vein, *Ann. Surg.*, 133, 588, 1951.

2. Leffert, R.D., Thoracic outlet syndromes, *Hand Clinics*, 8, 285, 1992.
3. Matsumura, J.S., Rilling, W.S., Pearce, W.H., Nemcek, A.A., Jr., Vogelzang, R.L., and Yao, J.S., Helical computed tomography of the normal thoracic outlet, *J. Vasc. Surg.*, 26, 776, 1997.
4. Ferguson, T.B., Buford, T.H., and Roper, C.L., Neurovascular compression at superior thoracic aperture: surgical management, *Ann. Surg.*, 167, 573, 1968.
5. Dale, A., Thoracic outlet compression syndrome, critique in 1982, *Arch. Surg.*, 117, 1437, 1982.
6. Molina, J.E., Surgery for effort thrombosis of the subclavian vein, *J. Thorac. Cardiovasc. Surg.*, 103, 341, 1992.
7. Molina, J.E., Need for emergency treatment in subclavian vein effort thrombosis, *J. Am. Coll. Surg.*, 181, 414, 1995.
8. Rutherford, R.B. and Hurlbert, S.N., Primary subclavian-axillary vein thrombosis: consensus and commentary, *Cardiovasc. Surg.*, 4, 420, 1996.
9. Machleder, H.I., Evaluation of a new treatment strategy for Paget-Schroetter syndrome: spontaneous thrombosis of the axillary-subclavian vein, *J. Vasc. Surg.*, 17, 305, 1993.
10. Puskas, J.D. and Gertler, J.P., Internal jugular to axillary vein bypass for subclavian vein thrombosis in the setting of brachial arteriovenous fistula, *J. Vasc. Surg.*, 19, 939, 1994.
11. Longley, D.G., Finlay, D.E., and Letourneau, J.G., Sonography of the upper extremities and jugular veins, *Am. J. Radiol.*, 160, 957, 1993.
12. Longley, D.G., Yedlicka, J.W., Jr., Molina, J.E., et al., Thoracic outlet syndrome: evaluation of the subclavian vessels by color duplex sonography, *Am. J. Roentgenol.*, 158, 623,1992.
13. Molina, J.E., Operative technique of first rib resection via subclavicular approach, *Vasc. Surg.*, 27, 667, 1993.
14. Molina, J.E., A new surgical approach to the innominate and subclavian vein, *J. Vasc. Surg.*, 27, 576, 1998.
15. Kock, H.J., Pietsch, M., Krause, U., et al., Implantable vascular access systems: experience in 1500 patients with totally implanted central venous port systems, *World J. Surg.*, 22, 12, 1998.
16. Lumsden, A.B., MacDonald, M.J., Isiklar, H., et al., Central venous stenosis in the hemodialysis patient: incidence and efficacy of endovascular treatment, *Cardiovasc. Surg.*, 5, 504,1997.

17. Jacobs, D.M., Fink, A.S., Miller, R.P., et al., Anatomical and morphological evaluation of pacemaker lead compression, *PACE Pacing Clin. Electrophysiol.*, 16, 434, 1993.

18. Magney, J.E., Flynn, D.M., Parsons, J.A., et al., Anatomical mechanisms explaining damage to pacemaker leads defibrillator leads and failure of central venous catheters adjacent to the sternoclavicular joint, *PACE Pacing Clin. Electrophysiol.*, 16, 445, 1993.

19. Hingorani, A., Ascher, E., Lorenson, E., et al., Upper extremity deep venous thrombosis and its impact on morbidity and mortality rates in a hospital-based population, *J. Vasc. Surg.*, 26, 853, 1997.

20. Bjarnason, H., Hunter, D.W., Crain, M.R., et al,. Collapse of a Palmaz stent in the subclavian vein, *Am. J. Radiol.*, 160, 1123, 1993.

21. Meier, G.H., Pollak, J.S., Rosenblatt, M., et al., Initial experience with venous stents in exertional axillary-subclavian vein thrombosis, *J. Vasc. Surg.*, 24, 974, 1996.

22. Sanders, R.J. and Roos, D.R., The surgical anatomy of the scalene triangle, *Contemp. Surg.,* 35, 11, 1989.

23. Makhoul, R.G. and Machleder, H.I., Developmental anomalies at the thoracic outlet: an analysis of 200 consecutive cases, *J. Vasc. Surg.*, 16, 534, 1992.

24. Urschel, H.C., Jr., Paulson, D.L., and McNamara, J.J., Thoracic outlet syndrome, *Ann. Thorac. Surg.*, 6, 1, 1968.

25. Urschel, H.C., Jr. and Razzuk, M.A., The failed operation for thoracic outlet syndrome: the difficulty of diagnosis and management, *Ann. Thorac. Surg.*, 42, 523, 1986.

26. Molina, J.E., Combined posterior and transaxillary approach of neurogenic thoracic outlet syndrome, *J. Am. Coll. Surg.*, 187, 39, 1998.

27. Roos, D.B., Transaxillary approach for 1st rib resection to relieve thoracic outlet syndrome, *Ann. Surg.*, 163, 354, 1966.

28. Cheng, W.K. and Stoney, R.J., Supraclavicular reoperation for neurogenic thoracic outlet syndrome, *J. Vasc. Surg.*, 19, 565, 1994.

29. Clagett, O.T., Presidential address: research and prosearch, *J. Thorac. Cardiovasc. Surg.*, 44, 153, 1962.

30. Melliere, D., Becquemin, J.P., Etienne, G., and LeCheviller, B., Severe injuries resulting from operations for thoracic outlet syndrome: can they be avoided?, *J. Cardiovasc. Surg.*, 32, 599, 1991.

20 Upper Extremity Arterial Disease

Thom W. Rooke

CONTENTS

20.1 Introduction 437
20.2 Conditions Affecting Arteries of the Upper Extremities.......438
    20.2.1 Atherosclerosis Obliterans...438
    20.2.2 Emboli 439
    20.2.3 Thrombosis..440
    20.2.4 Arterial Inflammation..441
    20.2.5 Trauma and Occupational Disorders 443
    20.2.6 Arterial Compression (Thoracic Outlet Syndrome).445
    20.2.7 Vasospasm 445
    20.2.8 Arteriovenous Malformations, Fistulas,
           and Vascular Tumors...447
    20.2.9 Miscellaneous Conditions of the Arteries 447
20.3 Strategies for Evaluation of Upper Extremity
    Arterial Diseases 448
    20.3.1 History...449
    20.3.2 Examination 449
    20.3.3 Vascular Testing 451
References...451

20.1 INTRODUCTION

Arterial disorders affect the upper extremities just as they do the lower extremities. However, some diseases are less common in the upper limbs. For example, significant atherosclerosis is roughly 20 times less common in the arms than in the legs.[1,2] Other disorders, such as vasospasm, appear to be much more common in the upper extremities. Still others, like occupational occlusive disease and thoracic outlet syndrome, are unique to the upper limbs. It is beyond the scope of this chapter to review all of the pathologic processes that can affect the arteries of the upper limb. Therefore, the focus will be on (1) selected major or unique conditions, and (2) strategies for the evaluation of upper extremity arterial diseases.

20.2 CONDITIONS AFFECTING ARTERIES OF THE UPPER EXTREMITIES

20.2.1 ATHEROSCLEROSIS OBLITERANS

Atherosclerosis in the upper extremities appears to be caused by the same factors that produce it in the lower extremities, although the incidence of atherosclerosis in the upper extremities is much lower. Proximal disease is more common than distal disease, with the highest incidence occurring in the subclavian and innominate arteries.[3]

Signs and symptoms of upper extremity atherosclerosis depend on the severity of the disease. Patients may be asymptomatic or have claudication (which is actually a misnomer in upper extremity disease—the word *claudication* comes from the Latin "to limp"), rest pain, or skin breakdown, ulceration, and gangrene. These signs and symptoms are not specific for atherosclerosis and may be found in patients with arterial obstruction from any cause.

Some manifestations of atherosclerosis obliterans are unique to the upper extremities. The subclavian steal syndrome is a rare and unusual symptom complex that occurs when arterial occlusion develops in the subclavian artery (the blockage must be distal to the origin of the carotid artery and proximal to the origin of the vertebral artery). When this happens, blood flows normally through the carotid artery into the circle of Willis, but then may move in a retrograde direction through the vertebral artery. This blood, which is "stolen" from the cerebral circulation, perfuses the upper extremity. Patients with "steal" are usually asymptomatic, and the finding of retrograde vertebral flow is typically an incidental one. However, during periods of upper extremity exercise (when the arm's demand for blood is high), the steal of blood from the cerebral circulation may be sufficient to produce intracranial ischemia. Atherosclerosis, along with other processes that damage the arterial wall, may also contribute to complications such as aneurysm formation, dissection, and acute thrombosis.

Atherosclerosis in the upper extremity is treated much the same as atherosclerosis in other arteries. Risk factors, including cholesterol, blood glucose, hypertension, and tobacco use, should be controlled or eliminated whenever possible. Interventional procedures including balloon angioplasty, intravascular stenting, surgical endarterectomy, and bypass operations are reserved for those patients with significant, usually symptomatic, disease. Careful postoperative follow-up, continued attention to risk factor reduction, and upper extremity exercise are important for long-term success.

20.2.2 EMBOLI

Emboli originating from the aorta are discussed elsewhere in this book. Emboli usually present in the upper extremity as acute or subacute arterial occlusions. Large emboli typically originate from the heart (or, less commonly, the aorta), whereas small (or micro) emboli may originate from the heart (these are often small clots, bacteria clumps, or other debris from diseased, infected, or otherwise abnormal valves) or from peripheral sources (such as atheroemboli from ruptured atherosclerotic plaques).[4] Less common sources of emboli include aneurysms of the heart or great vessels, and paradoxical emboli (which originate as clots in the venous system and pass through a patent foramen ovale or atrial septal defect into the arterial circulation).[5] Catheter procedures involving the heart or great vessels may also cause embolization. Both large and microemboli can produce significant tissue ischemia and infarction, although large emboli are more likely to result in limb loss than microemboli. Emboli may be recurrent, and the new emboli will frequently lodge in vessels affected by previous episodes of embolization.

When emboli are suspected, appropriate laboratory studies can help to document or identify the emboli and their source. Angiography is useful for diagnosing and localizing embolic occlusion, and may also serve as a stepping stone to interventional procedures such as thrombolysis. Ultrasound and magnetic resonance angiography may also be valuable in selected settings. It is important to search for the source of emboli. In many cases, evaluation will include a cardiac work-up with transthoracic or transesophageal echocardiography.

Unless contraindicated, the patient with large, thrombotic embolization is heparinized immediately. Whenever possible, the source, location, and extent of embolization should be identified with imaging studies. When ischemia is severe, this may not be possible; urgent intervention is sometimes needed. Thrombolysis, Fogarty catheterization, and revascularization surgery are potential options for large emboli. Microembolization (especially atheroembolization) is more difficult to treat. Anticoagulation may help, but often the damage is done and the small vessels cannot be readily reopened. Supportive measures to protect the tissues and promote healing are important if infarction occurs.

20.2.3   THROMBOSIS

Thrombosis *in situ* may occur because of extrinsic vascular compression, arterial damage, plaque rupture, intravascular catheterization, clotting disorders, or a variety of other causes. In some cases, the thrombosis appears to be spontaneous, although the history will often suggest that the patient was lifting, straining, or otherwise using the upper extremity at the time the clot occurred. Evaluation and treatment of spontaneous upper extremity arterial thrombosis are similar to those for emboli, although the subsequent work-up frequently includes a search for pathologic disorders, such as primary clotting disorders, systemic diseases (e.g., cancer or inflammatory bowel disease) that can predispose to clotting, and connective tissue disorders.

20.2.4 ARTERIAL INFLAMMATION

Inflammation of the arteries (arteritis or vasculitis) is relatively uncommon, but often affects the upper extremities when it occurs. The causes of most arterial inflammatory disorders are unknown, but some type of autoimmunity is probably involved. Vasculitis may affect large, medium-sized, or small upper extremity vessels. These diseases are covered elsewhere in this book.

Giant cell arteritis, a condition that primarily affects large vessels, is the most common inflammatory disorder of the upper extremity arteries. There are two forms: temporal arteritis, which tends to affect older individuals (over age 55) and Takayasu arteritis,[6] which tends to affect younger (below age 50) females. Both vessels can involve the aorta and great vessels, although Takayasu arteritis probably involves the arteries of the arm more often than temporal arteritis (Figure 20.21). Either disease can lead to arterial stenosis, occlusion, or aneurysm formation. The arteritides that affect small and medium-sized vessels include polyarteritis nodosa, Wegener granulomatosis, lymphomatoid granulomatosis, Kawasaki disease, Churg-Strauss syndrome, and a variety of connective tissue disorders such as lupus erythematosus, rheumatoid arthritis, dermatomyositis, mixed connective tissue disease, and scleroderma. Other conditions that may be associated with small-vessel inflammation include hypertension, cryoglobulinemia, drug reactions, and other forms of autoimmunity.

Thromboangiitis obliterans (TAO), or Buerger's disease, is another unusual form of arteritis. Unlike other vasculitides, TAO can affect both the arteries and the veins.[7] Giant-cell granulomas may be found within the clotted lumen of the vessels, whereas other vasculitic changes are apparent throughout all layers of the arteries. This disease is known to have a very strong association with tobacco use; a history of tobacco exposure, including secondhand smoke or smokeless tobacco products, is found in virtually every patient with TAO.

Definitive therapy of vasculitis is directed at the underlying condition. Whenever possible, a precipitating agent (e.g., drug or tumor) should be identified and removed. In many cases, immunosuppression

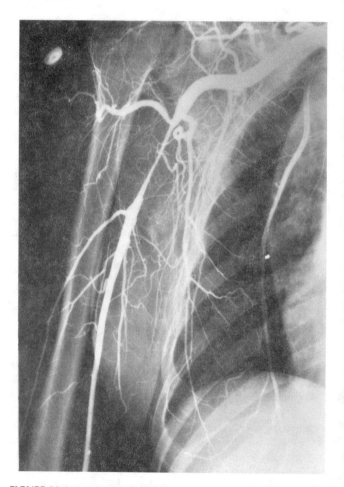

FIGURE 20.1 Arteriogram from a patient with advanced Takayasu arteritis. The figure shows a long, tapered stenosis in the brachial artery.

with prednisone or steroid-sparing agents is necessary. TAO is unlikely to make any therapeutic progress unless the patient discontinues all tobacco exposure.[8] Conversely, the disease may improve considerably when tobacco is discontinued, even without the use of any other therapy.

20.2.5 TRAUMA AND OCCUPATIONAL DISORDERS

The arteries of the upper extremities are frequently subjected to trauma that can be acute or chronic. Examples of acute trauma include penetrating injuries (e.g., from bullets or knives) and blunt trauma (e.g., due to high-speed deceleration or crush injuries). The arterial damage from penetrating wounds to an upper extremity may be occult in one fourth to one third of all penetrating injuries.[9] Even when acute trauma spares the arteries, it is possible to have arterial involvement because of entities such as fat embolization or extrinsic compression (as occurs with compartment syndrome).

Certain types of repeated injuries may also damage the arteries of the upper extremity. Any activity that causes repetitive trauma to the hand or digits may result in arterial occlusion. Two relatively common conditions deserve special attention. One is chronic vibration injury, which is seen in workers who use vibrating tools (e.g., drills, jackhammers, chain saws) for lengthy periods. The other is the hypothenar hammer syndrome, in which the ulnar artery develops occlusion or aneurysmal changes as it crosses the area near the hook of the hamate bone. Many types of chronic trauma will damage the vessel in this region (Figure 20.2). Patients with hypothenar hammer syndrome may develop symptoms from chronic ulnar artery occlusion, or, more likely, will experience microembolization from the diseased portion of the vessel.

The best form of treatment is to prevent arterial injury, especially in situations where chronic trauma occurs. A small change in the way the hands are used may prevent long-term complications. Surgical intervention may be necessary in the setting of acute trauma. Chronic trauma can produce aneurysmal or occlusive changes (such as those

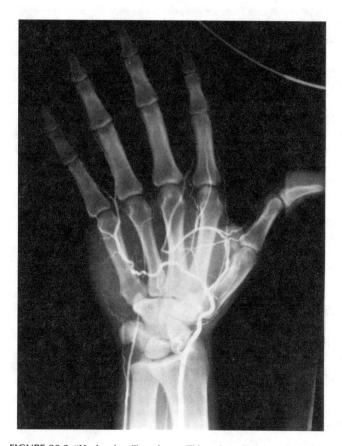

FIGURE 20.2 "Hockey-hand" syndrome. This variant of the hypothenar hammer syndrome occurred in a man who played goalie for a professional hockey team. Not only is the ulnar artery occluded as it crosses the hamate, but other vessels within the palm of the hand show evidence of traumatic damage.

seen in hypothenar hammer syndrome) that may be amenable to surgical reconstruction. Angiography is frequently necessary to identify the abnormalities in either acute or chronic trauma. When necessary, medical therapy that includes vasodilators (to prevent vasospasm) or anticoagulants (to prevent clotting) may be used as adjunct therapy to interventional treatments and preventive measures.

20.2.6 Arterial Compression (Thoracic Outlet Syndrome)

Thoracic outlet syndrome and other compression syndromes are discussed elsewhere in this book, but it is important to recognize that these are some of the most common problems affecting the upper extremity arteries. Positional compression of the subclavian or axillary artery as it passes through the thoracic outlet is so common that this phenomenon may almost be considered a normal variant; however, the number of patients who develop significant symptoms from this compression is small. Even when intermittent arterial compression can be documented, symptoms may actually result from nerve or venous compression. In some cases, intermittent arterial compression will produce structural arterial damage resulting in aneurysm formation, embolization, or even arterial occlusion.[10] This is most common when significant anatomic abnormalities are present, especially cervical ribs (Figure 20.3).

In many cases, thoracic outlet arterial problems can be treated by avoiding the maneuvers that precipitate problems (e.g., hyperabduction of the arms), or by following a physical medicine protocol that includes various stretching exercises. When prominent abnormalities such as cervical ribs are present, surgery is often required to decompress the thoracic outlet.[11]

20.2.7 Vasospasm

Vasospasm, or Raynaud phenomenon, is discussed in a separate chapter of this book, but it is such a common upper extremity disorder that it deserves a second mention. Vasospasm may be a primary occurrence

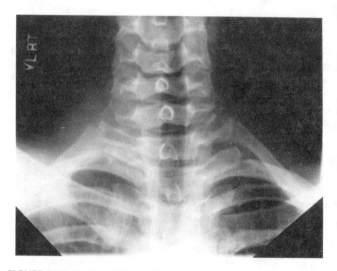

FIGURE 20.3 Cervical rib in a patient with severe thoracic outlet syndrome.

or it can be produced by secondary causes. In either case, episodes of intense vasospasm are typically precipitated by cold exposure, emotional stress, and certain types of exercise or activities. The condition may be bilateral and affect most of the digits (which is common in primary vasospasm), or may be limited to some or even a single digit (often seen in the secondary form). The causes of secondary vasospasm are numerous and include systemic disorders ,such as connective tissue disease, hyperviscosity syndromes, abnormal blood proteins, fixed obstructive disease of the upper extremity or digits, certain drugs (such as nicotine, β-blockers, or ergotamine), and many others. Although upper extremity skin breakdown is rare with primary vasospasm, ulceration and even gangrene with severe secondary cases may be seen.

The diagnosis of vasospasm can usually be made by history, and occasionally can be noted on examination. When the diagnosis is in doubt, specific noninvasive vascular laboratory testing (including provocative testing with ice-water immersion) may help clarify or document the presence of vasospasm.

The treatment of vasospasm should be directed against an underlying cause whenever possible. If no underlying cause is present (primary), or if the condition cannot be effectively treated (e.g., scleroderma), therapy will depend on conservative or medical means in most cases. Conservative measures include avoiding cold (which may precipitate the attacks), dressing warmly (including gloves and a hat), and avoiding drugs that may precipitate vasoconstriction, such as β-blockers and nicotine. Specific medical treatment with certain vasodilators (especially calcium channel blockers and α_1-blockers) may be helpful. Biofeedback will occasionally help. In severe cases, interruption of the sympathetic nerves has proven useful.

20.2.8 ARTERIOVENOUS MALFORMATIONS, FISTULAS, AND VASCULAR TUMORS

The arteries of the upper extremities may be involved with congenital malformations or acquired arteriovenous (AV) fistulae. In some cases, the malformations/fistulae take the form of tumors, such as benign hemangiomas (which may have a predominantly arterial component) or aggressive malignant tumors such as angiosarcomas. Acquired AV fistulae are usually the result of penetrating trauma such as gunshot wounds, surgical procedures, and bony fractures. Iatrogenic injuries, particularly those associated with catheter procedures, are seen with increasing frequency as interventional procedures become more common.

When therapy is necessary, surgery (to ligate or debulk the abnormal vessels) or embolization (to occlude vessels) may often be used. Postcatheterization problems such as AV fistula, and especially false aneurysm, can occasionally be treated with relatively conservative means, such as ultrasound-guided external compression.

20.2.9 MISCELLANEOUS CONDITIONS OF THE ARTERIES

Upper extremity arteries can be affected by a variety of unusual conditions such as degenerative arthropathies (e.g., as seen in the Marfan syndrome, Ehlers-Danlos syndrome andcystic medical necrosis), fibro-muscular dysplasia, medial calcification of the arteries, and a wide variety of coagulation problems, including various hypercoagulable states, platelet disorders, and thrombocytosis.

20.3 STRATEGIES FOR EVALUATION OF UPPER EXTREMITY ARTERIAL DISEASES

When a patient presents with an upper extremity problem, the signs and symptoms will often suggest the possibility of specific vascular abnormalities. For example, pain may be seen with virtually any vascular disorder (e.g., arterial, venous, or small vessel). Swelling suggests a venous or lymphatic disorder, but may complicate certain arterial conditions (for example, some patients with ischemic arms may keep them immobile and dependent, which causes edema formation) or small-vessel disorders (i.e., those associated with inflammation). Claudication usually indicates arterial obstruction, although exercise-induced symptoms may also occur in severe venous obstruction (so-called venous claudication). Discoloration can be seen in limbs with arterial disease, but may be even more spectacular in those with venous disorders and is especially dramatic in certain small-vessel conditions such as acrocyanosis, vasospasm, and micro-emboli. Episodic symptoms, produced by cold or emotional stress, suggest vasospasm, but may also be associated with "fixed" arterial occlusions from any cause. Cutaneous ulcerations and infarction imply advanced arterial or small-vessel diseases. Positional symptoms often reflect thoracic outlet syndrome or one of the other impingement syndromes.

Some clinical presentations are complicated by a confusing constellation of symptoms that reflect multiple vascular problems (i.e., multifactorial symptoms). Other presentations may involve unusual symptoms that are partially vascular in etiology (for example, the swollen, cold, painful, weak arm seen with advanced reflux sympathetic dystrophy[12]). Finally, some presentations are ultimately nonvascular in origin (e.g., pain and edema caused by connective tissue diseases, arthritis, dermatitis or trauma). The successful diagnosis of upper extremity signs and symptoms of vascular disease therefore requires careful evaluation of the history, physical examination, and, where appropriate, specific vascular testing (which may be invasive or noninvasive).

20.3.1 History

The usual symptoms of peripheral arterial disease have been described above. Briefly, the clinician must identify the cardinal complaint such as pain, swelling, cold sensation, discoloration, claudication, and skin breakdown. These questions should be considered:

- Was the onset acute or gradual?
- Have the symptoms ever occurred before?
- What circumstances precipitated the symptoms?
- Does the patient have any known medical conditions that might be involved?

The list is extensive. The examiner should search for specific factors that trigger or relieve the symptoms. For example, does any specific activity affect or precipitate symptoms? Do the symptoms change when the arm is elevated? When the limb is made dependent? In most cases, a good history will enable the investigator to determine if the symptoms are likely to be vascular in origin.

20.3.2 Examination

The pulse examination is the most important single component of the upper extremity vascular evaluation. It should include an assessment of the pulses during thoracic outlet maneuvers and the Allen test (Figure 20.4). The arms should also be assessed for color, edema, temperature, presence of an increased superficial venous pattern, strength, motor and sensory function, and other characteristics as clinically indicated.

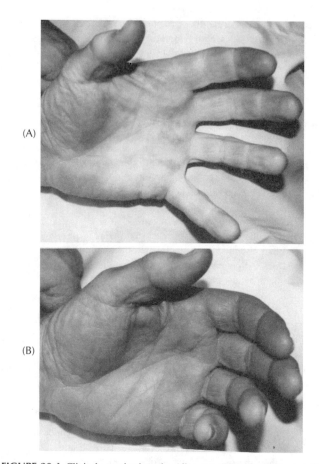

FIGURE 20.4 Clinical examination: the Allen test. To perform this test, the radial artery is manually compressed and the patient is asked to expel blood from the hand by performing a series of fist clenches. If the ulnar artery is occluded, the hand cannot reperfuse and distinct blanching will occur (A). When pressure is released from the radial artery (B) refilling will occur normally.

20.3.3 VASCULAR TESTING

In many patients, specific vascular testing is necessary to make a diagnosis of peripheral arterial disease. Even in those situations where the history or examination strongly suggests the correct diagnosis (i.e., the pulses are absent, thoracic outlet maneuvers are positive, the limb is swollen and plethoric with increased superficial venous pattern), objective testing may help to document, quantify, or otherwise assess the disease and its severity.[13]

It is beyond the scope of this chapter to discuss the details of noninvasive vascular testing for the upper extremity. An algorithm for the assessment of upper extremity arterial disease is provided in Figure 20.5. In brief, arterial disease is usually evaluated by (1) measuring arterial pressure at various levels along the upper extremity (including the digits), and (2) by assessing the Doppler signals at various levels. Transcutaneous oxygen is occasionally measured in some vascular laboratories. Venous disease is best assessed with duplex ultrasonography (plethysmography is notoriously unreliable in the upper extremity). Measurements of skin temperature and laser Doppler cutaneous blood flow may also provide valuable information about the circulation. Provocative studies may be extremely useful and include:

- measurement of digital flow or blood pressure during thoracic outlet maneuvers or Allen testing
- arm blood pressure before and after exercise
- effective ice-water immersion on skin blood flow or cutaneous rewarming time
- effective ambient warming on digital blood flow (as measured with laser Doppler)

REFERENCES

1. Welling, R.E., Cranley, J.J., Krause, R.J., et al., Obliterative arterial disease of the upper extremity, *Arch. Surg.,* 116, 1593, 1981.

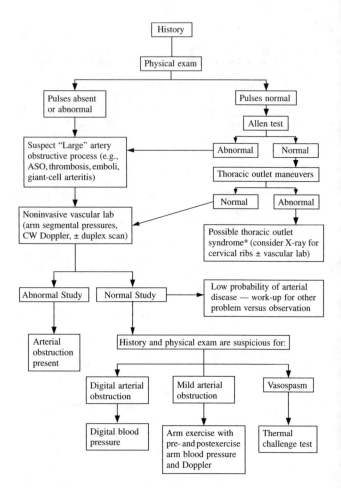

FIGURE 20.5 Algorithm for patients with suspected upper extremity arterial problems. ASO = atherosclerosis obliterans; CW = chest wall. *Clinical correlation is necessary to make a diagnosis of thoracic outlet syndrome.

2. Laroche, G.P., Bernatz, P.E., Joyce, J.W., et al., Chronic arterial insufficiency of the upper extremity, *Mayo Clin. Proc.*, 51, 180, 1976.

3. Crawford, E.S., De Bakey, M.E., Morris, G.C., Jr., et al., Thromboobliterative disease of the great vessels arising from the aortic arch, *J. Thorac. Cardiovasc. Surg.*, 43, 38, 1962.

4. Shoor, P.M., Fogarty, T.J., Acute arterial insufficiency, in *Diagnosis and Management of Peripheral Vascular Disease*, Miller, D.C. and Roon, A.S., Eds., Addison-Wesley Publishing Co, Inc., Menlo Park, CA, 1982, 119.

5. Meister, S.G., Grossman, W., Dexter, L., et al., Paradoxical embolism: diagnosis during life, *Am. J. Med.*, 53, 292, 1972.

6. Hall, S., Barr, W., Lie, et al., Takayasu arteritis, *Medicine*, 64, 89, 1985.

7. Shionoya, S., Diagnostic criteria of Buerger's disease, *Int. J. Cardiol.* 66, S243, 1998.

8. Shigematsu, H. and Shigemyatsu, K., Factors affecting the long-term outcome of Buerger's disease (thromboangiitis obliterans), *Int. Angiol.*, 18, 58, 1999.

9. Trunkey, D.D., Lim, R.C., Vascular trauma, in *Diagnosis and Management of Peripheral Vascular Disease*, Miller, D.C. and Roon, A.J., Eds., Addison-Wesley Publishing Company, Inc., Menlo Park, CA, 1982, 103.

10. Hood, D.B., Kuehne, J., Yellin, A.E., et al., Vascular complications of thoracic outlet syndrome, *Am. Surg.*, 63, 913, 1997.

11. Fantini, G.A., Reserving supraclavicular first rib resection for vascular complications of thoracic outlet syndrome, *Am. J. Surg.*, 172, 200, 1996.

12. Kurvers, H.A., Reflex sympathetic dystrophy: facts and hypotheses, *Vasc. Med.*, 3, 207, 1998.

13. Rooke, T.W., Arterial disease: noninvasive assessment, in *Current Management of Hypertensive and Vascular Diseases,* Cooke, J.P. and Frohlich, E.D., Eds., Mosby-Year Book, Inc., St. Louis, 1992, 1999.

Section VII

Integrated Vascular Care

21 The Vascular Health Care Team: Teamwork Devoted to the Optimal Care of Peripheral Arterial Disease

Alan T. Hirsch, Anthony J. Comerota, David Hunter, M. Eileen Walsh, Diane Treat-Jacobson, and Marsha Neumyer

CONTENTS

21.1 Introduction 458
21.2 The Vascular Physician 462
    21.2.1 Role of the Vascular Physician in the Care of Patients with Peripheral Arterial Disease 462
    21.2.2 Educational Preparation of the Vascular Physician..462
        21.2.2.1 Vascular Surgery 462
        21.2.2.2 Vascular Medicine......................................463
        21.2.2.3 Cardiology 464
        21.2.2.4 Vascular-Interventional Radiology.............465
    21.2.3 Professional Support for Vascular Physicians 466
    21.2.4 What Does the Future Look Like?............................467

0-8493-8413-3/01/$0.00+$1.50
© 2001 by CRC Press LLC

21.3 The Vascular Nurse 467
        21.3.1 Role of the Vascular Nurse in the Care of Patients
                   with Peripheral Arterial Disease..................................467
                   21.3.1.1 Vascular Rehabilitation 469
        21.3.2 Educational Preparation of the Vascular Nurse........470
        21.3.3 Professional Support for Vascular Nursing 471
        21.3.4 Professional Certification...472
        21.3.5 What Does the Future Look Like?..............................472
21.4 The Vascular Technologist 473
        21.4.1 Role of the Vascular Technologist in the Care
                   of Patients with Peripheral Arterial Disease 473
        21.4.2 Evolutionary Development of the Profession...........475
        21.4.3 Educational Preparation
                   of the Vascular Technologist.....................................475
        21.4.4 Professional Support for Vascular Technologists 476
        21.4.5 Professional Certification...476
        21.4.6 Accreditation of Vascular Laboratories 477
        21.4.7 What Does the Future Look Like?..............................479
References...480

21.1 INTRODUCTION

Optimal long-term care of patients with atherosclerotic peripheral
arterial diseases (PAD) is best achieved by an integrated medical
management program, coordinated by a vascular health care team.
This is essential, because patients require distinct health care interventions at different stages of their disease.

For those patients fortunate enough to have their PAD diagnosed
at an early stage, preventive interventions (e.g., atherosclerosis risk
reduction, antiplatelet therapies, exercise prescriptions, and foot care)
may predominate in the care plan to delay progression of atherosclerosis and prevent ischemic events and development of functional disability. Most patients with chronic symptomatic, but not limb-threatening, PAD are best managed by lifestyle and pharmacotherapeutic

interventions designed to decrease symptoms and reduce the rate of cardiovascular ischemic events. In patients with severe and usually multilevel occlusive disease that may cause ischemic rest pain or tissue necrosis, more-aggressive clinical efforts (including revascularization, either by endovascular or surgical techniques) are mandated during later PAD disease stages to decrease the likelihood of amputation and to prolong life.

These interventions and the overall care of these patients are often complex and demanding. An interdisciplinary team approach is required to offer each patient the best preventive, diagnostic, therapeutic, and rehabilitation options. The consistent, lifelong application of such a vascular therapeutic program is augmented by a partnership that involves the patients, their families, their primary care providers, and a dedicated vascular health care team. In this regard, this handbook can foster better care by acknowledging the various contributions of the members of the vascular health care team that are the foundation of clinical success.

Although creation of such a vascular health care team is desirable, it is important to recognize potential barriers to the delivery of effective collaborative care for PAD. First, many primary care and vascular clinicians alike continue to believe that "conservative care" is an adequate clinical strategy for PAD patients. Unfortunately, conservative care is frequently thought to be synonymous with either casual advice to "stop smoking and walk," or with any care that is "nonoperative." In the last decade, however, it has become clear that *all* patients with PAD, whether symptomatic or asymptomatic, suffer high rates of stroke, myocardial infarction, and death.

These outcomes can be reduced by appropriate medical therapies, but are often left "unmanaged" by conservative care. Similarly, such casual advice is ineffective in preventing deterioration of symptoms and in improving quality of life. Therefore, it is imperative that vascular clinicians be familiar, either individually or as a health care team, with those medical therapies that are known to be effective in blunting the adverse cardiovascular and limb symptoms and ischemic events that frequently occur in PAD patients.

Similarly, for patients to be offered an appropriate set of alternatives to ameliorate claudication, an adequate physician examination and careful use of noninvasive arterial imaging may be required to determine if either endovascular or surgical options would provide the best long-term outcome. Patients with critical limb ischemia similarly benefit from the clinical synergy that results when excellence in vascular technology is linked to excellence in the provision of percutaneous, surgical, and medical therapies. In addition, long-term risk factor reduction strategies are hard to achieve without effective partnering with vascular nursing colleagues. Quality of life can be improved when patients are offered the sympathetic and educational interventions that can be delivered by experienced vascular nurses.

Therefore, vascular nurses, vascular technologists, vascular surgeons, interventional radiologists, vascular medicine specialists, and cardiologists can deliberately work together as a team to coordinate care for PAD patients. An integrated multidisciplinary vascular health care team provides the PAD patient with optimal therapeutic choices, not only for a specific care episode, but also for the lifetime of the patient.

The patient is the ultimate partner in this collaboration. The success of all vascular therapies (e.g., smoking cessation; antiplatelet, lipid-lowering, antihypertensive, and diabetic therapies; revascularization interventions) requires a trusting, long-term therapeutic relationship. This relationship may encompass the physician, vascular nurse, rehabilitation staff, and many other vascular care professionals (Figure 21.1).

Long-term compliance with a treatment plan often requires patients to adopt major behavioral and lifestyle modifications that can affect their vocations, home relationships, social support, and life goals. Patients with PAD are sometimes perceived to be among the least motivated of patients with atherosclerotic syndromes to undertake such efforts. Motivation to adopt a healthier lifestyle is *not* a function of the disease or a specific patient population itself, and can be improved. PAD patients have rarely been offered adequate information that places their PAD in proper perspective as a major threat to life

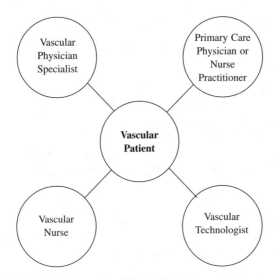

FIGURE 21.1 All patients with peripheral arterial disease will usually require the coordinated care of a dedicated primary care provider, vascular physician specialist, vascular nurse, and vascular technologist during their lifetime of care. Teamwork and ongoing communication between these clinicians is fundamental to the achievement of excellence in care outcomes.

and limb. This current lack of public vascular knowledge increases the challenge to all vascular clinicians to serve as educators of and advocates for public vascular awareness. All vascular health care professionals should be able to provide guidance on lifestyle improvements, the rationale for change, and specific tools for success.

This chapter describes the educational preparation and training of vascular specialists as they provide care for patients with PAD and the roles of such clinicians within the health care team. It also outlines both professional societal resources and selected online resources for vascular information. It is important to recognize that PADs are chronic and risk factor care is lifelong. Vascular teamwork is essential to the success of preventive strategies; early and accurate diagnosis; effective medical, endovascular, and surgical therapies to improve quality of life and prolong survival; and for beneficial outcomes from PAD vascular rehabilitation.

21.2 THE VASCULAR PHYSICIAN

ALAN T. HIRSCH, ANTHONY J. COMEROTA,
*   AND DAVID HUNTER*

21.2.1 ROLE OF THE VASCULAR PHYSICIAN IN THE CARE OF PATIENTS WITH PERIPHERAL ARTERIAL DISEASE

Physicians provide vascular specialty skills in vascular surgery, vascular medicine, interventional radiology, or cardiology. Traditionally, these four specialties have fulfilled rather distinct roles, and yet each type of physician could potentially provide diagnostic and therapeutic services beyond these particular traditions.

21.2.2 EDUCATIONAL PREPARATION OF THE VASCULAR PHYSICIAN

The traditional vascular specialties provide rather distinct pathways toward the achievement of competence and autonomy within their field. These pathways are outlined below.

21.2.2.1 Vascular Surgery

The specialty of vascular surgery has evolved from general surgery. Unlike most other surgical specialties, vascular surgeons have not traditionally had medical counterparts to assist in the management of patients with vascular diseases. Therefore, vascular surgeons have often assumed the responsibility for the nonoperative as well as the operative management of these patients. Fortunately, interest and progress in the creation of vascular medicine specialists are growing and are enthusiastically welcomed.

Vascular surgeons must complete an approved general surgery residency program of at least 5 years before acceptance into a vascular surgery residency (fellowship). As of this writing, there are 82 approved vascular surgical fellowships in the United States that graduate 150 vascular surgeons annually. Most vascular surgery programs are 2 years in duration and include basic science of vascular disease, noninvasive vascular technology with rotations through the noninvasive vascular laboratory, education and clinical experience in percutaneous and endovascular intervention, and the full spectrum of operative reconstruction techniques.

Board certification in vascular surgery is achieved after successful board certification in general surgery. Upon completion of an approved vascular fellowship and performing a requisite number of vascular reconstructive procedures, the candidate can apply to take the qualifying examination (written examination). After passing this qualifying examination, the candidate is admitted to the certifying examination (oral examination). On successful completion of the certifying examination, the vascular surgeon is board certified for a period of 10 years, at which time a written recertification examination must be successfully completed to maintain board certification.

21.2.2.2 Vascular Medicine

The vascular medicine specialist represents those physicians whose core training is derived from internal medicine and some of its subspecialties, such as hematology-thrombosis and cardiovascular medicine, which has been augmented by an advanced postgraduate vascular training program. Physicians can elect to become vascular medicine specialists after completion of either a 3-year postgraduate course of internal medicine training or on completion of any traditional medical fellowship (e.g., cardiology, hematology and thrombosis, pulmonary medicine, rheumatology). Most vascular medicine fellowships include a minimum of 1 year of devoted clinical training, and such an advanced vascular training program is focused on the study of vascular biology and acquisition of those skills required for expertise in clinical vascular care.

The vascular medicine curriculum includes didactic training (lectures, focused study, and knowledge of the medical literature); clinical and scientific mentorship (a partnership with an advanced vascular practitioner); and supervised clinical experience (both outpatient and inpatient care management of a broad array of diagnostic and therapeutic vascular conditions). This core triad of didactic training, mentorship, and clinical experience serves as the fundamental experiential core that is required by the vascular medicine specialist who will be expected to independently manage both common and unusual vascular disorders. This management must be performed with reference to the broadest scientific database and modified by both clinical experience and knowledge of local vascular care resources. Requisite components of vascular medicine fellowship training are outlined by the Society for Vascular Medicine and Biology. Although vascular medicine is recognized by the American Medical Association (AMA) as a "self-defined medical specialty," to date there is no specific board certification for vascular medicine specialists.

21.2.2.3   Cardiology

During their minimum 24-month postgraduate program, cardiology trainees currently receive extensive mentorship and clinical experience in the prevention of atherosclerosis and in the management of coronary atherosclerotic syndromes, but much less emphasis has traditionally been placed on a curriculum that encompasses care for noncoronary vascular diseases.

Cardiovascular training standards are prepared by the American College of Cardiology which, via the Core Cardiology Training Symposium document, outlines the recommendations for curricula in 10 areas of cardiovascular medicine, including vascular medicine and peripheral catheter-based interventions. Multiple levels of training intensity are outlined in this document, which is regularly updated to reflect the increasing interest in vascular medicine training. A basic level of vascular competence, usually offered as a minimum of 2 to 3 months of elective rotations, is expected of all cardiovascular fellows. This core training includes exposure to noninvasive vascular diagnostic modalities, evaluation and management of many common vascular diseases, and exposure to peripheral angiography and percutaneous procedures. The core training is not expected to lead to broad competence in vascular medicine.

A second level of training is designed for those who seek special expertise in the evaluation and management of patients with vascular disorders. This level of training is expected to require a minimum of 1 additional year and encompasses specific rotations in the noninvasive vascular laboratory, the peripheral catheterization laboratory dedicated to noncoronary diagnostic and therapeutic interventions, a continuity outpatient vascular clinic, and an inpatient vascular service. The trainee is also expected to actively participate in vascular educational conferences. This deeper level of training should permit the trainee to achieve general competence in vascular care and provides further exposure to the techniques of the peripheral vascular interventional laboratory. However, an additional year of training is required for those who seek expertise in endovascular diagnosis and peripheral vascular interventions.

21.2.2.4   Vascular-Interventional Radiology

Interventional radiologists currently have two pathways by which they can approach their specialty. Traditionally, after a year of internship, they must complete a standard 4-year radiology residency after which they complete a 1- or 2-year vascular or interventional radiology fellowship. Most fellowship programs are designed to provide a 1-year curriculum, with occasional programs offering a second year to outstanding candidates who are planning to continue as academic interventionalists and who desire either further training or time to complete research projects.

The other plan involves earlier exposure to interventional practice during a middle year of the residency and opportunities to participate in clinical specialty training that is designed to augment interventional radiology skills. Fellowship programs emphasize the areas of expertise of the facility or staff in which they are centered and, although all programs encompass both vascular and nonvascular procedures, many programs provide a distinct emphasis on one type of procedure.

An increasing number of fellowship programs also offer participants an opportunity to become involved in the noninvasive diagnosis of vascular disease by participating in, supervising, and interpreting studies in the noninvasive laboratory, or in vascular imaging services that use computed tomographic and magnetic resonance techniques. The spectrum of vascular diseases and procedures to which an interventional trainee can be exposed is vast. In addition to the large number of patients with peripheral, renal, and cerebrovascular atherosclerotic disease, trainees can also expect to see patients with vascular malformations, other congenital vascular abnormalities, trauma, and a broad range of nonatherosclerotic pathologies. The trainees learn to use the various imaging tools, not only for diagnosis, but also as guides to intervention. In this respect, many programs are beginning to plan for a time when many vascular interventions will likely be performed using magnetic resonance guidance.

On completion of the internship and 4 years of residency, radiology residents take their board certification examination and are allowed to perform interventional procedures. Individuals who elect to pursue an interventional radiology fellowship complete the 1 or 2 years of additional training and are then allowed to sit for the Certificate of Added Qualification examination in interventional radiology.

21.2.3 PROFESSIONAL SUPPORT FOR VASCULAR PHYSICIANS

Each respective vascular specialty is supported by a professional society that provides continuing medical education (CME), professional member services, and annual scientific sessions. These societies increasingly coordinate their educational activities and are forming a growing number of affiliations. It seems likely that this trend will continue. Appendix 1 includes a list of vascular professional societies and foundations.

21.2.4 WHAT DOES THE FUTURE LOOK LIKE?

It seems increasingly likely that skills that were traditionally reserved (or particularly emphasized) by a given vascular specialty will slowly become integrated into the postgraduate training of another related vascular specialty. For example, integration of endovascular skills into the curricula of vascular surgeons, cardiologists, and vascular medicine specialists is already under way. Similarly, the role of pharmacotherapies will be increasingly emphasized in all vascular training programs beyond those reserved for cardiovascular physicians. Of course, there are other alternatives to the creation of more intensive cross training. There is some speculation that the skills required for competence in a particular specialty would be diminished by broadening the curriculum for each physician vascular specialty. In lieu of emphasizing cross training as a means to provide a range of vascular clinical skills, it seems likely that vascular physician specialists will link their skills in "centers of excellence" that contain two or more vascular physician specialties as well as vascular nurses and technologists.

21.3 THE VASCULAR NURSE

DIANE TREAT-JACOBSON AND M. EILEEN WALSH

21.3.1 ROLE OF THE VASCULAR NURSE IN THE CARE OF PATIENTS WITH PERIPHERAL ARTERIAL DISEASE

Vascular nurses are particularly well suited to provide care for patients with PAD. These patients require complex care at most points along the care continuum, including disease prevention, screening, risk factor management, lifestyle modification, acute intervention, chronic disease management, and rehabilitation.

Vascular nurses serve in a variety of roles from direct care provider to consultant, typically coordinating the care of PAD patients from the hospital to the clinic to the rehabilitation setting to home. Through communication and collaboration with the patient, family, and health care team, vascular nurses help to ensure continuity and consistency of care across all settings. Vascular nurses use sound clinical judgment, established standards of care, and clinical pathways to guide care delivery. They facilitate care for the patient through the transition between health care settings, based on changing needs and available resources. Vascular nurses can initiate consultations with other health care providers, such as dietary, physical therapy, and home care specialists, to complement care.

Vascular nurses provide care to patients with PAD in a variety of clinical settings. Traditionally, they have provided care in the acute-care or hospital setting. Inpatient care can be delivered in the emergency room, operating room, intensive care unit, step-down unit, specialty vascular unit, or general medical or surgical unit. However, with today's increased emphasis on shorter hospital stays, more nurses are providing care in the outpatient setting.

There is great value derived from the expertise of the vascular nurse in the role of patient care coordinator. The nurse is often anchored in the outpatient clinic and can assist the patient in navigating through the complex web of care. This enhances continuity from the outpatient clinic to the noninvasive vascular laboratory, through percutaneous and surgical intervention, inpatient care, home care, and follow-up.

Vascular nurse coordinators can also serve as liaisons to the vascular health care team (including the primary care provider, vascular physicians, and vascular technologists) to help coordinate care from the outpatient to inpatient settings. The coordinator assists in communicating the plan of care to inpatient nurses, promotes adherence to clinical pathways, and serves as a resource for home care nurses and outpatient pharmacists, thereby facilitating transition of the patient back to the outpatient follow-up setting.

Advanced practice nurses (APNs), including clinical nurse specialists and nurse practitioners, may serve as primary care providers. APNs possess advanced knowledge and clinical expertise and provide care within the hospital, clinic, or office-based practice. Responsibilities typically include taking the patient history and performing the physical examination, pulse assessment, performance of the ankle-brachial index (ABI), identification of health care problems, and initiation of specific therapeutic interventions. These interventions may include aggressive modification of atherosclerosis risk factors (e.g., specific counseling about lipid control, blood pressure management, use of medications, exercise, and smoking cessation). The APN in the hospital setting manages vascular inpatients, conducts inpatient rounds, and provides education about the disease process, risk factors, treatment options, medications, and diet. The APN may also serve as a consultant to the nursing staff to address complex care needs of patients.

There is a distinct lack of public awareness of PAD, creating larger patient- and family-education challenges than exist for many other chronic diseases. This is compounded by the lack of awareness of PAD that remains common in the primary care setting. Recent heightened awareness of the increased risk of cardiovascular ischemic events and death associated with PAD has prompted the need for all vascular specialists to aggressively educate patients and primary care clinicians, modify risk factors, and provide timely intervention. Nurses play a vital role in the ongoing education of patients with PAD in all practice environments.

Educational interventions include explanation of the systemic nature of the disease process and the causal relation of risk factors to disease progression and incidence of cardiovascular ischemic events. Such educational interventions should review all available therapeutic options for claudication symptom relief and the importance of a PAD-focused exercise rehabilitation program. In addition to educating patients, vascular nurses are essential in working with patients to translate these educational interventions into real-world, lifelong behavioral change so that such theoretical knowledge is used to actually modify risk and fundamentally alter the course of PAD through better, more consistent patient care.

21.3.1.1   Vascular Rehabilitation

Vascular nurses have the requisite skill to lead in the creation and function of the vascular rehabilitation program. In this environment they have a unique opportunity to help patients with PAD make

significant lifestyle and behavioral changes. Throughout the PAD rehabilitation program, frequent contact with the patient opens a window
of opportunity to provide specific educational interventions. These
should include information on:

- claudication
- the role of the ABI in following disease progression
- atherosclerosis risk factors
- exercise and nutrition
- lipid and blood pressure management
- the need to maintain antiplatelet therapy
- the mandate to achieve complete smoking cessation

This information is provided one-to-one or through interactive
group classes. As most inpatient and outpatient care has recently been
characterized by increasingly brief interactions between clinicians and
patients—with a consequent deterioration of patient education—the
PAD vascular rehabilitation setting may provide a uniquely therapeutic
environment for achieving lifestyle behavioral improvements.

Patients with PAD who take part in a rehabilitation program learn
specific exercise strategies to improve claudication symptoms and
increase functional status. Patients receive an exercise prescription
based on both the severity of their PAD and their personal functional
goals. This information is readily translated into a home exercise
program, so that the benefits of the supervised setting can be continued
long after the formal supervised vascular rehabilitation program has
been completed.

21.3.2   Educational Preparation of the Vascular Nurse

Vascular nurses come from a variety of educational backgrounds.
Undergraduate education qualifying a student to sit for the state board
examination for licensure as a registered nurse (RN) can be obtained
through a diploma, associate, or bachelor's degree program. Special-
ization in vascular nursing usually occurs on the job and is augmented
by continuing or higher education.

Nursing curricula, like those of our medical colleagues, currently contain little specific education about PAD. However, there are several areas within the undergraduate nursing curricula that prepare nurses to positively impact the care of patients with PAD. These content areas include:

- patient education
- principles of adult teaching and learning
- behavior modification
- assistance of patients and families through all phases of health and illness
- family dynamics
- emphasis on the patient as a whole, with a focus on care options with consideration for individual life goals.

This educational preparation is very helpful in the care of PAD patients. The chronic long-term nature of PAD, and the often cyclical course of the disease and its treatment through many phases of the health care continuum, are ideally suited to the specific expertise of the vascular nurse.

Nurses may choose to complete an APN program, either as a nurse practitioner or a clinical nurse specialist. These programs often include a master's degree and prepare nurses to function more independently in the areas outlined above. APNs receive specific education that prepares them to identify research questions and conduct clinical research. APNs contribute to the dissemination of new clinical knowledge to the practice setting and may also report research findings through publication and presentations.

Some nurses obtain a doctoral degree (Ph.D., Ed.D., or D.N.Sc.). These nurses receive extensive clinical or research training and may choose to focus their research and clinical efforts on the broad area of vascular care delivery and patient outcomes.

21.3.3 Professional Support for Vascular Nursing

The Society of Vascular Nursing (SVN) is a not-for-profit international professional association dedicated to promoting excellence in the compassionate and comprehensive management of persons with vascular disease (see Appendix 1). Through the SVN, vascular nurses have developed and disseminated educational materials for patients on vascular topics. The SVN designed and implemented the first community-based PAD screening programs, such as the "A Step Ahead" program, to detect PAD. These PAD-screening events provide the opportunity for patient education and distribution of educational materials. Vascular nurses have also been in the forefront of developing vascular rehabilitation programs for patients with PAD.

21.3.4 PROFESSIONAL CERTIFICATION

Through the Vascular Nursing Certification Board, a subsidiary of the SVN, a nurse in vascular practice can become certified as a vascular nurse. Certified vascular nurses (CVNs) must have an active RN licensure equivalent and practice in vascular nursing. Certification is valid for 3 years, and CVNs can maintain their status by examination or meeting continuing education requirements.

21.3.5 WHAT DOES THE FUTURE LOOK LIKE?

There are many opportunities for vascular nurses to play a greater role in educating primary care providers, including physicians, about all available diagnostic and treatment options for patients with PAD. In addition, vascular nurses possess a unique perspective that would greatly contribute to the development of new knowledge related to the care of PAD patients. They should begin to play an increasing role in the design and implementation of vascular clinical trials and other clinical research in this patient population. In addition, the importance of PAD—including its high prevalence, morbidity, and mortality—should be brought to the attention of those who are designing nursing curricula so that awareness of this disease is promoted early in the education process. It might also be beneficial to overlap with medical education and form combined educational programs.

21.4   THE VASCULAR TECHNOLOGIST

MARSHA NEUMYER

21.4.1   Role of the Vascular Technologist in the Care Of Patients with Peripheral Arterial Disease

Vascular technologists are an important part of the team approach to the care of patients with PAD. As noted elsewhere in this book, the initial diagnosis of vascular disease can often be made based on a review of the patient's medical history and a thorough physical examination. The patient may then be referred to the vascular laboratory. The role of the laboratory is to confirm the clinical impression, determine the location and severity of disease, and help define the therapeutic options.

The vascular technologist will perform a limited physical examination and review the presenting symptoms, appropriate medical history, and any past or planned revascularization procedures. The technologist may advise the referring physician regarding selection of the ideal vascular testing procedures, in part based on the clinical presentation and initial diagnostic data, and will usually provide a preliminary interpretation of the test results. Additional time is used to explain these results in the context of the patient's particular presentation of PAD, and this discussion will, again, often include information about its causes and treatments.

For patients who have undergone revascularization procedures, the importance of ongoing surveillance may be discussed. Diagnostic testing may be performed in the hospital clinic or office setting, or the technologist may provide service in the emergency room (e.g., to evaluate the patient with deep vein thrombosis or acute arterial ischemia); in the operating room to confirm patency of a bypass graft; in the angiography suite to direct placement of arterial catheters and assess the results of percutaneous dilatation procedures; or in postendovascular intervention to confirm appropriate blood flow patterns.

The vascular technology specialty is represented by a professional organization, the Society of Vascular Technology (SVT), which has joined with members of the Sonography Coalition to develop a "Scope of Practice" document for diagnostic ultrasound professionals.[1] This document defines the role of the technologist in today's health care settings. A key component of the "Scope of Practice" is a focus on the vascular technologist's function as a member of the health care team who collaborates with other health care professionals to optimize patient care.

In most vascular laboratories, there is a close working relationship between the technologists and the vascular laboratory physicians. Although the medical director is responsible for assuring appropriate high-quality testing and ongoing quality assurance, all members of the technical and medical staff of the laboratory share this responsibility. Together, they review patient histories, develop testing protocols and diagnostic criteria, and commit to ongoing correlation with other validated vascular test modalities.

Residency programs in general surgery and vascular surgery, radiology, and emergency medicine increasingly recognize the important role of noninvasive vascular testing in the diagnostic algorithms for patients with PAD. As a result, components of their core curricula address vascular testing and are often co-taught by the technical and medical directors of the vascular laboratory. Local, regional, and national educational conferences commonly feature both physician and technologist faculty to emphasize the importance of this team approach to the care of the patient with vascular disease.

Because vascular technologists have knowledge of the disease process and its associated risk factors, they share responsibility with the physicians and nurses for patient education. The SVT supports this practice by publishing patient education pamphlets that illustrate vascular symptoms and discuss the role of noninvasive diagnostic testing and the treatment of PAD. Additionally, the vascular laboratory can serve as a site where educational pamphlets from many sources—whether from a vascular society, vascular foundation, or local health care institution—can be made available to patients at the time of their initial laboratory or office visit.

21.4.2 EVOLUTIONARY DEVELOPMENT OF THE PROFESSION

The specialty of vascular technology, which is still in its infancy, was developed in response to the need for accurate noninvasive diagnosis of vascular disorders. Before the introduction of this specialty in the early 1960s, the clinical impression of vascular disease was confirmed primarily by invasive techniques such as arteriography. Today, PAD can be detected, and its location and severity determined, noninvasively by using technology that ranges from the simple handheld continuous wave Doppler to complex and sophisticated ultrasound systems that offer 2- and 3-dimensional imaging and Doppler display of blood flow patterns. To meet the demands of the profession, the vascular technologist must be able to function independently and as a member of the vascular team; have a broad understanding of vascular anatomy, physiology, and disease processes; have a working knowledge of ultrasound physical principles, tissue perfusion, and pressure and volume measurements; and be skilled in the performance of multiple examination procedures.

Initially, the specialty was closely affiliated with vascular surgery, but in recent years the field has expanded to include cardiothoracic surgery, radiology, vascular medicine, cardiology, neurology, and internal medicine physicians. As a result, there is increasing focus on education, certification of technologists, standardization of practices, and accreditation of testing facilities.

21.4.3 EDUCATIONAL PREPARATION OF THE VASCULAR TECHNOLOGIST

Many vascular technologists gain their initial skills through a limited period of apprenticeship in a laboratory. Short-term programs of didactic instruction and supervised hands-on applications are offered nationally to augment this training. The education committee of the SVT has compiled a list of guidelines and recommendations for training centers and publishes a list of these facilities that details the contents and objectives of each site.[2] Instrument manufacturers have recognized the growing demand for quality education and have developed both on-site instruction that is instrument specific and web-based programs that address a wide range of subjects relevant to the field. Many technologists are graduates of associate degree programs in cardiovascular technology and some may be accredited by the Committee on Allied Health Education and Accreditation of the AMA. On completion of such an educational program, the student must have acquired training in one or more of the following specialty areas: invasive cardiology, noninvasive cardiology, and noninvasive peripheral vascular studies. However, at present, there is only a single program that offers a bachelor's degree in vascular technology (Oregon Institute of Technology, Klamath Falls, OR). Despite a significant increase in the number of short-term programs, the need for quality education remains critical in the face of increasing demands for certification of vascular technical personnel.

21.4.4 PROFESSIONAL SUPPORT FOR VASCULAR TECHNOLOGISTS

The SVT is a not-for-profit international professional organization dedicated to providing CME and maintaining a central educational source for vascular professionals (see Appendix 1). The SVT conducts an annual scientific and educational meeting; offers registry review courses, physician interpretation tutorials, and legislative and regulatory programs; and publishes a professional journal and numerous educational publications and videotapes. Additionally, the SVT is proactive in legislative endeavors that impact health care reimbursement and the quality of care provided in vascular testing facilities

21.4.5 PROFESSIONAL CERTIFICATION

After technologists have received appropriate training, they should pursue certification. Candidates for certification must satisfy clinical and educational prerequisites and pass a two-part examination. The prerequisites differentiate the number of years of clinical experience and CME required for candidates whose training ranges from high school graduation to graduation from an accredited ultrasound/vascular technology program. There is a minimum requirement of 24 months of full-time clinical experience and 24 clock hours of CME. On successful completion of examinations in vascular physical principles and instrumentation, and the specialty examination in vascular technology, the candidate is awarded the title "registered vascular technologist" (RVT).

Increasing numbers of vascular laboratory physicians are obtaining certification in vascular technology as evidence of competency in the field. The certificate is required for completion of a vascular surgical fellowship by several of the leading national programs. This certificate ensures that technologists and physicians meet minimum requirements for the practice of noninvasive vascular diagnostics.

The RVT maintains active status for 3 years after certification. This requires proof of CME to ensure continued competence in the field. The technologist must submit documentation of 30 hours of relevant CME every 3 years. Failure to obtain ongoing CME credits results in a provisional rather than active status.

21.4.6 ACCREDITATION OF VASCULAR LABORATORIES

Despite more than a decade of efforts to provide quality education and a mechanism for certification of vascular technologists, there is still variability of quality assurance and standardization of instrumentation, test procedures, and interpretive criteria in many laboratories. In 1989, several members of the SVT, the Joint Vascular Societies, and the American Institute of Ultrasound in Medicine met to address the need for a mechanism to provide voluntary accreditation of vascular testing facilities. Health care professionals were becoming increasingly aware that such a mechanism was necessary to forestall imposition of regulations by government agencies seeking to restrict availability of testing. The proposed restrictions were based largely on financial considerations, without emphasis on the quality of patient care. The Intersocietal Commission for Accreditation of Vascular Laboratories (ICAVL) was formed to meet this need. The ICAVL includes two delegates from each organization representing the medical specialties involved in noninvasive vascular testing (Table 21.1). The primary goals of the ICAVL are to recognize testing facilities performing

TABLE 21.1
Vascular Society Sponsors of the Intersocietal Commission for the Accreditation of Vascular Laboratories

- American Academy of Neurology/American Society of Neuroimaging
- Joint Section on Cerebrovascular Surgery/American Association of Neurological Surgeons and Congress of Neurological Surgeons
- American College of Cardiology
- American Institute of Ultrasound in Medicine
- North American Chapter of the International Society of Cardiovascular Surgery
- Society of Cardiovascular & Interventional Radiology
- Society for Vascular Medicine and Biology
- Society for Vascular Surgery
- Society of Diagnostic Medical Sonographers
- Society of Vascular Technology

appropriate high-quality studies, to issue certificates of recognition of quality service, and to maintain a registry of accredited laboratories.

The Essentials and Standards for Accreditation of Vascular Laboratories includes:

- qualifications of medical and technical personnel
- instrumentation
- testing protocols
- diagnostic criteria
- quality assurance
- patient safety
- facilities.

The impact of accreditation has been:

- improved quality of testing; increased standardization of testing protocols and diagnostic criteria
- improved quality assurance procedures

- an increase in the number of certified technologists
- improved educational opportunities
- increased job security for certified staff in accredited laboratories

The ICAVL serves as a central example of the success that can be achieved in maintaining vascular care standards when a strong interdisciplinary consensus is established.

21.4.7 WHAT DOES THE FUTURE LOOK LIKE?

Rapid advances in technology have propelled the vascular technology field forward during the past 2 decades. Noninvasive testing is now considered an important part of the diagnostic algorithm for most vascular patients and is central to effective long-term follow-up care of the patient with PAD. In recent years, ultrasound imaging has replaced venography as the primary diagnostic modality for detection of deep vein thrombosis. Similarly, in some institutions, patients may be selected for carotid endarterectomy based on the results of a duplex ultrasound examination without requiring the additional risk of preoperative contrast arteriography. Recent studies in high-volume vascular surgical laboratories have shown that this practice may also be applied to lower-extremity arterial bypass grafting.

With increasing emphasis placed on this technology, there is a concomitant demand for accreditation of laboratories, improved educational programs, and certification of technologists by health care and government agencies. To date, Medicare has mandated accreditation of laboratories in several states, with additional emphasis placed on certification of technologists. It is very likely that all vascular testing facilities will need to obtain accreditation to receive reimbursement for testing. The ICAVL has recently revised the standards for training of laboratory medical staff to include relevant education, experience in the performance and interpretation of test procedures, and documented hours of observation in an accredited facility. As a consequence, residency and fellowship programs will mandate vascular laboratory experience.

The professional organizations representing the field of vascular technology are committed to high standards of education and training, as well as advancement of the profession. The Society of Diagnostic Medical Sonographers has spent several years designing a career ladder that recognizes clinical excellence and appropriate standards of education, training, and certification in sonography and vascular technology. The new designations "ultrasound practitioner" and "advanced practice sonographer" require master's and bachelor's degrees, respectively, in addition to specialty certification, ongoing CME, and contributions to the field through research, publication, and education.

REFERENCES

1. Sonography Coalition, *Scope of Practice for the Diagnostic Ultrasound Professional*, Society of Diagnostic Medical Sonographers, Dallas, TX, 1993-2000.
2. Society of Vascular Technology, *Training Center Directory*, The Society of Vascular Technology, Lanham, MD, 1991.

Appendix 1
Selected Professional and Educational Resources for Vascular Professionals

SPECIFIC EDUCATIONAL RESOURCES FOR THE VASCULAR PHYSICIAN

PROFESSIONAL SOCIETIES AND WEBSITES

Society for Vascular Medicine and Biology
13 Elm Street
Manchester, MA 01944-1314
Phone: 978-526-8330
Fax: 978-526-7521
E-mail: svmb@prri.com
Website: http://www.svmb.org

Society of Cardiovascular & Interventional Radiology
10201 Lee Highway, Suite 500
Fairfax, VA 22030
Phone: 703-691-1805 or 800-488-7284
Fax: 703-691-1855
E-mail: info@scvir.org
Website: http://www.scvir.org/

Society for Vascular Surgery
13 Elm Street
Manchester, MA 01944-1314
Phone: 978-526-8330
Fax: 978-526-4018
E-mail: svs@prri.com
Website: http://www.vascsurg.org/

American Association for Vascular Surgery
13 Elm Street
Manchester, MA 01944-1314
Phone: 978-526-8330
Fax: 978-526-4018
E-mail: aavs@prri.com
Website: http://www.vascsurg.org/

Peripheral Vascular Surgical Society
824 Munras Avenue, Suite C
Monterey, CA 93940
Phone: 831-373-0508
Fax: 831-373-0460
E-mail: suzanne@dmc2000.com
Website: http://www.vascsurg.org/doc/849.html##.htm

American College of Cardiology
Heart House
9111 Old Georgetown Road
Bethesda, MD 20814-1699
Phone: 301-897-5400 or 800-253-4636
Fax: 301-897-9745
Website: http://www.acc.org/

American Heart Association
National Center
7272 Greenville Avenue
Dallas, TX 75231
Phone: 800-AHA-USA1 (242-8721)
Website: http://www.americanheart.org

Vascular Disease Foundation
3333 S. Wadsworth Boulevard #B-104-37
Lakewood, CO 80227
Phone: 303-949-8337
Fax: 303-989-6522
E-mail: info@vdf.org
Website: http://www.vdf.org

Journals

Vascular Medicine
Publisher: Arnold
338 Euston Road
London NW1 3BH
U.K.
Phone: +44 (0) 20 7873 6000
Fax: +44 (0) 20 7873 6325
E-mail: susan.aitkenhead@hodder.co.uk
Website: http://www.arnoldpublishers.com/Journals/Journpages/1358863x.htm
Editorial offices:
Mark A. Creager, M.D., Senior Editor
Vascular Medicine & Atherosclerosis Unit
Cardiovascular Division
Brigham & Women's Hospital
75 Francis Street
Boston, MA 02115

Journal of Vascular Surgery
Publisher: Mosby Press
Subscription and Customer Relations Department:
6277 Sea Harbor Drive, Fifth Floor
Orlando, FL 32887-4800
Phone: 800-654-2452 or 407-345-4066
Fax: 407-363-9661
E-mail: hhspcs@harcourt.com
Website: www.mosby.com/jvs
Editorial offices at:
K. Wayne Johnston, Editor-in-Chief
Toronto General Hospital
200 Elizabeth Street
Eaton Wing, 5th Floor, Room 312
Toronto, ON M5G 2C4
Canada
Phone: 416-340-3722
Fax: 416-340-4903
E-mail: jvascsurg@aol.com

Journal of Vascular and Interventional Radiology
Publisher: Lippincott, Williams & Wilkins
Subscriptions at:
P.O Box 1600
Hagerstown, MD 21741
Phone: 301-223-2300 or 800-777-2295
Fax: 301-223-2320
Editorial offices at:
530 Walnut Street
Philadelphia, PA 19106
Phone: 215-521-8300
Fax: 215-521-8902

SPECIFIC EDUCATIONAL RESOURCES FOR THE VASCULAR NURSE

Professional Societies and Websites:
Society for Vascular Nursing
7794 Grow Drive
Pensacola, FL 32414
Phone: 888-536-4SVN (4786)
Fax: 850-484-8762
E-mail: svn@puetzamc.com
Website: http://www.svnnet.org

Council of Cardiovascular Nursing, American Heart Association
National Center
7272 Greenville Avenue
Dallas, TX 75231
Phone: 800-AHA-USA1 (242-8721)
Fax: 214-691-6342
Website: www.americanheart.org/Scientific/council/cvn

JOURNALS

Journal of Vascular Nursing
Publisher: Mosby, Inc.
Subscription services at:
11830 Westline Industrial Drive
St. Louis, MO 63146-9988
Phone: 314-453-4351 or 800-453-4351
Editorial offices at:
Cindy Lewis, R.N., M.S.N.
St. Luke's Medical Center
2900 West Oklahoma Avenue
Milwaukee, WI 53215
Phone: 414-649-7821
Fax: 414-649-5081
E-mail: Cindy_Lewis@aurora.org

SPECIFIC EDUCATIONAL RESOURCES
FOR THE VASCULAR TECHNOLOGIST

Professional Societies and Websites:
American Institute of Ultrasound in Medicine
14750 Sweitzer Road, Suite 100
Laurel, MD 20707-5906
Phone: 301-498-4100 or 800-638-5352
Fax: 301-498-4450
Website: http://www.aium.org

Intersocietal Commission for the Accreditation of Vascular Laboratories
8840 Stanford Boulevard, Suite 4900
Columbia, MD 21045
Phone: 410-872-0100
Fax: 410-872-0030
E-mail: katanick@intersocietal.org
Website: http://www.icavl.org

Society of Diagnostic Medical Sonographers
12770 Coit Road, Suite 708
Dallas, TX 75251-1314
Phone: 972-239-7369 or 800-229-9506
Fax: 972-239-7378
Website: http://www.sdms.org

Society of Vascular Technology
4601 Presidents Drive, Suite 260
Lanham, MD 20706
Phone: 301-459-7550
Fax: 301-459-5651
E-mail: info@svtnet.org
Website: http://www.svtnet.org

JOURNAL

Journal of Vascular Technology
Publisher: Allen Press
All questions to the Society for Vascular Technology at:
4601 Presidents Drive, Suite 260
Lanham, MD 20706
Phone: 301-459-7550

Index

A

AAA, *see* Abdominal aortic
    aneurysms
Abdominal aorta
  aneurysms, *see* Abdominal aortic
    aneurysms
  atherosclerosis of, 300
Abdominal aortic aneurysms
  algorithms for
  diagnostic, 263
  treatment, 264
  aortoiliac disease and, 258
  computed tomography of,
    256–257, 269
  definition of, 243–244
  diagnosis of, 255–258, 263
  epidemiology of, 244, 246–248
  evaluation of, 255–258
  expansion of, 252–253
  familial factors, 247, 252
  gender predilection, 244
  incidence of, 248
  magnetic resonance imaging of,
    257–258
  mortality rates, 248
  natural history of, 249–253
  pathogenesis of, 253–255
  racial predilection, 246
  risk factors, 246–247
  rupture of
    diagnostic tests, 256–257
    economic costs, 261–262
    risks, 249–253

    signs and symptoms,
      255–256
    treatment, 262–265
  screening, 258–262
  size of, 249–250, 258–260
  transmural inflammatory
    responses associated with,
    254–255
  treatment of
  algorithm, 264
  arteriography use, 268–269
  costs, 261
  endoluminal approach, 270–271
  historical descriptions of,
    242–243
  risk assessments, 265
  study findings, 266–267
  surgical, 266–268
  symptomatic patient, 262–265
  ultrasonography of, 257
ABI, *see* Ankle–brachial index
Acetylcholine, 35
Acrocyanosis, 405
Acute arterial ischemia, *see* Acute
    limb ischemia
Acute intestinal ischemia
  causes of, 195
  clinical presentation of, 195
  diagnostic tests, 197–198
  mortality rates, 195–196
  nonocclusive, 202–203
  pathophysiology of, 195
  superior mesenteric artery
    angioplasty of, 198–199

embolectomy of, 199–201
embolism, 197, 199
revascularization of,
    199–202
thrombosis, 196, 199
treatment of
    bowel resection
        considerations, 202
    bypass surgery, 201–202
    colonic ischemia after,
        204–206
    embolectomy, 199–201
    laparotomy, 199
    management after, 202
    percutaneous transluminal
        angioplasty, 198–199
Acute limb ischemia
    algorithms for
        evaluative, 152
        treatment, 158
    angiographic evaluations, 155
    categories of
        I, 153
        IIa, 153
        IIb, 153–154
        III, 154–157
    definition of, 148
    diagnosis of, 152
    embolus as cause of, 159–161
    epidemiology of, 148–149
    etiology of, 148
    natural history of, 149–150
    outcome of, 149–150
    pathophysiology of, 150–151
    popliteal artery aneurysm as
        cause of, 163
    thrombosis as cause of
        graft, 161–162

native artery, 161
treatment of
    algorithm, 158
    anticoagulants, 157
    complications, 165
    embolectomy, 149, 159–161
    etiology-specific, 152–153,
        159–163
    goals, 157
    outcome after, 149–150
    revascularization, 165
    severity-specific, 157–158
    thrombectomy, 161–162
    thrombolysis, 163–164
Adhesion molecules, 5
Advanced practice nurse, 468–469
Aging
    endothelium-dependent
        vasodilation and, 38
    oxidative stress and, 7
ALI, *see* Acute limb ischemia
Allen test, 328–329, 449–450
Aneurysm
    abdominal aortic, *see* Abdominal
        aortic aneurysms
    classification of, 244–246
    definition of, 243
    epidemiology of, 244, 246–248
    historical descriptions of,
        241–243
    in polyarteritis nodosa patient,
        346–347
    popliteal artery
        description of, 150, 153
        evaluation of, 157
        historical descriptions of,
            242
        treatment of, 163

Angiography
    acute limb ischemia evaluations,
        155
    critical limb ischemia
        evaluations, 130
    magnetic resonance
    carotid artery disease
        evaluations, 175
    renal artery stenosis evaluations,
        225–226
Angioplasty, *see* Percutaneous
        transluminal angioplasty
Angiotensin-converting enzyme
        inhibitors, 42–43,
        226–227, 380
Angiotensin II, 39, 43
Ankle–brachial index
    in calcified ankle arteries, 87
    cerebrovascular disease risks
        and, 69
    criteria for using, 84–85
    critical limb ischemia
        evaluations, 123
    equipment for obtaining, 84
    exercise, 89
    intermittent claudication
        diagnosed using, 60–61,
        100
    normal, 87
    peripheral arterial disease
        diagnosed using, 69, 100
    procedure, 84–86
    results of, 87
Anticoagulants, *see also* Heparin;
        Thrombolysis; Warfarin
    acute limb ischemia treated
        using, 157

atheroembolism syndrome
    secondary to, 308
    subclavian vein compression
        treated using, 420, 422
    thrombosis and, 25
Antioxidants, 40
Antiplatelet therapy
    atheroembolism, 313
    carotid artery disease, 185
    critical limb ischemia, 136
    ischemia prevention using,
        97–98
Antiplatelet Trialists' Collaboration,
        97–98
Antithrombin, 25
Aortic dissection
    algorithms for, 293–294
    aortic involvement
        determinations, 286, 288
    treatment based on, 294–295
        types of, 286–287
    computed tomography of, 292
    diagnosis of, 291–292
    epidemiology of, 283
    evaluation of, 291–293
    ischemic complications, 290
    morbidity and mortality
        associated with, 286,
        288–289, 295–296
    natural history of, 289–291
    pathophysiology of, 283–289
    predisposing factors, 285
    rupture of, 289
    symptoms of, 290
    treatment of, 292, 294–295
Aortobifemoral bypass, 137
Aortoiliac disease, 137, 258
Apoptosis, 6

Arterial calcification diseases
  chronic renal failure, 401–402
  idiopathic infantile arterial
    calcification, 401
  Mönckeberg arteriosclerosis,
    400–401
Arterial compression, 425–427, 445
Arterial duplex ultrasonography, 90,
    92, see also Duplex
    ultrasonography
Arteries, see specific artery
Arteriography
  abdominal aortic aneurysm
    repair, 268–269
  carotid artery disease, 176
  cystic adventitial disease,
    396–397
  intestinal ischemia, 197–198,
    208–209
  lateral aortography, 208–209
  popliteal artery entrapment
    syndrome, 392–394
  thromboangiitis obliterans,
    330–332
Arteriovenous fistula, 447
Ascorbic acid, 40
Aspirin, 98, 185, 357, 409
Asymmetric dimethylarginine, 10,
    39
Asymptomatic Carotid
    Atherosclerosis Study, 180,
    182–183
Atheroembolism, see also
    Embolism;
    Thromboembolism
  anticoagulant effects, 308
  clinical features of, 300,
    309–310
  description of, 299–300

diagnosis of, 309–311
epidemiology of, 301
evaluation of, 309–311
natural history of, 301–302
pathophysiology of, 306,
    308–309
symptoms of, 301–302
thrombolytic therapy and, 308
transesophageal
    echocardiography of, 307,
    310
treatment of, 311–314
Atherosclerosis
  antiatherogenic mechanisms,
    8–11
  in chronic renal failure patients,
    402
  definition of, 31–32
  description of, 3–4
  intermittent claudication and,
    388, 396
  mortality rates associated with,
    3–4
  pathogenesis of
    endothelial dysfunction, 5–7
    neovascularization of plaque,
    7–8
  risk factors, 4
  summary overview of, 15–16
  upper extremity, 438–439
Atherosclerosis obliterans, 438–439
Atherosclerotic plaque, see Plaque
Azathioprine, 356

B

Behçet syndrome
  characteristics of, 353

diagnostic criteria, 353–354,
354t
etiology of, 353
pathophysiology of, 353
treatment of, 354–357
Betamethasone, 355
Brachial plexus compression
description of, 427
surgical treatment of, 432
Buerger's disease
algorithm, 333
Allen test, 328–329
arteriographic findings, 330–332
clinical features of, 323–324,
327–331
definition of, 323
epidemiology of, 324
etiology of, 325
histopathologic findings,
326–327
laboratory findings, 330
pathogenesis of, 325–326
signs and symptoms of, 328
treatment of, 331, 333–335
upper extremity, 441
in women, 324
Bypass graft surgery
acute intestinal ischemia,
201–202
atheroembolism, 313
chronic intestinal ischemia,
211–214
critical limb ischemia, 137–138
intermittent claudication,
110–111, 113

C

CAD, *see* Coronary artery disease

Calcifying vascular cells, 6–7
Calciphylaxis, 402
Calcium channel blockers, 377–378
Captopril, 380
Cardiovascular disease, 70–71
Carotid artery disease
causes of, 170
clinical presentation of, 173
description of, 169–170
evaluation of
arteriography, 176
duplex ultrasonography,
173–175
magnetic resonance
angiography, 175
pathology of, 172–173
treatment of
algorithm, 179
antiplatelet agents, 185
asymptomatic stenosis,
178–181
carotid endarterectomy,
178–181
percutaneous transluminal
angioplasty, 184–185
risk factor modification,
185–186
symptomatic stenosis,
176–179
Carotid endarterectomy
asymptomatic stenosis treated
using, 179–181
contraindications, 181
symptomatic stenosis treated
using, 177–178
technologist's role in, 479

Carotid Surgery Versus Medical
 Therapy in Asymptotic
 Carotid Stenosis, 179–180
Carpal tunnel syndrome, 371–373
CBVD, *see* Cerebrovascular disease
Celiac artery, 192–193, 209
Cerebrovascular disease
 peripheral arterial disease risk
 for, 69–70, 72
 risk factors, 61
Chemokines, 5
Chilblains, *see* Pernio
Chlorambucil, 356
Chronic intestinal ischemia
 abdominal pain findings, 194
 diagnosis of, 207–208
 natural history of, 206–207
 pathophysiology of, 193–194
 treatment of
 bypass surgery, 211–214
 percutaneous, 208, 210
 surgical, 208, 211–216
 weight loss associated with,
 194–195
Chronic limb ischemia, 83
Chronic renal failure, arterial
 calcification associated
 with, 401–402
Churg-Strauss syndrome, 348, 350
Cigarette smoking, *see* Smoking
Cilostazol, 109–110, 113
Claudication, *see* Intermittent
 claudication
CLI, *see* Critical limb ischemia
Clopidrogel Versus Aspirin for the
 Prevention of Ischemic
 Events, 98, 185
Cogan syndrome, 344

Colchicine, 356
Colonic ischemia
 acute, 203
 postoperative, 204–206
Computed tomography
 abdominal aorta aneurysm,
 256–257, 269
 aortic dissection, 292
 atheroembolism, 310
 cystic adventitial disease, 396
 plaque rupture, 14
Connective tissue disorders, 372
Coronary arteries
 acetylcholine effects, 35
 atherosclerosis of, 128, *see also*
 Atherosclerosis
 vasoconstriction of, 36
 vasomotor tone of, 35–36
Coronary artery disease
 peripheral arterial disease and,
 70–71, 74
 risk factors, 61
Corticosteroids, 355–356
C-reactive protein, 13
Critical limb ischemia
 algorithms for
 evaluation, 132
 treatment, 140
 amputation risks, 122, 138–139
 ankle–brachial index, 122
 aortoiliac disease, 137
 definition of, 120
 diagnostic and evaluative tests
 angiography, 130
 ankle–brachial index, 127
 Doppler velocity waveform,
 128
 electrocardiogram, 128–129

pulse volume recordings, 128
segmental limb systolic
pressure, 127–128
segmental plethysmography,
128
transcutaneous partial
pressure of oxygen,
129–130
differential diagnosis, 131–132,
134
epidemiology of, 121
evaluation of
history-taking, 124–125
physical examination,
126
pulses, 126
signs and symptoms,
125–126
tests, 127–130
incidence of, 121
infrainguinal disease, 138
intermittent claudication
progression to, 121
laboratory tests, 129
microcirculatory findings,
123–124
natural history of, 121–123
pain control, 133
pathophysiology of, 123–124
prognosis for, 122, 124
risk factors
description of, 121–123
modification of, 135
signs and symptoms of, 125–126
thrombosis prophylaxis, 133
treatment of
algorithm, 140
amputation, 138–139

antibiotics, 133
antiplatelet agents, 136
aortobifemoral bypass, 137
bypass grafts, 137–138
immediate, 133
long-term, 135
pharmacologic, 136
prostanoids, 136
revascularization, 136–137
risk factor modification, 135
surgical, 136–138
surveillance program after,
139, 141
CVC, see Calcifying vascular cells
CVD, see Cardiovascular disease
Cyclophosphamide, 356
Cyclosporine, 356
Cystic adventitial disease, 395–398

D

Dapsone, 356
Deep venous thrombosis, 150
Dexamethasone, 355
Diabetes mellitus
critical limb ischemia and, 121
management of, 135
Diabetic sensory neuropathy, 131
Diet, 4
Diltiazem, 378
Dipyrimadole, 357
Doppler velocity waveform, 128
Duplex ultrasonography
arterial compression evaluations,
426
carotid artery disease
evaluations, 173–175

chronic intestinal ischemia
    evaluations, 207
critical limb ischemia
    evaluations, 130, 139, 141
mesenteric artery evaluations,
    207–208
percutaneous transluminal
    angioplasty assessments,
    230
peripheral arterial disease
    evaluations, 90, 92
renal artery stenosis evaluations,
    222, 224–225
subclavian vein compression
    evaluations, 419, 421
Dyslipidemia, 66

E

EDRF, *see* Endothelium-derived
    relaxing factor
Effort thrombosis of subclavian vein
    causes of, 417–418
    diagnosis of, 419–421
    signs and symptoms of, 418–419
    treatment of, 420, 422–423
Ehlers-Danlos syndrome, 247
Embolectomy, 149, 159–161,
    199–200
Embolism, *see also*
    Atheroembolism;
    Thromboembolism;
    Thrombosis
    acute limb ischemia caused by,
    159–161
    anticoagulant therapy for, 440
    carotid artery disease caused by,
    170

definition of, 150
ischemic stroke caused by, 170
sources of, 439
superior mesenteric artery, 197
thrombosis *vs.*, 155
upper extremity, 439–440
Endarterectomy
    asymptomatic stenosis treated
    using, 179–181
    contraindications, 181
    symptomatic stenosis treated
    using, 177–178
    technologist's role in, 479
Endoaneurysmorrhaphy, 243
Endothelial cells
    tissue plasminogen activator
    production by, 8
    transcription factor activation, 5
Endothelium
    anatomy of, 31
    antioxidant benefits for, 40
    disruption of, 22
    dysfunction of
    description of, 5–7
    mechanisms, 37–41
    treatment, 41–44
    estrogen replacement therapy
    effects, 41–42
    functions of, 31
    inflammation of, 32
    lipid-lowering therapies, 40–41,
    43
    macrophage adhesion, 5–6, 32
    oxygen-derived free radicals, 5
    platelet adhesion and
    aggregation to, 23
    receptors, 34
    summary overview of, 44

thromboangiitis obliterans, 326
tissue factor pathway inhibitor
production by, 25
treatments for, 41
Endothelium-derived nitric oxide
angiotensin-converting enzyme
inhibitor effects, 42
atherogenic protective
mechanisms of, 36
description of, 44
discovery of, 33–34
hypercholesterolemia effects,
8–9
platelet adhesiveness and
aggregation reduced by, 35
superoxide anion effects, 39
synthesis of, 34–35, 37
vasomotor tone regulation by,
35–36
Endothelium-derived relaxing
factor, 33–34
End-stage renal disease, 221
Ergotamine, 374
Ergotism, 403
Erythromelalgia, 407–409
Estrogen, 41–43
European Carotid Surgery Trial, 177
Exercise
ankle–brachial index, 89
benefits of, 72
intermittent claudication treated
using, 105, 107–108, 113
performance measurements, 103
Extracellular matrix, 12
Extracranial carotid artery disease,
see Carotid artery disease

F

Factor VII, 27
Factor V Leiden, 25
Factor Xa, 24
Fatty streaks, 6
Felodipine, 378
Femoral pulse, 126
Fibrin, 28
Fibrinogen, 27
Fibrinolysis, 25–26
Fibromuscular dysplasia
carotid artery dysplasia caused
by, 172
characteristics of, 398–400
renal artery stenosis caused by,
220–221
treatment of, 231–232
types of, 221
FMD, see Fibromuscular dysplasia
Foam cells, 6

G

Gangrene, 126
Giant-cell arteritides
description of, 340, 342
Takayasu arteritis, 342–343,
441–442
temporal arteritis, 342, 441
upper extremity, 441
Glycoprotein IIb/IIIa, 22–23
Guanethidine, 379

H

Health care team, see Vascular health
care team

Hemostasis
    coagulants involved in, 25
    risk factors for peripheral arterial
        disease, 27–28
    summary overview of, 28
Henoch-Schönlein purpura, 351
Heparin, 357, *see also*
        Anticoagulants
High-density lipoprotein, 8, 66, 110
HMG-CoA reductase inhibitors, 41,
        186, 313–314
Homocysteine, 7
3-Hydroxy-3-methylglutaryl
        coenzyme A reductase
        inhibitors, *see* HMG-CoA
        reductase inhibitors
Hypercholesterolemia
    description of, 8–9
    endothelium-dependent
        vasodilation abnormalities,
        39
    L-arginine–NO pathway
        abnormalities, 9–10
    peripheral arterial disease risks,
        66
    treatment of, 41
Hyperhomocysteinemia, 36
Hypersensitivity vasculitis, 350–351
Hypertension
    abdominal aneurysm ruptures
        and, 252
    in aortic dissection patient,
        291–292
    management of, 135, 185–186
    peripheral arterial disease risks
        and, 61, 66
    renal artery stenosis, 226

    in Takayasu arteritis patient,
        342–343
Hypertriglyceridemia, 121
Hypocomplementemia, 310
Hypothenar hammer syndrome,
        443–444

I

Idiopathic infantile arterial
        calcification, 401
Indomethacin, 357
Infection, plaque rupture secondary
        to, 13
Inferior mesenteric artery, 193
Inflammatory cells
    collagen synthesis reductions
        caused by, 12
    description of, 8
    macrophages, *see* Macrophages
Infrainguinal disease, 138
Intercellular adhesion molecule-1,
        32
Interferon-α, 357
Interferon-γ, 12
Intermittent claudication
    aging and, 58–59
    ambulatory effects, 105
    ankle–brachial index, 60–61
    atherosclerosis and, 388, 396
    in atherosclerosis obliterans
        patient, 438
    clinical features of, 82
    critical limb ischemia and, 121
    definition of, 82, 96
    diagnosis of, 100–102
    differential diagnosis, 83–84,
        100, 102
    epidemiology of, 96

evaluation of, 99–100
foot, 329
functional status effects,
    104–105
gender predilection, 58, 60
history-taking findings, 99–100
incidence of, 57–58
natural history of, 96
prevalence of, 58–60
questionnaires for assessing,
    61–65, 104
severity assessments, 102–104
thromboangiitis obliterans, 328
treatment of
algorithm, 106
cilostazol, 109–110, 113
exercise rehabilitation, 105,
    107–108, 113
goals, 105
limb bypass surgery, 110–111,
    113
pentoxifylline, 108–109
percutaneous transluminal
    angioplasty, 111–112
pharmacologic, 108–110, 113
Internal carotid artery, 173
Intersocietal Commission for
    Accreditation of Vascular
    Laboratories, 477–478
Intestinal ischemia
acute, *see* Acute intestinal
    ischemia
chronic, *see* Chronic intestinal
    ischemia
colonic ischemia
acute, 203
postoperative, 204–206
diseases and conditions that
    cause, 192

nonocclusive, 202–203
pathophysiology of, 193–195
Ischemic colitis, *see* Colonic
    ischemia
Israpidine, 378

K

Kawasaki disease, 347–348

L

Large-vessel vasculitis
    algorithm for, 341
Cogan syndrome, 344
Takayasu arteritis, 342–343,
    441–442
    temporal arteritis, 342, 441
L-arginine, 9–10, 37
LDL, *see* Low-density lipoprotein
Limb bypass surgery, 110–111, 113
Limb ischemia, *see* Critical limb
    ischemia
Lipid-lowering therapies, 40–41, 43
Livedoid vasculitis, 404
Livedo reticularis, 403–404
Losartin, 380
Low-density lipoprotein, 5–6, 66
Lumbar sympathectomy, 381–382

M

Macrophages
    endothelial adhesion of, 5–6, 32
    in plaque rupture, 12
Magnetic resonance angiography
    carotid artery disease
        evaluations, 175

renal artery stenosis evaluations,
        225–226
Magnetic resonance imaging
    abdominal aorta aneurysm
        assessment, 257–258
    aortic dissection evaluations, 292
    plaque rupture assessments, 14
Marfan syndrome, 247
Matrix metalloproteinases, 12, 254
Medium-vessel vasculitis
    algorithm, 345
    Kawasaki disease, 347–348
    polyarteritis nodosa, 346–347
Metastatic calcification, 402
Methotrexate, 356
Methylarginines, 10
Methylprednisolone, 355
MMP, *see* Matrix metalloproteinases
Mönckeberg arteriosclerosis,
        400–401
Monocyte chemoattractant protein,
        32
Myocardial infarction
    antiplatelet therapy for
        preventing, 98
    circadian patterns associated
        with, 15
    diet and, 4
    incidence of, 3–4
    postoperative, 268
    precipitating events, 15
    stress and, 15

N

Nerve root compression, 131

Neurogenic thoracic outlet
        syndrome
    anatomy of, 429
    description of, 427–428
    diagnosis of, 429–431
    differential diagnosis, 431
    electromyography evaluations,
        428
    etiology of, 428–429
    symptoms of, 430–431
    tests, 428, 431
    treatment of, 431–432
Nifedipine, 377–378
Night cramps, 131
Nitric oxide, endothelium-derived
    angiotensin-converting enzyme
        inhibitor effects, 42
    atherogenic protective
        mechanisms of, 36
    description of, 44
    discovery of, 33–34
    hypercholesterolemia effects,
        8–9
    platelet adhesiveness and
        aggregation reduced by, 35
    superoxide anion effects, 39
    synthesis of, 34–35, 37
    vasomotor tone regulation by,
        35–36
Nitric oxide synthase
    description of, 10, 34
    HMG-CoA reductase inhibitor
        effects, 41
Nitroglycerin, 379
North American Symptomatic
        Carotid Endarterectomy
        Trial, 176–177, 182–183
Nurse, *see* Vascular nurse

O

Oxidative stress
  aging and, 7
  description of, 32
  endothelial dysfunction
      secondary to, 5, 32, 40
  schematic representation of, 33
Oxygen-derived free radicals, 5

P

PAD, *see* Peripheral arterial disease
Paget-Schroetter syndrome,
      416–419
Patient
  compliance with treatment plan,
      460–461
  quality of life improvements for,
      460
Peak systolic velocity, 225
Peak walking time, 103
Pentoxifylline, 108–109, 356
Percutaneous transluminal
      angioplasty
  duplex ultrasonography
      assessments, 230
  indications
    carotid artery disease,
      184–185
    chronic intestinal ischemia,
      208, 210
    intermittent claudication,
      111–112
    renal artery stenosis,
      229–230
    superior mesenteric artery,
      198–199

subclavian vein obstruction
    contraindications, 425
Peripheral arterial disease, *see also*
      specific disease or
      condition
  aging and, 58–59
  ambulatory effects of, 72, 74
  definition of, 57–58, 71–72
  diagnosis of, 100–102
  evaluative approach
    ankle–brachial index, 84–87,
      100
    arterial duplex
      ultrasonography, 90, 92
    differential diagnosis, 83–84
    Doppler waveforms, 89, 92
    history-taking, 82
    laboratory tests, 87–93, *see*
      also Ankle–brachial index
    overview, 81
    physical examination, 82–83
    pulse volume recordings, 88,
      91
    segmental limb pressures,
      88, 91
  exercise benefits, 72, 105,
      107–108
  gender predilection, 58, 60
  healthcare barriers for, 459
  health care team for, *see* Vascular
      health care team
  hemostatic risk factors for,
      27–28
  incidence of, 57
  mortality risks, 70–71
  prevalence of, 58–60, 74, 96
  public awareness of, 469
  risk factors

modification of, 97
types of, 61, 66–68, 72
treatment of, 72–73, 458–460
vascular risks and predictions
 associated with
cardiovascular disease, 70,
 96–99
cerebrovascular disease,
 69–70, 72
coronary artery disease, 69,
 72
description of, 68–69, 73
Pernio
clinical manifestations of,
 406–407
description of, 405
differential diagnosis, 407
treatment of, 407
Physician, *see* Vascular physician
Plaque
formation of, 6
growth of, 7–8
illustration of, 171
inflammatory cells, 8
intraplaque hemorrhage
 effects, 170
necrotic core of, 6, 11
neovascularization of, 7–8
rupture vulnerability
imaging of, 13–14
infection effects, 13
macrophage effects, 12
pathophysiologic factors,
 308–309
signs of, 11–12
transesophageal
echocardiography of,
 302–305

Plasmin, 25–26
Plasminogen activator inhibitor-1,
 27
Platelets
activation of, 22–23
adhesion of, 23
aggregation of, 23
endothelium-derived nitric oxide
 effects, 35
phospholipid surface of, 23
thrombosis caused by, 21–23
Polyarteritis nodosa, 346–347
Popliteal aneurysm
description of, 150, 153
evaluation of, 157
historical descriptions of, 242
treatment of, 163
Popliteal artery
cystic adventitial disease of,
 395–398
entrapment syndrome of
arteriography evaluations,
 392–394
classification of, 389–391
clinical presentation of,
 391–392
gender predilection, 391
historical descriptions of,
 388
pathology of, 388–389
treatment of, 392, 395
Prazosin, 378
Prednisolone, 355
Prostacyclin, 8, 381
Prostaglandins, 381
Prostanoids, 136
Protein C, 25
Protein S, 25

Pseudoaneurysms, 92–93
Pseudoclaudication, 102
PTA, *see* Percutaneous transluminal angioplasty
Pulse volume recordings
    critical limb ischemia evaluations, 128
peripheral arterial disease evaluations, 88, 91
PVRs, *see* Pulse volume recordings

Q

Quinapril, 43

R

RAS, *see* Renal artery stenosis
Raynaud's phenomenon
    age of onset, 365–366
    carpal tunnel syndrome and, 371–373
    clinical presentation of, 364–365
    diagnostic criteria, 368–370, 446–447
    drugs that cause, 374
    epidemiology of, 365–366
    evaluation of, 368–370
    gender predilection, 366
    hereditary factors, 367
    natural history of, 364–365
    pathophysiology of, 366–368
    prognosis for, 364
    secondary causes of, 371–375
    syndromes associated with, 364–365
    tests for, 369–370

thoracic outlet syndrome and, 373
thromboangiitis obliterans and, 329, 374–375
treatment of
    algorithm, 376
    angiotensin preparations, 380
    calcium channel blockers, 377–378
    cryotherapy, 375, 377
    nitroglycerin preparations, 379
    nonpharmacologic, 375, 377, 447
    prostaglandins, 381
    sympathectomy, 381–382
    sympatholytic agents, 378–379
    thyroid preparations, 380
    upper extremity, 445–447
    vasospastic disease and, 373–374
Reflex sympathetic dystrophy, 131
Renal artery stenosis
    algorithms for
        evaluative, 224
        treatment, 227
    diagnosis of, 223–226
    duplex ultrasonography evaluations, 222, 224–225
    end-stage renal disease secondary to, 221–222
    epidemiology of, 219–220
    fibromuscular dysplasia
        description of, 220–221
        treatment of, 231–232

magnetic resonance angiography
    evaluations, 225–226
natural history of, 221–223
racial predilection, 220
treatment of
algorithm, 227
endovascular stents, 230–231
nonpharmacologic, 222
overview of, 232
percutaneous transluminal
    angioplasty, 229–230
pharmacologic, 226–227
restenosis after, 231
revascularization, 221, 228–231
surgery, 228–231
Reperfusion syndrome, 165
Reserpine, 378–379
Revascularization
acute limb ischemia treated
    using, 165
complications of, 165
critical limb ischemia treated
    using, 136–137
vascular physician's role in, *see*
    Vascular physician
Risk factors
atherosclerosis, 4
cerebrovascular disease, 61
coronary artery disease, 61
peripheral arterial disease, 61,
    66–68, 97
Rose questionnaire, 61
Rupture of plaque
imaging of, 13–14
infection effects, 13
macrophage effects, 12
signs of, 11–12

S

Scleroderma, 372
Segmental limb pressures
critical limb ischemia
    evaluations, 127–128
peripheral arterial disease
    evaluations, 88, 91
Segmental plethysmography, 128
Sjögren syndrome, 372
SMA, *see* Superior mesenteric artery
Smoking
abdominal aneurysm ruptures
    and, 252
cessation of, 72–73, 135, 333
critical limb ischemia and, 121
thromboangiitis obliterans and,
    325, 331
Sneddon syndrome, 404
Society of Diagnostic Medical
    Sonographers, 480
Society of Vascular Technology, 473,
    475–476
Stents
aortic dissection treated using,
    295
renal artery stenosis treated
    using, 230–231
Stroke
hemorrhagic, 170
hypertension and, 186
incidence of, 169
ischemic, 170
sequelae of, 169–170
thromboembolism cause of, 306
warfarin prophylaxis, 314–315
Subclavian vein compression or
    obstruction
causes of, 416–417, 424

contraindicated treatments, 425
description of, 415–416
diagnosis of, 419–420
effort thrombosis, 417–419
symptoms of, 417
treatment of, 420, 422–423, 425
Subendothelial matrix, 22
Sulfasalazine, 357
Superior mesenteric artery
  angioplasty of, 198–199, 210
  bypass surgery of, 212–214
  description of, 192–193
  embolectomy of, 199–201
  embolism, 197, 199
  revascularization of, 199–202
  thrombosis, 196, 199
Superoxide anion, 9, 39
Superoxide dismutase, 39
Sympathectomy, 381–382
Sympatholytic agents, 378–379
Syndrome X, 66
Systemic calcinosis, 402

T

Takayasu arteritis, 342–343,
    441–442
TcPO$_2$, see Transcutaneous partial
    pressure of oxygen
Technologist, see Vascular
    technologist
Temporal arteritis, 342, 441
Tetracycline, 356
Thalidomide, 356
Thoracic outlet syndromes
  algorithm, 433
  anatomy of, 414–415

arterial compression, 425–427,
    445
description of, 413–414
neurogenic
  anatomy of, 429
  description of, 427–428
  diagnosis of, 429–431
  differential diagnosis, 431
  electromyography
    evaluations, 428
  etiology of, 428–429
  symptoms of, 430–431
  tests, 428, 431
  treatment of, 431–432
Raynaud phenomenon associated
    with, 373
subclavian vein compression or
    obstruction, see Subclavian
    vein compression or
    obstruction
upper extremity, 445
Thrombectomy, 161–162
Thrombin, 23–24
Thromboangiitis obliterans
  algorithm, 333
  Allen test, 328–329
  arteriographic findings, 330–332
  clinical features of, 323–324,
    327–331
  definition of, 323
  epidemiology of, 324
  etiology of, 325
  histopathologic findings,
    326–327
  laboratory findings, 330
  pathogenesis of, 325–326

Raynaud's phenomenon
  associated with, 329,
    374–375
signs and symptoms of, 328
smoking and, 325, 331
treatment of, 331, 333–335
upper extremity, 441
in women, 324
Thromboembolism, *see also*
    Embolism; Thrombosis
  algorithms for
    diagnostic, 312
    treatment, 316
  description of, 300–301
  diagnosis of, 311
  epidemiology of, 301
  evaluation of, 311, 312
  natural history of, 302, 306
  pathophysiology of, 306,
    308–309
  recurrent, 306
  stroke secondary to, 306
  treatment of
    algorithm, 316
    medical, 314–315, 440
    surgical, 315–317
    thoracic aorta surgery, 315
Thrombolysis, *see also*
    Anticoagulants
  atheroembolism and, 308
  description of, 163–164
Thrombosis, *see also*
    Thromboembolism
  anticoagulant factors, 25
  carotid, 171
  deep venous, 150
  effort, of subclavian vein
    causes of, 417–418

diagnosis of, 419–421
signs and symptoms of,
    418–419
treatment of, 420, 422–423
embolus vs., 155
fibrinolysis, 25–26
fibrin-rich, 23–25
mechanisms of, 21, 28
pathophysiology of, 150
plaque rupture and, 11
platelet-dependent, 21–23
prognosis, 149
summary overview of, 28
superior mesenteric artery, 196
thrombin's role in, 23–24
upper extremity, 440
Ticlodipine, 98
Tissue factor, 24
Tissue factor pathway inhibitor, 25
Tissue plasminogen activator, 8,
    25–26
Tobacco, *see* Smoking
α-Tocopherol, 39
Transcutaneous partial pressure of
    oxygen, 129–130
Transesophageal echocardiography,
    300, 302–305, 310
Traumatic vasospastic disease,
    373–374
Treadmill test, 103
Triamcinolone acetonide, 355
Triglycerides, 66
Triiodothyroxine, 380

U

Ulcers, 134

Ultrasonography, *see* Duplex
ultrasonography
Upper extremity arterial disease or
conditions
algorithm, 452
arterial compression, 445
arterial inflammation, 441–443
arteriovenous fistula, 447
atherosclerosis obliterans,
438–439
clinical presentation of, 448–449
description of, 437–438
emboli, 439–440
evaluation of
algorithm, 452
history-taking, 449
physical examination,
449–450
signs and symptoms, 448
vascular testing, 451
occupational disorders, 443–445
Raynaud's phenomenon, 445–447
thrombosis, 440
trauma, 443–445
vasospasm, 445–447
Urokinase-like plasminogen
activator, 26

V

Vascular cell adhesion molecule-1,
32
Vascular health care team
description of, 459–460
multidisciplinary approach, 460
nurse, *see* Vascular nurse
physician, *see* Vascular
physician

schematic representation of, 461
technologist, *see* Vascular
technologist
Vascular laboratory, 477–479
Vascular medicine, 463–464
Vascular nurse
certification of, 472
educational preparation of,
470–471
future of, 472
professional support of, 471–472
rehabilitation program
administered by, 469–470
role and responsibilities of,
467–470
Vascular physician
educational preparation of
cardiology, 464–465
fellowship programs, 465–466
vascular-interventional
radiology, 465–466
vascular medicine, 463–464
vascular surgery, 462–463
future of, 466
professional support of, 465
role of, 462
Vascular smooth muscle cells
apoptosis of, 12
description of, 6
Vascular surgery, 462–463
Vascular technologist
certification of, 476–477
educational preparation of,
475–476
future of, 479–480
laboratory accreditation,
477–479
patient education by, 474

professional support of, 476
profession development, 475
role and responsibilities of,
    473–474
Vasculitis
    classification of, 340
    definition of, 339
    etiology of, 340
    large-vessel
        algorithm for, 341
        Cogan syndrome, 344
        Takayasu arteritis, 342–343,
            441–442
        temporal arteritis, 342, 441
    medium-vessel
        algorithm, 345
        Kawasaki disease, 347–348
        polyarteritis nodosa,
            346–347
    small-vessel
        algorithm for, 349
        Behçet syndrome, 353–357
        Churg-Strauss syndrome,
            348, 350
        hypersensitivity vasculitis,
            350–351

Wegener granulomatosis,
    351–353
Vasospasm, *see* Raynaud's
    phenomenon
Vasospastic disease, 373–374
Veterans Administration
        Cooperative Study of
        Symptomatic Carotid
        Stenosis, 177
Vitamin C, 40
Vitamin E, 40
von Willebrand factor, 22, 28
vWF, *see* von Willebrand factor

W

Walking
intermittent claudication effects,
    104–105
    percutaneous transluminal
        angioplasty benefits, 112
Walking impairment questionnaire,
    104
Warfarin, 314, 357, *see also*
        Anticoagulants
Wegener granulomatosis, 351–353